Early-Onset Scoliosis

Guidelines for Management in Resource-Limited Settings

T0136197

Edited By

Dr Alaaeldin (Alaa) Azmi Ahmad, MD

Paediatric Orthopaedic Surgeon
Associate Professor, Faculty of Medicine, An-Najah University, Nablus, Palestine
Adjunct Faculty, Medical University of South Carolina, Charleston, South Carolina
Adjunct Faculty, Biomedical Engineering Department, University of Toledo, Toledo, Ohio

Dr Aakash Agarwal, PhD

Director of Research, Spinal Balance Inc., Toledo, Ohio
Adjunct Professor of Bioengineering, University of Toledo, Toledo, Ohio

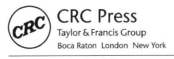

CRC Press

Taylor & Francis Group
Boca Raton London New York

CRC Press is an imprint of the
Taylor & Francis Group, an **informa** business

First edition published 2021
by CRC Press
6000 Broken Sound Parkway NW, Suite 300, Boca Raton, FL 33487-2742

and by CRC Press
2 Park Square, Milton Park, Abingdon, Oxon, OX14 4RN

ISBN: 9780367370312 (hbk)
ISBN: 9780429352416 (ebk)

Typeset in Times
by Deanta Global Publishing Services, Chennai, India

To all the children with spine deformities I treated in Palestine and globally, and to their families, who motivate me to provide better care. To my wife, Fatima, and my children, Amal and Azmi, for their love and support.
—Alaa

Dedicated to the children around the world who deserve conscientious care and the opportunity to heal and flourish. I hope the result of this work will ultimately help in our unified goal of providing young patients with better care and reduced morbidity. As Bob Brown said, 'The future will either be green or not at all.'
—Aakash

Contents

Preface

Early-onset scoliosis (EOS) is a deformity of the growing spine in children, usually 10 years of age and younger, with potentially life-threatening consequences if left untreated. Over the past 2 decades, EOS management has evolved to try to understand the cause, identify coexisting problems and morbidities, and surgically manage the issue while maintaining the growth of the spine and lung. Numerous protocols have been established within a multidisciplinary framework, and growth-friendly implants have been developed to achieve the best results with the fewest complications.

Unfortunately, the science of EOS management has centred on case studies in advanced economies and has largely sidestepped the particular issues of regions with limited resources, where many, if not most, children with EOS cannot access treatment because of a lack of experts and weak organisational frameworks. This book is a humble effort to provide guidelines to implement this important service within a limited-resources setting, by highlighting realistic, on-the-ground experiences of pioneering spine surgeons from developing and developed countries who have succeeded in establishing EOS programmes that not only serve patients directly, but also educate young spine surgeons and promote EOS research in developing countries. Besides addressing surgeons, the book will also provide guidelines to global organisations interested in paediatric spine deformity programmes and highlight the issues that must be prioritied and tackled to enable the development of sustainable EOS programmes in limited-resources economies. It will explain the difference between short-term volunteer missions and long-term educational programmes and advocate for the latter as an important vessel of EOS service provision in developing countries.

The book is not meant to provide formulaic solutions for all problems related to the spine in regions with limited resources but, rather, to draw attention to the particular problems facing developing countries in this regard and to provide rough roadmaps based on previous successful experiences for interested actors. It is meant to promote an understanding of the clinical, educational, and organisational problems for the surgeons, global organisations, and local governments dealing with paediatric spine deformity in limited-resources regions, as well as an appreciation for the importance of context-based solutions to these problems.

This book is possible owing to the valuable contributions of our authors, from various parts of the world, who are drawing on their knowledge and experience to explain how to best overcome the difficulties of promoting EOS service in developing regions. In these times that highlight the connectivity of global public health, as well as the importance of equal rights for all, it is our collective hope that this book contributes to a more egalitarian world where children from all social and economic backgrounds can receive quality care and where surgeons and organisations, especially in the advanced economies, use their various privileges to help materialise such a vision.

Acknowledgments

This book is possible owing to the valuable contributions of our authors, who are drawing on their knowledge and experience from various parts of the world to explain how to best overcome the difficulties of promoting EOS services in developing regions. I also sincerely acknowledge the invaluable help of the publishing team Shivangi Pramanik and Himani Dwivedi for their support and hard work to get this book published.

Editors

Dr Alaaeldin Azmi Ahmad, M.D

A paediatric orthopaedic surgeon by training, Dr Ahmad entered the field of paediatric orthopaedic surgery 18 years ago following a 1-year fellowship at Shriner's Hospital in Los Angeles, California. Since then, he has initiated paediatric spine surgery and education services in Palestine as well as other countries with limited resources. In his role as a surgeon and professor, he holds the position of Professor at An-Najah Medical School, Head of The Pediatric Orthopedic and Spine Unit at An-Najah University Hospital, Consultant Paediatric Orthopaedic Surgeon at Saint Joseph Hospital, Jerusalem, Palestine, and Visiting Consultant Paediatric Spinal Surgeon in Abdali Hospital, Amman, Jordan. He also holds an adjunct faculty appointment at the Orthopedic Department in University of South Carolina in Charleston and in the biomedical engineering department at the University of Toledo in Ohio.

As a paediatric orthopaedic surgeon, Dr Ahmad possesses extensive experience in the management of children with spine deformity, with a special interest in early-onset scoliosis (EOS) cases. He invented a new surgical technique that is more affordable than prevailing techniques that avoids current surgeries for the growing spine through posterior tethering called active apex correction (APC). Dr Ahmad has presented this technique in numerous international congresses and has published papers in peer-reviewed journals discussing its efficiency in the surgical management for children with EOS. Currently, this technique is being used in Palestine, Jordan, India, and Mozambique with positive results. Overall, Dr Ahmad has been published in more than 35 international journals and books, most of them related to EOS management. He shares editorial responsibilities as editorial board member in *JOP B* and as a reviewer board member in *GSJ, SICOT J*, and *Journal of Clinical Orthopaedics and Trauma*.

Dr Ahmad has been active in spinal orthopaedic education initiatives, both locally and globally. In Palestine, he has trained residents in the orthopaedic residency programme and is a member of the orthopaedic committee of the Palestinian Board for nine years. He also became head of the orthopaedic programme at the Palestine International Cooperation Agency (PICA), in charge of developing a paediatric spine surgery programme in Mozambique and Nicaragua as well as paediatric spine missions in Pakistan and Rwanda. Globally, he is a member of Scoliosis Research Society's Growing Spine Committee, the North American Spine Society's International Outreach Work Group, and the AO Spine's Education Strategy Task Force; he also serves as the Spine Committee chair and secretary general of World Orthopaedic Concern-International Society of Orthopaedic Surgery and Tramautology, and an international fellow at the College of Surgeons of East, Central, and Southern Africa (COSECSA). In addition, he is involved in the Weil Cornell Spine education programme in Tanzania. He possesses a global vision and a drive to collaborate with colleagues toward the development of education and training programmes that can improve spine surgery services in countries with limited resources.

Dr Aakash Agarwal

Aakash Agarwal, PhD, is the Director of Research at Spinal Balance Inc., in Toledo, Ohio, and an Adjunct Professor of Bioengineering at University of Toledo in Ohio. Dr Agarwal is a prolific researcher in the field of preventive and predictive science of spinal pathology and postoperative complications, such as spinal deformity, surgical site infection, hardware failure, and spinopelvic imbalance. Dr Agarwal's primary expertise lies in new preventative measures to combat spinal surgery complications, including surgical site infection and implant failures associated with EOS. His major interests include translational research with immediate bench-to-bedside applicability. He has been a major contributor to several important projects that have been recognised as significant. He uses combinatory knowledge of biomedical engineering, clinical medicine, mechanical engineering, and biomechanics to study surgical failures and new treatments to mitigate the risk of complications and infections. He is the inventor of a two-step asepsis process that involves providing spinal implants in an individual sterile tube and a preloaded intraoperative sheath allowing implants to be handled hygienically that aims to reduce surgical site infection and biofilm formation. Dr Agarwal has also extensively explored the mechanism behind the failure of scoliosis spinal implants in children. Through human trial studies and biomechanical simulations, he identified the high failure rate of certain distraction-based rods and growth-guided systems and provided guidelines on how to reduce such failure modes. Dr Agarwal holds several national and international patents. He is an editorial board member for the journals *Clinical Spine Surgery* and *Spine* by Lippincott Williams & Wilkins. Dr Agarwal also serves as an advisory board member for the Center for the Disruptive Musculoskeletal Innovation (CDMI) under the aegis of the National Science Foundation (NSF).

List of Contributors

Ahmed Shawky Abdelgawaad
Spine Center
Erfurt, Germany
and
Assiut University Hospitals
Assiut, Egypt

Emre Acaroglu
Ankara Spine Center
Ankara, Turkey

Aakash Agarwal
Department of Bioengineering
University of Toledo
Toledo, Ohio
and
Colleges of Engineering
University of Toledo
Toledo, Ohio

Alaaeldin Azmi Ahmad
An-Najah University
Nablus, Palestine
and
Medical University of South Carolina
Charleston, South Carolina
and
Biomedical Engineering Department
University of Toledo
Toledo, Ohio

Amal Ahmad
Department of Economics
University of Massachusetts
Amherst, Massachusetts

Kaustubh Ahuja
Department of Orthopaedics
All India Institute of Medical Sciences
New Delhi, India

Behrooz A. Akbarnia
San Diego Spine Foundation and Global Spine
    Outreach
San Diego, California

Shahid Ali
Doctors Hospital & Medical Centre
Lahore, Pakistan
and
Orthopaedic Unit 1
Jinnah Hospital
Lahore, Pakistan

Amer Alkot
Al-Azhar University, Assiut Branch
Assiut, Egypt

Sri Vijay Anand
Department of Spine Surgery
Ganga Hospital
Coimbatore, India

Rashid Anjum
Acharya Shri Chander College of Medical
    Sciences and Hospital
Jammu, India

Amer Aziz
Ghurki Trust Teaching Hospital
Lahore, Pakistan

Mohit Bhandari
Division of Orthopaedic Surgery
McMaster University
Hamilton, Ontario, Canada

François Bonnel
Laboratory of Anatomy
University of Montpellier
Montpellier, France

Federico Canavese
Pediatric Surgery Department
University Hospital Estaing
Clermont-Ferrand, France

Mary Crocker
Pulmonary and Sleep Medicine Division
University of Washington School of Medicine
and
Department of Pediatrics
University of Washington School of Medicine
Seattle, Washington

Ujjwal Kanti Debnath
Fortis Hospital
Kolkata, India
and
AMRI Hospitals
Kolkata, India

Alain Dimeglio
Pediatric Orthopedic Department
Clinique St. Roch
Montpellier, France

Laura Ellington
Pulmonary and Sleep Medicine Division
University of Washington School of Medicine
and
Department of Pediatrics
University of Washington School of Medicine
Seattle, Washington

Mohammad M. El-Sharkawi
Assiut University
Assiut, Egypt

Meric Enercan
Istanbul Spine Center
Istanbul Florence Nightingale Hospital
Istanbul, Turkey

Bhavuk Garg
Department of Orthopaedics
All India Institute of Medical Sciences
New Delhi, India

Michael Grevitt
Nottingham University Hospitals
Nottingham, United Kingdom

Yong Hai
Department of Orthopedic Surgery
Beijing Chaoyang Hospital
Beijing, China

Azmi Hamzaoglu
Istanbul Spine Center
Istanbul Florence Nightingale Hospital
Istanbul, Turkey

Damarla Haritha
Department of Anaesthesiology, Pain Medicine
    and Critical Care
All India Institute of Medical Sciences
New Delhi, India

Ashok N. Johari
Enable – International Centre for Paediatric
    Musculoskeletal Care
Mumbai, India

Rishi Mugesh Kanna
Department of Spine Surgery
Ganga Hospital
Coimbatore, India

Mohamed Fawzy Khattab
Ain Shams University,
Cairo, Egypt

Souvik Maitra
Department of Anaesthesiology, Pain Medicine
    and Critical Care
All India Institute of Medical Sciences
New Delhi, India

Gregory M. Mundis, Jr.
San Diego Spine Foundation and Global Spine
    Outreach
San Diego, California

Aixing Pan
Department of Orthopedic Surgery
Beijing Chaoyang Hospital
Beijing, China

Samuel Pantoja
Clinica Las Condes Private Hospital
and
Dr. Roberto Del Río Children's Hospital
Santiago, Chile

Devin Peterson
Division of Orthopaedic Surgery
McMaster University
Hamilton, Ontario, Canada

Vrushali Ponde
Children's Anaesthesia Services
Children's Ortho Centre
Surya Children Hospital
Hinduja Healthcare Surgical Hospital
and
Holy Spirit Hospital
Mumbai, India
and
Holy Family Hospital
New Delhi, India

S. Rajasekaran
Department of Spine Surgery
Ganga Hospital
Coimbatore, India

Gregory Redding
Pulmonary and Sleep Medicine Division
University of Washington School of
    Medicine
and
Department of Pediatrics
University of Washington School of Medicine
Seattle, Washington

Fernando Rios
San Diego Spine Foundation and Global Spine
    Outreach
San Diego, California

Alpaslan Senkoylu
Department of Orthopaedics and Traumatology
Gazi University
Ankara, Turkey

Abdullah Shah
Ghurki Trust Teaching Hospital
Lahore, Pakistan

Ajoy Prasad Shetty
Department of Spine Surgery
Ganga Hospital
Coimbatore, India

Harwant Singh
Spine and Joint Centre
Pantai Hospital
Kuala Lumpur, Malaysia

Muhammad Tariq Sohail
Pakistan Academy of Medical Sciences
Islamabad, Pakistan
and
Doctors Hospital & Medical Center
Lahore, Pakistan

Patrick Thornley
Division of Orthopaedic Surgery
McMaster University
Hamilton, Ontario, Canada

List of Abbreviations

Accelerated discharge (AD)
Acid-fast bacilli (AFB)
Acquired immunodeficiency syndrome (AIDS)
Active apex correction (APC)
Acute normovolemic haemodilution (ANH)
Adolescent idiopathic scoliosis (AIS)
Alanine aminotransferase (ALT)
Annual progression ratio (APR)
Anteroposterior (AP)
Antidiuretic hormone (ADH)
Anti-retroviral therapy (ART)
Anti-tubercular chemotherapy (ATT)
Apical vertebra rotation (AVR)
Apical vertebral distance (AVD)
Artificial intelligence (AI)
Bispectral index (BIS Index)
Blended learning (BL)
Bone mineral density (BMD)
Breath holding time (BHT)
C-reactive protein (CRP)
Central sacral vertical line (CSVL)
Central sterile services department (CSSD)
Cerebral palsy (CP)
Classification for early-onset scoliosis (C-EOS)
Closing opening wedge osteotomy (COWO)
College of Surgeons of East,
    Central and Southern Africa (COSECSA)
Compound muscle action potential (CMAP)
Computerised tomography (CT)
Countries with limited resources (CLRs)
Diagnosis-related groups (DRGs)
Disc bone osteotomy (DBO)
Distal junctional kyphosis (*DJK*)
Early-onset scoliosis (EOS)
Electrocardiogram (ECG)
Elongation, derotation, and flexion (EDF)
End tidal carbon dioxide (ETCO2)
Endotracheal (ET)
Epsilon-aminocaproic acid (*EACA*)
Erythrocyte sedimentation rate (ESR)
Estimated blood loss (EBL)
Evidence-based medicine (EBM)
External remote controller (ERC)
Face to face (F2F)
Fellow of College of Physicians
and Surgeons Pakistan (FCPS)

Forced expiratory volume in the
first second (FEV1)
Forced vital capacity (FVC)
Foundation of Orthopedics and
Complex Spine (FOCOS)
Functional residual capacity (FRC)
Global outreach programmes (GOPs)
Global Spine Care Initiative (GSCI)
Global Spine Outreach (GSO)
Gross domestic product (GDP)
Gross national income (GNI)
Growth guidance system (GGS)
Growth rods (GRs)
Halo-gravity traction (HGT)
Health-related quality of life (HRQoL)
Hemoglobin A1c (HbA1C)
High-dependency unit (HDU)
High-income countries (HIC)
Human immunodeficiency viruses (HIV)
Intensive care unit (ICU)
International classification of
diseases (ICD)
International normalised ratio (INR)
Intraoperative neuromonitoring (IOM)
Intravenous (IV)
Learning management system (LMS)
Learning outcomes (LO)
Leg length discrepancy (LLD)
Limited resources (LR)
Low- and middle-income countries (LMICs)
Magnetic Expansion Control MAGEC
Magnetic growth rod (MGR)
Magnetic resonance imaging (MRI)
Magnetically controlled
    growing rods (MCGR)
Managed care (MC)
Maputo Central Hospital (MCH)
Maximum expiratory pressures (MEP)
Maximum inspiratory pressures (MIP)
Mean arterial pressure (MAP)
Memorandum of agreement (MOA)
*Methicillin-resistant Staphylococcus
aureus* (*MRSA*)
Minimum alveolar concentration (*MAC*)
Ministry of Health (MOH)
Motor evoked potentials (MEP)

National Health Services	**(NHS)**	Rib vertebral sternal complex	**(RVSC)**
Neural axis abnormality	**(NAA)**	Scoliosis Research Society	**(SRS)**
Neurofibromatosis	**(*NF*)**	Scoliosis Research Society Global	
Neurophysiologic monitoring	**(NM)**	Outreach Mission Programs	**(SRS-GOP)**
Nongovernmental organisations	**(NGOs)**	Scoliosis Research Society	
Noninvasive blood pressure	**(NIBP)**	questionnaire	**(SRS-22r)**
Nonprofit organisations	**(NPOs)**	Self-contained surgical platforms	**(SCSPs)**
Nonsteroidal anti-inflammatory		Self-sliding growth guidance	**(SSGG)**
drugs	**(NSAIDs)**	Selling, general, and administrative	**(SG&A)**
North American Spine Society	**(NASS)**	Shared decision-making	**(SDM)**
Occult spinal dysraphism	**(OSD)**	Short-term surgical mission trips	**(STSMs)**
Online learning	**(OL)**	Slipped capital femoral epiphysis	**(SCFE)**
Operating time	**(OT)**	Society on Scoliosis Orthopaedic	
Operation Straight Spine	**(OSS)**	and Rehabilitation Treatment	**(SOSORT)**
Outpatient department	**(OPD)**	Somatosensory evoked potentials	**(SSEP)**
Oxygen saturation	**(SPO2)**	Space available for lung	**(SAL)**
Palestine International Cooperation		Spring distraction system	**(SDS)**
Agency	**(PICA)**	Syndrome of inappropriate	
Partial thromboplastin time	**(PTT)**	antidiuretic hormone release	**(SIADH)**
Patient controlled analgesia	**(PCA)**	Target controlled infusion	**(TCI)**
Patient-reported outcomes measures	**(PROMs)**	Three dimensional	**(3D)**
Pedicle subtraction osteotomy	**(PSO)**	Total intravenous anaesthesia	**(TIVA)**
Physical medicine and rehabilitation	**(PM&R)**	Total lung capacity	**(TLC)**
Polyvinyl chloride	**(PVC)**	Traditional growth rod	**(TGR)**
Posteroanterior	**(PA)**	Triradiate cartilage	**(TRC)**
Postoperative nausea vomiting	**(PONV)**	Tuberculosis	**(TB)**
Postoperative pain management	**(POPM)**	Two dimensional	**(2D)**
Preoperative autologous donation	**(PAD)**	U.S. Food and Drug Administration	**(FDA)**
Prothrombin time	**(PT)**	United Nations Development	
Proximal junctional failure	**(PJF)**	Programme	**(UNDP)**
Proximal junctional kyphosis	**(PJK)**	University Hospital of Wales	**(UHW)**
Pulmonary functional tests	**(PFT)**	Vertebral column resection	**(VCR)**
Queens Medical Centre	**(QMC)**	Vertical expandable prosthetic	
Randomised controlled trials	**(RCTs)**	titanium rib	**(VEPTR)**
Rapid eye movement	**(REM)**	Virtual reality	**(VR)**
Red blood cells	**(RBCs)**	World Health Organization	**(WHO)**
Research and developmental	**(R&D)**	World Spine Care	**(WSC)**
Resource-limited settings	**(RLS)**		
Rib vertebral angle difference	**(RVAD)**		

1 Introduction

Alaaeldin Azmi Ahmad

CONTENTS

INTRODUCTION

Early onset scoliosis (EOS) includes all scoliotic deformity for children under 10 years of age. It is a life-threatening disease, unlike adolescent idiopathic scoliosis, which makes early intervention crucial. Most of the patients in this category have complex spine problems with associated comorbidities. These patients require a multidisciplinary approach in a resource abundant facility with management subspecialised in spine deformity. Ironically, the incidences of EOS are higher and more widespread in countries with limited resources (CLRs), and except for a very sporadic provision of exemplary management of such patients in Asia, Africa, and Latin America, these patients have no access to solutions with which developed nations are equipped. None of the previously published books on EOS has a theme dedicated to this problem and the accompanying solutions to this vacuum. This book will be the first to give guidelines based on the successful programmes run by the most experienced doctors and global thinkers. The upcoming chapters will lay out a roadmap on how to implement this service within the context of a limited-resource region, unlike the past publications dealing with the assumption that you have all the resources within your reach and the only missing link is the surgical technique; clearly this is not the case here. Below are several reasons explaining why there is a lack of publications about EOS services in CLRs.

1. The treatment two decades ago for EOS was similar to the management undertaken for adolescent deformity, i.e. correction and fusion under the concept that a straight, shorter spine is better than a long, crooked spine. Accordingly, there was no need to explore and write about EOS as a separate problem that demands a specific management, until it became known that pulmonary function would be compromised unless certain nonfusion techniques were employed.

2. The heterogenicity of this population with different etiological backgrounds presented unique challenges in management for these patients. Many authors refrained from writing about the management of this particular problem because there is still a lack of consensus as too few evidence-based studies have been conducted.

3. A long-standing myth that a very small number of children suffer from this problem; we know now that 20% of adolescent children with scoliosis had juvenile idiopathic scoliosis, which is a part of EOS. If we now calculate 20% of adolescent idiopathic scoliosis cases in the United States, for example, juvenile idiopathic scoliosis refers to 20%

of 6 million or 1.2 million cases. We would think this magnitude of occurrence needs more attention, especially when management is a life saving measure.

4. Surgery was relegated as a low-priority status in global health and was viewed as an expensive measure that would compromise other large-scale global health initiatives.

5. Many short-term missions were used as an alternate (excuse) to not implement permanent EOS management services and thus EOS management were discounted from the aegis of global health initiatives.

6. Misconception of high per unit cost of pedicle screws making surgery infeasible, inability of local surgeons to learn and implement the treatment, wait and watch approach, and reduced relative priority in the spine training programs, from surgeons or organisations that deal with spine surgery across the globe.

All these factors were a reason for the unavailability of a book focussing on implementing this service in low- and middle-income countries (LMICs). Even with the evolved interest in this service, most of the publications were about the updated management for EOS concerning developed countries and written mostly by experts in these countries. This is the first book that will give guidelines for the surgeons and global organisations that are interested in improving global health concerning EOS in LMICs.

DISCUSSION

Why Is This Book Necessary Now?

1. An increased awareness of the importance of the problem, experiencing a higher rate of than was thought, and the benefits of early management in these cases and thus reducing complexities and complications of late intervention is evidenced in the increase in symposiums related to EOS in the annual international congresses, such as the Scoliosis Research Society (SRS),

the North American Spine Society (NASS), AO Spine, Eurospine, etc.

2. The added advantage of the nonfusion techniques on adolescent idiopathic scoliosis and the role of tethering in preserving spine mobility has attracted attention to the nonfusion techniques, which are now a mainstay principle for the management of EOS.

3. The epidemiological shift with the global industrialisation gave importance to surgery as an important health factor. In addition, people living in LMICs are now less likely to die from communicable diseases, and they live to an age at which cancer and cardiovascular problems are more prevalent [1].

4. Recently, international societies have shifted their attention, making surgical care a fundamental component of global health [2].

5. Global activity has changed from short-term missions with a focus on service to capacity building through long-term sustainable programmes with special focus on education.

6. The change of perception of highly specialised surgery has changed. Whereas such procedures were considered to be cost-inefficient global activity, they are now viewed as a necessary activity that augments other health facilities (such as laboratory services, radiology development, blood banking services, anaesthesia services, etc.).

7. Awareness of the effects of globalisation, especially with coronavirus affecting the world, developed countries fear that the vulnerable health systems in the developing world would increase the chance of reemergence of infectious diseases. This necessitates the global community to uniformly improve the health system for developing countries and approaches for sub-specialised surgeries.

What Makes This Book Important?

This book will provide guidelines instead of a prescription because we are dealing with a complicated and heterogenous health problem within a context of limited resources that varies from region to region. We were keen to look at the problem holistically, and any discussion on the surgical aspect is futile without understanding the capabilities of individual regions. Furthermore, aspects such as industry and its relationship with the facility, economic status, education, and training process are pertinent to this subject matter. This book shares experiences of the pioneers who have worked in LMICs, making the information relevant to the readers working in LMICs around the world. Most of the chapters are from authors practising in Asia, Africa, Latin America, and a few selected surgeons from developed countries working to implement this programme in developing countries. An important thing to be discussed is the training process to improve the surgical skills of the local surgeons through newly evolved teaching methods that include artificial intelligence (AI). With the spread of digital education and worldwide internet access, we have new training tools that were not established before, such as YouTube videos, webinars, discussion groups, and blended learning, that efficiently share knowledge without financial burden in limited-resource settings. Recently, there has been a move toward using augmented simulation and virtual-reality training programmes, though they are still expensive for most limited-resource regions. However, given its potential, companies are trying to make these new learning tools accessible to surgeons in limited-resource settings, thereby exposing them to pre-, intra-, and postoperative protocols and eliminating the need for frequent travel. Also, the readers will be informed of legal issues related to the licenses that are of a concern to surgeons and organisations dealing with these programmes. We think this book is mandatory for any surgeon, health worker, nongovernmental organisation, and other health officials in developing countries who are interested in implementing this important service. If you are based in an LMIC, this book will provide you with a holistic guideline to assist in building a road map toward implementing this service within the region of interest. It will provide you with necessary platform and background information to further customise an execution plan,

such as the hospital plan, access to instruments, relations with international organisations, and the impact of this service on the health system in your area. If you are a surgeon or an officer in a global organisation interested in implementing surgical services in LMICs, this book will give you an overview of the problem that doctors and health workers involved in this activity face, the auxiliary factors in play, and the limitations within their practices. This will give you realistic guidelines that will overcome many problems during implementation of this service and will help to avoid duplication of services and unnecessary efforts toward management of EOS in LMICs. With these guidelines, we hope that the dynamics of the relationships between the surgeons from developed countries and LMICs will evolve, from being a one-sided exchange to a two-way street of positive feedback and comprehension. This will help to position local orthopaedic surgeons as a central part of the planning and execution of global EOS surgery initiatives. This requires durable training programmes that help surgeons relegate increasing responsibilities to local doctors with each visit [3].

CONCLUSION

This book is the first to address the challenges involved in the management of EOS services in a limited-resource setting, i.e. LMICs. It provides guidelines for the local surgeon on how to deal with the EOS cases effectively while overcoming specific preoperative, operative, and postoperative difficulties that come with the dearth of financial and organisational resources. It aims not only to enhance the medical and surgical skill of the local surgeon in this challenging setting, but also to boost the self-confidence necessary for overcoming the numerous institutional barriers. This book also addresses surgeons travelling to these countries, explaining how to best understand this challenging logistical, legal, and organisational context and how to most effectively contribute to the elevation and support of local surgeons through sustainable mentoring and other partnership programmes. By providing the various guidelines based on real-life experiences and successful programmes, this book ultimately aims to facilitate the improvement and expansion of paediatric spine deformity service in these underserved communities.

REFERENCES

1. Mathers CD, Loncar D. Projections of global mortality and burden of disease from 2002 to 2030. *PLOS Medicine*. 2006;3(11):e442.

2. DeVries CR, Price RR. *Global Surgery and Public Health: A New Paradigm*. Jones & Bartlett Publishers; Sudbury, MA, 2012.

3. Ahmad AA. What's important: Recognizing local power in global surgery. *Bone & Joint Surgery*. 2019;101(21):1974.

2a Economics and Implementing Early-Onset Scoliosis in Limited-Resources Facilities

Ahmed Shawky Abdelgawaad

CONTENTS

INTRODUCTION

Tremendous challenges present themselves in developing countries throughout the world in which infrastructure for healthcare is limited. Two-thirds of the world's population live in developing countries, however, 80% of all orthopaedic surgeons reside in the 26 developed nations in the world [1, 2].

Management of early-onset scoliosis (EOS) is associated with particular psychological, social, and economic burdens for patients and families as well as economic costs for the society itself. Treatment evaluation must be concerned with this total cost effectiveness. While this applies to developed as well as developing countries, developing nations are in need of assistance on many fronts in order to address current healthcare needs and to prepare for the health problems of the near future. Spinal deformity surgeons have the ability to assist in direct care of EOS patients and, more importantly, educate and train existing surgeons and medical personnel and help establish infrastructure by which patients can be evaluated and subsequently treated [3].

The total cost of paediatric spinal deformity in developing countries is difficult to determine because both direct (hospital expenditures) and indirect expenditures are not available in the databases. These countries usually even lack databases. In addition to direct and indirect costs, children afflicted with spinal deformity experience a reduced quality of life, which may include major constraints on their mobility, activity, and quality of life.

PROBLEMS IN MANAGEMENT OF EOS WITH LIMITED RESOURCES

Limited resources (LR) is defined as a basic condition in which the quantity of available labour, capital, land, and entrepreneurship used for services are finite. It means that the economy has only so many resources that can be used at any given time to produce services [4].

EOS represents a challenge to developed countries, but this challenge heightened for countries or facilities with limited resources. The availability of experienced surgeons, capital, infrastructure, and entrepreneurship is limited. The most common problems include:

1. Limited human resources:
   - Lack of experienced medical teams; not limited to surgeons but also anaesthesiologists,

neuromonitoring technicians, nursing staff, and physiotherapists.
- The low educational level of parents and children in rural, underserved areas is responsible in part for late presentation and causes difficulty with shared decision-making (SDM) (Figure 2a.1).
2. Limited financial resources:
    - Deficient infrastructure of health providers; lack of well-equipped hospitals, scarcity of intensive care unit beds, lack of cell-savers and intraoperative neuromonitoring devices.
    - Unavailability of high-quality recent implant systems:
    - Geographical scarcity of specialised centres also contributes to late presentations and more severe deformities. It also adds to the transportation costs of the children and their families.

The geographical placement of hospitals is particularly crucial in the context of the considerable financial burdens imposed on families required to visit patients at a typically distant specialist hospital. Many patients live in distant rural areas where public transport is inadequate. Even relatively moderate distances could entail high financial costs when visiting is regular and frequent over a long period. Distances of more than 100 kilometres are quite common. Added to these difficulties are the problems of finding time for visiting without losing wages and of providing alternative care for other children in the family. Parents typically make great sacrifices to stay with or visit their children regularly, usually daily. The greater the effort to support the patient by visiting, the greater the costs incurred.

For the vast majority of patients and families, financial aid for visiting is nonexistent and difficult to obtain even in extreme cases. In principle, patients may be directed to distant hospitals and admitted for prolonged hospital stay, but

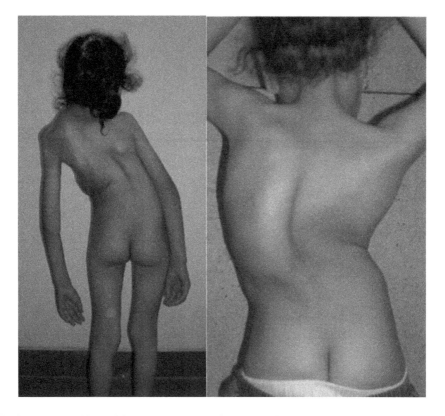

FIGURE 2A.1   Two children with late presentation of severe EOS.

the government or insurance (if present) take no responsibility for the financial burden imposed on the family. The idea that hospital treatment is 'free', therefore, requires considerable reevaluation [3, 4].

Other aspects of treatment evaluation relevant to long- vs. short-stay alternatives include the problem of how scarce hospital resources should be most efficiently employed, taking into account the effects on the rate of patient throughput. Consultants commonly report waiting lists for scoliosis treatment.

Limited resources also lead to longer waiting lists. A recently published study on international disease severity that included data from Ghana, Egypt, and Pakistan concluded that larger curve magnitudes for patients living in countries with the least access to orthopaedic care correlated to a higher number of levels fused, longer occupational therapy (OT), and greater estimated blood loss (EBL), indicating that an increased curve magnitude at the time of surgery could explain the difference in operative morbidity between countries with low and high access to orthopaedic care. With OT as the prevailing predictive factor of complications, we suggest that increased curve magnitude leads to longer OT and more complications. A lack of access to orthopaedic care may be the largest contributor to the postponement of treatment [5].

3. Deficient entrepreneurship:
- Deficient administrative experiences.
- Deficient national registries and databases.
- Lack of regular public health screening programmes for early detection.
- Nongovernmental organisations (NGOs) commonly overtake responsibilities of the government to organise missions or even develop specialised centres for treatment.

COSTS OF EOS MANAGEMENT

Costs of EOS management can be classified in two main categories: direct costs and indirect costs.

- **Direct costs [6]**
  - Hospital stays: Most limited-resources facilities in developing countries do not follow a standard International Classification of Diseases (ICD) or Diagnosis-Related Groups (DRGs). Commonly, there is no official Diagnosis-Related Groups (DGRs) tariff for scoliosis surgery (i.e. cost of standard hospital stay with a low-grade of severity, cost of standard hospital stay with a mid-grade of severity).
  - Implantable medical devices: Costs are estimated based on official fares that differ from one country to another, knowing that conventional devices are sometimes reimbursed in addition to hospital stay tariffs, depending on the type of construct (e.g. rod, screw, hook, connector). For special implants such as VEPTER or MCGR, tariffs are also variable (tariffs for MAGEC system single MCGR, and dual MGCGs include the provision of the external remote controller by the local distributor). Many developing countries do not have these recent implants; they depend on locally produced modified systems that sometimes lack optimal quality.
  - Spinal bracing: For orthosis and the moulding.
  - Medical and physiotherapy visits.
  - Full spine radiographs.
  - Medical transportation: Cost is estimated taking into account the most frequently observed proportion of transportation modes (ambulance – sanitary vehicle – taxi – or other) [6].
- **Indirect costs**
  - Transportation costs: This means the nonmedical transportation. Also, transportation of parents if they accompany the child.
  - Lost wages: If one or both parents accompany the child to the hospital

visit or during the hospital stay. This can be calculated according to the following equation: Maternal Lost Wages = [(Driving time) + (Wayfinding time) + (Length of Clinic Appointment)] × (Mother's hourly wage estimate) × (Probability mother was present at the appointment).

- Clinic or hospital overhead costs [7].

MANAGED CARE CONCEPTS AND IMPLEMENTATION OF EOS MANAGEMENT

Although managed care (MC) has its pros and cons in the developed countries, applying its quality-control instruments to the problems of EOS in LR countries may be of the utmost value. The principles of MC quality-control instruments help to improve management of EOS in limited-resources countries. MC could improve costs of the medical service in many developed countries, and applying the same principles may improve costs in developing nations [8, 9]. MC Quality-control instruments include structure quality, process quality, and results quality.

1. **Structure Quality.** Indicators of structure quality include, for example, training level of the medical personnel and preventive measures. Limited-resources countries lack experienced surgeons trained to manage EOS. Treatment is mainly concentrated in main cities. Frequently, deficiency in trained teams is managed by missions of international organisations or through surgeons travelling from their home countries to help during short visits. Examples of international organisations supporting global outreach programmes are the Scoliosis Research Society, Setting Scoliosis Straight, and Doctors without Borders
   - Preventive measures for EOS may be primary, secondary, or tertiary. Primary prevention includes all measures taken to prevent the

disease itself. As EOS is mostly genetic, primary prevention should include premarital screening programmes. These are still not routine and not obligatory in many countries. Secondary prevention includes early diagnosis and management of EOS in children. Under this category include measure such as screening programmes for children at school and by primary care physicians. Tertiary prevention involves mainly minimising complications and long-term negative effects of EOS on those children.

- All the three forms of prevention are deficient in limited-resources countries because of:
- The infrastructure and equipment of clinics and hospitals.
- Availability of documentation systems and databases. Databases and national registries are of utmost importance to collect, retrieve, analyse, and report data. They are also very important for future publications.
- The availability and safety of treatment.

2. **Process Quality.** Process quality means delivering high-quality medical service to children with EOS. The focus of process quality is the adherence to known medical standards. Indicators of process quality include the quality of the diagnostic procedures and the length of the hospital stay.

One of the problems with EOS is that the treatment and follow-up plan is usually tailored for each child. There are no universally available guidelines to follow. Even globally available protocols may be difficult to follow in limited-resources facilities. Frequency of follow-up visits and X-ray images are not standard. Patients need to travel long distances to reach a specialised hospital, which they commonly pay out of their own pockets.

In limited-resources countries, waiting for the surgical procedure in a specialised hospital commonly exceeds 6 months. Delaying surgery for more than six months for adolescent idiopathic scoliosis (AIS) patients who are premenarchal, TRC (triradiate cartilage) open, or Risser 0 are at risk of clinically significant Cobb angle progression, which is statistically greater than their more mature peers. Skeletally mature patients do not progress rapidly, allowing elective timing of surgical intervention [10].

The length of hospital stay is also influenced by many other factors. Availability of experienced surgeons, availability of intensive care beds, even availability of implants and neuromonitoring teams. Managing all these interdisciplinary issues is sometimes very difficult. If these are not well-coordinated, the hospital stay will be lengthened.

Shared Decision-Making (SDM). EOS is a condition in which SDM plays a very important role because children are legally vulnerable subjects. Commonly, parents decide on diagnostic and surgical procedures to be done. The surgeons are sometimes foreign and do not speak the local language. The information is propagated from the doctor to the family and the child. Modality, frequency, and importance of diagnostic measures should be discussed as well as the short- and long-term goals of treatment. Goals include partial correction of the curve, maintenance of vertebral and trunk growth, and maintenance of lung development. The follow up protocols, frequency of hospital visits and possibly frequent anaesthesia are important concerns. Graduation and definitive fusion or implant removal after skeletal maturity should be discussed. Data regarding graduation after skeletal maturity after recent implants are still scarce.

Positive effects of SDM include tailored patient-specific management, higher compliance, better treatment results, rapid recovery, better informed

family and children where realistic expectations and reduced fears are supported. Ensuring good communication is important because the longer the child (and family) become adjusted to living with the deformity, the weaker may become the incentive to accept a costly and stressful hospital treatment when offered [3]

Guidelines and Evidence-Based Medicine. Globally accepted guidelines for EOS do not exist. Even management protocols and algorithms applied in developed countries may not be applicable in developing ones. This is usually due to different cultural, social, and economic issues. Guidelines are developed in quality circles and focus on medical service with less interest in the economic and financial side. Adapted protocols and management plans should be developed for limited-resources countries and facilities that take into consideration the best available evidence, surgical experience, patient and family expectations, and available resources. Evidence-based medicine (EBM) is also adapted to available resources. For example, evidence strongly recommends the use of intraoperative neuromonitoring (IOM), however, such equipment is in short supply in limited-resources facilities. The pool of patients for which surgeries are performed requires the most complex procedures. Spinal cord injuries are certain to happen give enough operations. Complex surgical procedures in paediatric deformities should be done under IOM even in underserved countries. This can be organised through global outreach programmes (GOPs) or mobile IOM devices [11].

IOM is of the utmost importance to provide safety to complex surgical procedures. This is especially true for missions and GOPs in situations in which there is insufficient time for staged procedures, the full instruments or implants are unavailable (ad hoc surgical team), and surgeons are operating in a foreign theatre and communicating with local nurses and anaesthesiologists is suboptimal.

Many technicians are interested in being involved in an outreach programme. Most of them would be delighted to cover some or all of the cost of their trips as part of their philanthropic endeavours. Often their employer is willing to cover their activity. Salaries and expenses are sometimes covered for global outreach services.

The value of IOM was highlighted in the recently published study 'Comprehensive Assessment of Outcomes from Patients with Severe Early-onset Scoliosis Treated with a Vertebral Column Resection: Results from an SRS Global Outreach Site (FOCOS) in Ghana'. The authors concluded that vertebral column resection (VCR) in the setting of EOS has excellent radiographic outcomes but a high complication profile. Half of their cases had intraoperative neuromonitoring changes that improved without lasting neurological deficit [12].

3. **Results Quality.** The quality of the results is the evaluation scale of the whole medical service process. Short- and long-term treatment goals should be determined in the early management process. They should be presented in a target-performance manner. Radiographic, functional, and patient-reported outcomes measures (PROMs) should be identified. For PROMs and quality of life questionnaires, cross-culture translated and validated versions should be used.

In many limited-resources countries, translated cross-cultural validated outcome measures for EOS are not available. This makes the validity of the used instrument questionable.

POSSIBLE SOLUTIONS

1. Global outreach programmes (GOPs) and missions organised by NGOs:

Regular visits are organised through international organisations in coordination with local doctors. Patients requiring surgery are asked to pay a relatively nominal fee if they are able, and spinal implant manufacturers donate implants. Surgeons with appropriate expertise volunteer their time and often their financial resources, while local orthopaedic surgeons observe and participate in operations. Local clinics are established to evaluate patients and determine surgical candidates for subsequent visits [13].

2. Governments should build geographically well-distributed healthcare facilities to treat these children. Political and economic stability is mandatory for this development.

3. Increased public awareness about the value of early intervention and compliance to reduce possible complications.

4. Surgeons adapt techniques and implants to manage these cases. Also planning intervals between elongations of expandable implants to the longest possible to minimise exposure to anaesthetics and hospital admissions.

5. Adoption of screening programmes: Many studies support the efficacy and cost effectiveness of public health screening for scoliosis. Early intervention sometimes with casting and bracing may reduce the complexity of surgical intervention and possibly subsequent complications.

6. Building specialised teams including orthopaedic specialists, spinal surgeons, anaesthesiologists, neuromonitoring physicians and technicians, orthotists, operative room and ward nurses, and physiotherapists.

CONCLUSION

The economic burden related to management of EOS on the health systems in limited-resources countries should not be underestimated. The best scenario is to develop the health systems in these countries as a part of national programmes aiming at education, health, and economy development. Implementation of managed care concepts may be a helpful solution to decrease and justify costs of EOS management. International global outreach programmes and building local specialised teams is mandatory to help in the current situation.

REFERENCES

1. Dormans JP, Fisher RC, Pill SG. Orthopaedics in the developing world: Present and future concerns. *J Am Acad Orthop Surg.* 2001;9(5):289–96.
2. Levine AM. Can we make a difference? *J Am Acad Orthop Surg.* 2001;9(5):279.
3. Clough F. The relevance of social and clinical criteria in making decisions for scoliosis treatment. *Soc Sci Med.* 1978;12(4A):219–28.
4. Ruffin RJ, Gregory PR. *Principles of Economics.* 5th ed. New York: HarperCollins College Publishers; 1993.
5. Toombs C, Lonner B, Fazal A, et al. The adolescent idiopathic scoliosis international disease severity study: Do operative curve magnitude and complications vary by country? *Spine Deform.* 2019;7(6):883–9.
6. Charroin C, Abelin-Genevois K, Cunin V, et al. Direct costs associated with the management of progressive early onset scoliosis: Estimations based on gold standard technique or with magnetically controlled growing rods. *Orthop Traumatol Surg Res.* 2014;100(5):469–74.
7. Meirick T, Shah AS, Dolan LA, Weinstein SL. Determining the prevalence and costs of unnecessary referrals in adolescent idiopathic scoliosis. *Iowa Orthop J.* 2019;39(1):57–61.
8. Sekhri NK. Managed care: The US experience. *Bull World Health Organ.* 2000;78(6):830–44.
9. Fairfield G, Hunter DJ, Mechanic D, Rosleff F. Managed care. Origins, principles, and evolution. *BMJ.* 1997;314(7097):1823–6.
10. Ramo B, Tran D-P, Reddy A, et al. Delay to surgery greater than 6 months leads to substantial deformity progression and increased intervention in immature adolescent idiopathic scoliosis (AIS) patients: A retrospective cohort study. *Spine Deform.* 2019;7(3):428–35.
11. Haynes B, Devereaux P, Guyatt G. Physicians' and patients' choices in evidence based practice. *Br Med J.* 2002;324(7350):1350.
12. Verma K, Slattery C, Duah H, et al. Comprehensive assessment of outcomes from patients with severe early-onset scoliosis treated with a vertebral column resection: Results from an SRS global outreach site (FOCOS) in Ghana. *J Pediatr Orthop.* 2018;38(7):e393–ee8.
13. Verma K, Slattery CA, Boachie-Adjei O. What's important: Surgeon volunteerism: Experiences with FOCOS in Ghana. *J Bone Joint Surg Am.* 2019;101(9):854–5.

2b Mismatch in Expectations between Industry and Countries with Limited Resources

Aakash Agarwal

CONTENTS

INTRODUCTION

Early-onset scoliosis (EOS) is not a new spinal pathology, yet countries with limited resources are left with yesterday's solutions. The root of this problem lies in a mismatch of expectations between healthcare providers in countries with limited resources and the industries whose innovations are focused on the reimbursement available in developed nations. Further exacerbating the issue is the relatively smaller market opportunity in EOS for orthopaedic and spinal industry members than other comparative areas, making the competition slower.

However, unlike many speculative 1–2 level spinal fusion procedures conducted in adult patients with nonspecific low back pain, the problem of EOS is distinct and well identified in candidates for surgical intervention. Nevertheless, the point of care where the surgical intervention fails in the field of EOS is the

regulatory impasse for newer technology, which takes decades of development and validation, and the economic unattainability of such technologies in countries with limited resources. However, this could be used to the advantage of emerging economies via reduced burden of proof for manufacturers to conduct a clinical trial, thus choosing the lesser of two evils.

Furthermore, the healthcare field is burgeoning with several new technologies and methods. It represents advancement in medicine, but it also makes choices and applicability from a user's standpoint very obscure. More often than not its a result of lopsided marketing, in which one or more technologies are well known and advertised whereas its direct and indirect substitutes are not. It presents an obvious disadvantage for countries with limited resources, as the limited resources that exist regionally may very well be misspent on technologies that are commonplace and do not require a larger allotment for procurement.

Cost of Doing Business

The medical device industry funnels a lot of resources into research and development (R&D), distribution channels and commissions, patents protection, legal and regulatory undertaking, and marketing. The cost of these activities defines the final cost of the device, eventually making the selling price of medical devices ten- to thirtyfold the cost of manufacturing. The other factor that is equally important in determining final cost is the production volume, i.e. the real-life usage of the device in question. If the device is used in high volume, a lower profit margin may still justify long-term profitability. However, the problem persists if the device is a low-volume product. In such cases the cost must be offset via a much higher mark up to justify its continued supply; sometimes, such devices are auxiliary products and are sustained via higher mark ups on the main products. The average selling, general, and administrative (or SG&A) expenses incurred by medical device manufacturers are a vast majority of the total revenues, and thus also the reason for higher final device prices. **Figure 2b.1** shows a pie chart distribution of the total revenue for Nuvasive, and it is

evident that SG&A is significantly higher than other cost brackets. This is typical for high-volume companies with relatively lower expense on R&D activities. Alternatively, for startups, technology and innovation are differentiating factors, and thus R&D expenses remain a significant cost component. However, to balance the equation, at the successful maturity of technology or commercial availability, it most likely is acquired by large medical device manufacturers with lower internal R&D cost and higher SG&A cost. Lately, there has been a push to reduce SG&A for long-term productivity with a few medical device manufacturers launching sales models in which trained hospital staff replaces the medical device manufacturer's sales representatives. These trained hospital staff members are often present at the physician's invitation in the operating room during procedures and may help the physician make a final decision about which devices to use [1, 2]. This has enabled significant SG&A expense reduction, although the majority of medical devices have yet to go that direction. Such changes would definitely help countries with limited resources.

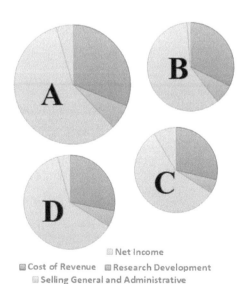

☒ Net Income

☒ Cost of Revenue ☒ Research Development
☒ Selling General and Administrative

FIGURE 2B.1 A pie chart distribution of total revenue for Nuvasive (a publicly traded orthopaedic company) in the years A. 2019, B. 2018, C. 2017, and D. 2016. The graphs show that SG&A has consistently been significantly higher than other cost brackets.

Poor Competition Due to 'Make-Believe' Product Differentiation

Contrary to popular belief, the degree of competition between manufacturers in the spine industry is often limited. Manufacturers of devices that can demonstrate clinical superiority over competing products may be in a stronger position to increase prices or at least keep them stable. In contrast, prices for a specific model can decline over time if other manufacturers enter the market or launch newer versions of existing products [3]. Manufacturers also have an incentive to lower prices and reduce their inventory of devices that will soon be replaced by a newer model. The manufacturer then typically launches the new model at a higher price. Manufacturers of implants differentiate their devices from those made by competing firms. For example, one manufacturer's spinal implant may have features or capabilities (more often than not, clinically unproven) different from a competitor's spinal implant, and physicians may need to use different techniques to implant each device. The short life cycles that are common in the medical device industry help manufacturers keep their products differentiated over time. Some differences among competing devices may have a clinical or therapeutic benefit, but in most cases, the benefits are unclear. However, because of the time required to learn how to use a new device properly, this kind of product differentiation makes it harder for physicians to switch suppliers and helps limit the extent to which manufacturers have to compete on price. Physician preferences can also reduce competition. Although hospitals are the entities that actually purchase implants, physicians have traditionally had significant influence on their purchasing decisions. Most physicians prefer to use a particular manufacturer's devices in their procedures, and hospitals have been willing to accommodate those preferences because of physicians' ability to control where their patients are admitted and the profitability of surgical lines such as orthopaedic procedures [4]. Physicians typically have had little incentive to consider differences in cost when deciding which devices to use because the hospital bears the cost [5].

FINANCIAL RELATIONSHIP BETWEEN PRACTISING SURGEONS AND INDUSTRY

The medical device industry is particularly notable for the substantial relationships that often exist between manufacturers and physicians. These ties are often deeper and more extensive than those between physicians and drug makers [6]. These relationships can take many different forms, such as royalty payments, consulting fees, funding for research, and medical education activities. In many instances, these relationships can benefit the public by fostering the development and improvement of new medical devices and educating physicians about how medical devices can be used safely and effectively. However, physicians have substantial influence over the purchase and use of many medical devices, and device manufacturers have a strong incentive to cultivate close relationships with physicians and encourage the use of their products. Manufacturers can also use their relationships with physicians to implicitly reward physicians for using their products, which has led to persistent concerns that these relationships may affect physicians' judgment about the best way to treat their patients [4, 7].

Figure 2b.2 shows the analyses of open payments (under the Sunshine Act), i.e. the payments received by physicians and teaching hospitals in the year 2018 across categories such as general, research, and in form of ownership across the United States. More specifically, **Figure 2b.3** shows payments made by Nuvasive Specialized Orthopedics, a division of Nuvasive focussed on the design and innovation of disruptive orthopaedic solutions, including its proprietary platform of magnetically adjustable implant systems (e.g. MAGEC). These general payments include consulting fees, royalty or license, travel and lodging, food and beverage, education, and services other than consulting (such as noncontinued educational speaking arrangements) in the years 2016–18. These data show the existence of

Entity Type	Number of Entities	$ General Payments	⚖ Research Payments	⬈ Value of Ownership or Investment Interest
Physicians	Receiving Payments 627,000	Amount $2.18 Billion	Amount $83.12 Million*	Amount $1.33 Billion
Teaching Hospitals	Receiving Payments 1,180	Amount $830.77 Million	Amount $1.20 Billion	Amount N/A**
Companies	Making Payments 1,583	Amount $3.01 Billion	Amount $4.89 Billion	Amount $1.33 Billion

FIGURE 2B.2   The aggregate analyses of open payments (under the Sunshine Act), i.e. the payments received by physicians and teaching hospitals in the year 2018 across categories such as general, research, and in the form of ownership across the United States.

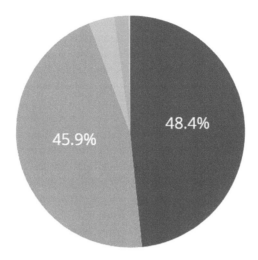

Nature of Payment	Amount	Payments	Amount (%)
▉ Consulting Fee ❶	$1,130,371.63	253	48.4%
▦ Royalty or License ❶	$1,071,750.93	51	45.9%
▦ Travel and Lodging ❶	$84,103.86	389	3.6%
▦ Food and Beverage ❶	$48,004.25	663	2.1%
▦ Education ❶	$2,823.07	8	0.1%
▦ Services other than consulting... ❶	$250.00	1	0.0%

FIGURE 2B.3   The analyses from open payments (under the Sunshine Act) made by Nuvasive Specialized Orthopedics, which include consulting fees, royalty or license, travel and lodging, food and beverage, education, and services other than consulting (such as noncontinued educational speaking arrangements) in the years 2016–2018.

extensive financial relationships between practising surgeons and industry. [8, 9].

CHANGING LANDSCAPE

Purchase prices for medical devices could equal 30%–80% of an insurer's payment to a hospital for a procedure [6]. Furthermore, as explained in an earlier section, because of reduced competition and higher 'make-believe' product differentiation, each manufacturer has some degree of control over the prices it charges for its products [10]. However, this landscape is now changing because of mergers and acquisitions in recent years, and many individual US hospital systems now control a very large volume of purchases and employ numerous physicians [11, 12]. The shift toward hospital employment has reduced the influence of physician preferences and given hospitals greater control over device purchases.

Hospitals are increasingly trying to negotiate lower prices on implants by purchasing from only two or three manufacturers. These efforts are often overseen by a 'value analysis committee' composed of hospital management and physicians from the relevant specialties that consider both cost of purchase and the perceived clinical benefit in their decision-making. Hospitals are more likely to negotiate favourable prices when they can promise significant sales in return. Hospitals have typically tried to do this by negotiating longer contracts and limiting the number of suppliers they use for a particular device, but the latter strategy may not be feasible for hospitals where physicians still have strong preferences. This shift may help reduce prices on many spinal technologies through manufacturer's incentive to uphold their profit margin and dissolution of make-believe product differentiation [13].

NEED FOR PATIENT ADVOCACY IN COUNTRIES WITH LIMITED RESOURCES

As described in previous sections, work on new spinal product development in developed countries such as the United States is driven by the possibility of reimbursement from a third party (public or private insurer) that pays the healthcare provider for costs or payments the provider incurred while using a medical device or performing a surgical procedure. Unfortunately, herein lies the problem in using these devices in countries with limited resources, regions that were not the focus when developing the device. Although new ways to reduce costs are always on the horizon because of rekindled competition in the medical device industry, there still exist problems concerning the medical devices used for EOS. EOS accounts for a very small percentage of all paediatric scoliosis cases, and scoliosis, by itself, is a small subsection of the massive number of 1–2 level spine surgeries being performed these days [14–16]. Consequently, the vast majority of resources from the industry members are focussed on other spine surgeries [17–21].

A ground up approach is needed to make sure the countries with limited resources do not fall behind in access to healthcare. Although scoliosis screening has helped reduce surgical intervention in developed countries, the countries with limited resources seldom have a regular scoliosis screening embedded in the school or healthcare curriculum. As a result, the majority of clinical presentations have already progressed to a point where surgical intervention becomes necessary. The most practical solution would be to establish regular screening procedures for children via advocacy of local surgeons and local, national, and international scoliosis societies. Such patients should be given appropriate attention and education to stay compliant with bracing and various aspects of physiotherapy. Ability for patients to share experiences directly or through indirect means also helps them remain focussed on this preventative measure. Nevertheless, there will be patients who will eventually be considered for surgical intervention [22].

In this regard, EOS surgeons should consider versatility in following any surgical philosophy for EOS, so as to not limit themselves and their patients to fewer options when cost is a real factor. For example, limitations to only distraction-based surgeries would reduce the choice to traditional growth rods, when MAGEC (MAGnetic Expansion Control, Nuvasive) rods are not available for economic reasons. However, if the surgeon is versatile, he or she could use a guided-growth technique that is cost efficient, i.e. SHILLA (performed using domino and not the proprietary screws) or a hybrid of multiple surgical philosophies, such as active apex correction (APC) (a hybrid of guided-growth and compression-based system) or spring distraction system (SDS) (a hybrid of guided-growth and distraction-based system). Practise in all possible techniques also allows the surgeon to make other patient-specific choices. For example, for a very stiff patient, distraction-based growth rods are more likely to result in fracture, autofusion, and clinically unsatisfactory results. In such patients, principles of guided-growth and compression-based systems should be considered.

SPONSORSHIP, COLLABORATIVE EFFORT, AND REGIONAL INNOVATION

A long-held view of innovation is that producers are motivated to innovate by the expectation of profits. These profits will disappear if anyone can simply copy producers' innovations, and, therefore, producers must be granted subsidies or intellectual property rights that give them exclusive control over their innovations for some period of time. However, the producers' model is only one mode of innovation; there are several alternatives to this model, as exemplified by single-user firms, individuals, and open collaborative innovation. Each of these three forms represents a different way to organise human effort and investments aimed at generating valuable new innovations [23, 24]. Approaching the respective industry member supplying the device for sponsorship or subsidy for patients who are unable to afford it seem like an impasse. If it is a multinational organisation (e.g. Nuvasive for MAGEC rods, Medtronic for SHILLA screws), it can easily afford to serve such patients and use it as a marketing tool to enhance their mission in advancement and availability of quality healthcare throughout the world. Another way to demonstrate value for the industry member is to begin a prospective study involving these patients, giving the industry member access to long-term clinical data in exchange for sponsoring such patients. In resource-limited settings such as India, public sector employees, private sector employees with health insurance, and upper middle class (out-of-pocket expense) constitutes 30% of all the patients who undergo MAGEC rod distraction-based surgery. The other 70% of patients undergoing traditional rod distraction-based surgery are people who cannot afford MAGEC and/or have congenital scoliosis, which is not covered by most medical policies. There lies an acceptance of traditional growth rod surgery among the people who have no means to afford surgeries or rely on medical loans, nongovernmental organisations, welfare funding, etc. This reflects the misunderstanding that MAGEC is a premium (i.e. unnecessary) product, and because traditional growth rods have been used in the past, underprivileged patients do not deserve any better. It is unknown why SHILLA (using domino-rod interface) or APC etc. have not be used instead of traditional growth rods in this majority of underprivileged patients. One may argue that there could be long-term complications with use of SHILLA leading to one or two revision surgeries, however repeated surgeries (5–15) with traditional growth rods is a bigger source of morbidity for patients with EOS.

There exists a gap between advancement in growth rod technology and affordability of such in developing countries. An ideal solution would be to provide the advanced technology at a lower cost, through government subsidies and affordable healthcare insurance. However, in the absence of such a programme or subsidies, a pragmatic approach should at least include provision of a bridging technology. A regional or locally developed source of such devices would avoid this problem because the development of such devices will, by design, consider the economy of the region. An opportunity exists to either innovate a distinct technology with the freedom to operate commercially or reproduce and build upon an existing technology when the parent industry or inventors does not deem it worthy of protection in a given economic system. By law, a disclosed technology is

public knowledge when not protected as per the countries' patent regulations within a given time frame. Efforts should also be directed toward collaborative work with the industry member to develop a bridging technology. Many external grants exist from large industry members, such as Medtronic, who support individual research conducted by surgeons.

When fostering innovation, surgeons should be careful of companies (nonpractising entities) that find ways to make money on patent-infringement lawsuits. These are entities who buy cheap patents from bankrupt companies, universities, and researchers affiliated to these institutions through superficially appealing agreements; however, they never actually produce anything. Instead, they find companies or individuals who appear to have infringed upon a patent they own and exploit them. They exploit the patent-infringers by demanding licensing fees and then threaten them with lawsuits if they will not comply [25].

REDUCING REGULATORY HURDLES

Exacting regulatory processes fosters micro-innovation (mini-innovation) to such a great extent that patients are exposed to passive forms of medical abuse. The model regulatory environment that exists today in developed nations, and is gradually being adopted in developing nations, penalises technological advancement in the form of delay and capital investment. Although it is necessary to guard public interest by governing bodies, such a stringent method also harms the public by reducing the rate of access to newer medical treatments and technologies [26, 27]. The regulation should be limited to a framework necessary to carry innovation with precision and safety without stifling the rate at which it is undertaken. Unlike a systematic drug development process, most spinal medical instrumentation achieves its objective via a mechanical mode of action. Most material and the wear particulates from these materials do pose a biological response, however, the focus of device development and the improvement cycle should be on reducing it rather than on drawing a hard line of acceptance and rejection. Nevertheless, this climate in developed nations could drive industry members to conduct clinical trials of their latest medical technology in countries with limited resources where there are fewer regulatory hurdles. The utmost safety and affordability may not coexist in countries with limited resources and thus remain open to new technologies in pursuit of better clinical data, which may provide a backdoor entrance to long-term clinical trials without the question of affordability. Just as Europe is well-known for conducting clinical trials of new technology, the cost of which are fully funded by the industry seeking long-term data, countries with limited resources could also encourage this with proper patient consent and the existence of credible preliminary data.

COMPARING VALUE OF MEDICAL TECHNOLOGIES

This section serves to provide a systemic tool to identify key parameters that distinguish and quantify the absolute value of a new technology or methodology. This could also be employed for comparison among various technologies or methods, either in the same category or different. Above all, it helps the healthcare professionals in countries with limited resources make a conscientious and judicious use of current best evidence, technologies, and methods for economical clinical care. Understanding the value or impact of a technology requires the collection of discretised parameters, such as the severity of the problem, the affected population, efficacy of the technology or the method in question, and its adoption and relative viability over other substitute technologies produced regionally or in developed nations [28–30]. The key and the traditional identifier of the impact of an innovation has always been the problem it solves, or the severity it reduces, with population of affected people being a close second. The problem and severity can be classified using different metrics such as rate of mortality, reduced quality of life, progression of disease, etc. The population considered here should be representative of the actual subset that are candidates for the technology and not the entire population which is affected by the disease or pathology. For example, scoliosis in children by itself affects a larger population, however they can further be divided into patient populations who will successfully be treated with conservative methods

such as bracing, while the remaining may have to undergo surgery. Therefore, if the technology under consideration is a growth rod system (surgical correction), then the population size should only account for the patients undergoing surgery instead of the entire population of children with scoliosis. In contrast, a bracing technology may consider the entire population of children with scoliosis as its affected population because surgery remains the second choice of treatment. Thus, consideration should be given to where the technology lies in terms of its applicability in the current diagnostics and treatment philosophy. Nevertheless, this data will never be accurate, but the sensitivity toward this data (along with adoption, cost of undertaking, and compliance to the technology) will help to guide the comparison between two very similar technologies or methodologies.

An equally important identifier is the effect of size, or the observed difference due to the technology's implementation. The technology or method in question should exemplify its efficacy via controlled studies, real-life studies, case series either employing the exact technology or appropriate analogous sources, and expert opinion where reasonable. Expert opinion should be in a form of an objectively answered questionnaire from multiple sources, however, its scope and usefulness are limited to ergonomic tools or methodology. Risks and side effects should also be part of efficacy evaluation for a technology or method. Based on current evidence, risk and benefit are very sensitive to the patient selection criteria employed [31]. For example, many clinicians and researchers would argue that more spinal fusion surgeries are being performed than needed. For evaluation purposes, one can choose to reduce the affected population (via more stringent patient selection criteria or considering the appropriate diagnoses and prognosis), thereby increasing the clinical efficacy or increasing the affected population (by generalisation) and reducing average efficacy. A slightly different approach may consider varying clinical efficacy parameters over many subsets of a population to find a balance of mass applicability and clinical efficacy.

Quantifying the problem, severity, affected population, and clinical efficacy as described above is relatively straightforward when compared to understanding the adoption of the technology. The adoption discussed here considers only the socioeconomical and legal aspects inherent to the technology and does not delve into the matter of awareness (marketing and advertisement), economics (micro and macro), management (execution and leadership) etc. Understanding the adoption helps in accounting for an auxiliary error in overestimation of the affected population, reduced because of economic, legal, or regulatory barriers. In past 5 years, MAGEC rod was considered the best, technically advanced option for most patients with scoliosis. The technology was approved by the US Federal Drug Administration (FDA) in 2014 and became the only distraction-based device used in the United States; however, this same technology was used less than 30% of time in countries with limited resources. Most patients, in lieu of the high upfront cost of the device, had to undergo traditional growth rod surgery. The cost assessment in countries with limited resources shows that the magnetic growth rod was at least 65% more expensive than the traditional growth rod and at the most 310% more expensive than traditional growth rods [32]. During the assessment, it was also found that the cost of treating EOS is substantially higher than the cost of a late-onset scoliosis with magnetic growth rod. This scenario does not affect the developed nations because of the availability of initial funds or credit from insurance or other healthcare programmes [33]. In such countries, repeated outpatient distraction compared to invasive procedures levels the economic ground long term, though a high rate of noninvasive distraction failure, up to 50%, is resurfacing the clinical and economic concerns, even for developed nations [34]. Like adoption but more varied, is the cost of establishing use and gaining patient compliance for the technology. Many technologies or methods would require the user to be trained in the appropriate use of the technology or technique or provision of resources for realising its potential. This is what the cost of establishing use entails. For example, the unavailability of well-trained endoscopic surgeons in a region requires an influx of resources for training [35]. Related, but more process- and design-based, is the patient compliance to the technology or method, i.e. how easy,

effortless, independent, error-proof, accountable etc. is the technology or method for the patient to use effectively. For example, traditional bracing technology shows moderate to poor results, which some experts and researchers claim is because of poor patient compliance [36, 37].

CONCLUSION

A vigilant approach to cost and technology procurement is the key to sustainable use of resources in developing nations. The method described here underlines the key principles required for a clinician to quickly evaluate an existing technology or ask relevant questions to themselves or the presenter. The impact being determined is specific to the problem being addressed. Sometimes a technology may solve multiple problems or could be used in different ways, and thus each should be assessed separately. Understanding the changing landscape in the field of healthcare may also play a crucial role in addition to the above-presented rationale and methodical evaluation of the impact. Furthermore, assessing the role of complementary tools and techniques that are under development or currently exist may also help determine the favorability or lack of thereof toward adoption of a technology. Nevertheless, quantified differentiation is the key to understanding the impact of a technology or tool.

A lot of disadvantages exist in a resource-limited setting, and thus providing optimal patient care in such a region requires multifaceted approach, such as early intervention, up-to-date training on all possible modes of surgical intervention (e.g. distraction-based, guided-growth, and compression-based) and the hybrids, regionally appropriate innovation, collaborative work, and sponsorship programmes.

REFERENCES

1. Lee J. Devicemaker sales reps being replaced in the OR. *Modern Healthcare*. 2014, 1–6.
2. Freed J. *Taking Back the OR Introducing a Direct-Access™ Model*, Western States Healthcare Materials Management Association (WSHMMA), Tacoma, WA.
3. Smith B. An empirical investigation of marketing strategy quality in medical markets. *Journal of Medical Marketing*. 2003;3(2):153–162.

4. Robinson JC. *Purchasing Medical Innovation: The Right Technology, for the Right Patient, at the Right Price.* University of California Press; 2015, Oakland CA.

5. Okike K, O'Toole RV, Pollak AN, et al. Survey finds few orthopedic surgeons know the costs of the devices they implant. *Health Affairs.* 2014;33(1):103–109.

6. Robinson JC. Value-based purchasing for medical devices. *Health Affairs.* 2008;27(6):1523–1531.

7. Chatterji AK, Fabrizio KR, Mitchell W, et al. Physician-industry cooperation in the medical device industry. *Health Affairs.* 2008;27(6):1532–1543.

8. Marshall DC, Jackson ME, Hattangadi-Gluth JA. Disclosure of industry payments to physicians: An epidemiologic analysis of early data from the open payments program. Paper presented at: *Mayo Clinic Proceedings*; 2016;91(1):84–96.

9. Iyer S, Derman P, Sandhu HS. Orthopaedics and the Physician Payments Sunshine Act: An examination of payments to US orthopaedic surgeons in the Open Payments Database. *Journal of Bone and Joint Surgery.* 2016;98(5):e18.

10. Pauly MV, Burns LR. Price transparency for medical devices. *Health Affairs.* 2008;27(6):1544–1553.

11. Beaulieu ND, Dafny LS, Landon BE, et al. Changes in quality of care after hospital mergers and acquisitions. *New England Journal of Medicine.* 2020;382(1):51–59.

12. Treat TF. *A Study of the Characteristics and Performance of Merging Hospitals in the United States.* Texas A&M University Libraries; College Station, Texas, 2020.

13. Miller FA, Lehoux P, Peacock S, et al. How procurement judges the value of medical technologies: A review of healthcare tenders. *International Journal of Technology Assessment in Health Care.* 2019;35(1):50–55.

14. Hedequist D, Emans J. Congenital scoliosis: A review and update. *Journal of Pediatric Orthopaedics.* 2007;27(1):106–116.

15. Akbarnia BA. Management themes in early onset scoliosis. *Bone and Joint Surgery.* 2007;89(suppl_1):42–54.

16. Carter OD, Haynes SG. Prevalence rates for scoliosis in US adults: Results from the first National Health and Nutrition Examination Survey. *International Journal of Epidemiology.* 1987;16(4):537–544.

17. Weinstein JN, Lurie JD, Olson P, et al. United States trends and regional variations in lumbar spine surgery: 1992–2003. *Spine.* 2006;31(23):2707.

18. Jancuska JM, Hutzler L, Protopsaltis TS, et al. Utilization of lumbar spinal fusion in New York State: Trends and disparities. *Spine.* 2016;41(19):1508–1514.

19. Lubelski D, Williams SK, O'Rourke C, et al. Differences in the surgical treatment of lower back pain among spine surgeons in the United States. *Spine.* 2016;41(11):978–986.

20. Kristiansen J-A, Balteskard L, Slettebø H, et al. The use of surgery for cervical degenerative disease in Norway in the period 2008–2014. *Acta Neurochirurgica.* 2016;158(5):969–974.

21. Li Y, Zheng S, Wu Y, et al. Trends of surgical treatment for spinal degenerative disease in China: A cohort of 37,897 inpatients from 2003 to 2016. *Clinical Interventions in Aging.* 2019;14:361.

22. Morais T, Bernier M, Turcotte F. Age-and sex-specific prevalence of scoliosis and the value of school screening programs. *American Journal of Public Health.* 1985;75(12):1377–1380.

23. von Hippel E, Jin C. The major shift towards user-centred innovation. *Journal of Knowledge-Based Innovation in China.* 2009;1(1):16–27.

24. Baldwin CY, von Hippel EA. Modeling a paradigm shift: From producer innovation to user and open collaborative innovation. *Harvard Business School Finance Working Paper.* 2010(10-038):4764–4709.

25. Uzoigwe CE, Shoaib A. Patents and intellectual property in orthopaedics and arthroplasty. *World Journal of Orthopedics.* 2020;11(1):1.

26. Buch B. FDA medical device approval: things you didn't learn in medical school or residency. *American Journal of Orthopedics-Belle Mead.* 2007;36(8):407.

27. Samuel AM, Rathi VK, Grauer JN, et al. How do orthopaedic devices change after their initial FDA premarket approval? *Clinical Orthopaedics and Related Research®.* 2016;474(4):1053–1068.

28. Lakdawalla DN, Phelps CE. *Evaluation of Medical Technologies with Uncertain Benefits.* National Bureau of Economic Research; 2019:0898-2937.

29. Fasterholdt I, Krahn M, Kidholm K, et al. Review of early assessment models of innovative medical technologies. *Health Policy.* 2017;121(8):870–879.

30. Ho M, Saha A, McCleary KK, et al. A framework for incorporating patient preferences regarding benefits and risks into regulatory assessment of medical technologies. *Value in Health.* 2016;19(6):746–750.

31. Smith WD, Gupta K, Kelesis M, et al. Selection of appropriate patients for outpatient spine surgery. In: *Minimally Invasive Spine Surgery.* Springer; 2019:605–617.

32. Agarwal A. TO THE EDITOR: Letter to Editor for: Harshavardhana NS, Noordeen MH, Dormans JP. Cost analysis of magnet-driven growing rods for early-onset scoliosis at 5 years. *Spine*. 2019;44(18):E1108–E1108.

33. Harshavardhana NS, Noordeen MH, Dormans JP. Cost analysis of magnet-driven growing rods for early-onset scoliosis at 5 years. *Spine*. 2019;44(1):60–67.

34. Joyce TJ, Smith SL, Rushton PR, et al. Analysis of explanted magnetically controlled growing rods from seven UK spinal centers. *Spine*. 2018;43(1):E16–E22.

35. Lin G-X, Kotheeranurak V, Mahatthanatrakul A, et al. Worldwide research productivity in the field of full-endoscopic spine surgery: A bibliometric study. *European Spine Journal*. 2019:1–8.

36. Karavidas N. Bracing in the treatment of adolescent idiopathic scoliosis: Evidence to date. *Adolescent Health, Medicine and Therapeutics*. 2019;10:153.

37. Rahimi S, Kiaghadi A, Fallahian N. Effective factors on brace compliance in idiopathic scoliosis: A literature review. *Disability and Rehabilitation: Assistive Technology*. 2019:1–7.

2c Organisational Deficiencies in Developing Countries and the Role of Global Surgery

Amal Ahmad

CONTENTS

INTRODUCTION

Surgical care in developing countries faces the dual challenge of limited financial and organisational resources. Limited financial resources imply a dearth of funds for necessary materials, such as surgical equipment, while limited organisational resources imply a limited ability to best combine and utilise existing material and human resources.

The predominant view, at least in advanced economies, is that the financial needs of developing countries are dire, without equally appreciating other institutional and organisational deficiencies that characterise economic underdevelopment. As a result, largely financial fixes, such as material donations and doctors from developed countries volunteering to perform surgeries for free, are popular. However, in the absence of a more holistic vision, such assistance remains temporary, operating more as a stopgap measure than a purveyor of structural change. Donor- and volunteer-exhaustion is not uncommon, and when funds dry up, it becomes clear that the local surgical system is still stagnant, with little lasting improvement to surgical care quality or outcomes.

This chapter offers a different viewpoint, which is that a big part of the problem stems from the underutilisation and poor organisation of the most valuable medical resource in any country – human capital – and that while additional funding can help, it cannot automatically or mechanistically fix this problem. The reality for many local doctors in developing countries is that they must perform their standard medical duties in a healthcare system that offers them little support. This involves not just material support in the form of equipment and other necessities, but also organisational support in the form of incentivised and effective training; equipped nursing and assisting staff; clear guidelines and protocols regarding medical error, accountability, and liability protection; clear protocols about communication with different healthcare institutions; incentives for data collection and research; and many more.

This weak organisational environment imposes numerous burdens on the local surgeon, a primary one of which relates to training and learning. Surgeons are unlikely to be motivated or able to engage in high-risk surgeries, such as spine surgeries, or to keep up with continually evolving global best practices, and surgical care quality is likely to remain poor. Funding and sporadic international volunteer missions do not fix this problem either, as some of the skills fundamental to improving surgical outcomes must be learned by actively and consistently engaging and supporting the local doctor.

For this particular need, global surgery can make a lasting difference: missions that not only provide clinical service but also train doctors and advance their long-term capabilities would work around some of the local organisational deficiencies, thereby facilitating structural change in a challenging environment and complementing financial assistance. This chapter focusses on why these programs matter and what they could look like.

The chapter is structured as follows. The 'Organisational Challenges in Developing Countries' section expands on the concept of 'organisational deficiency' in healthcare systems and argues that this has been not been at the forefront of global surgery concerns in dealing with developing countries. The 'Learning and the Local Surgeon' section explains why and how limited organisational resources impede learning and training, especially in highly demanding surgical fields, such as spine and early-onset scoliosis (EOS) surgery, and the repercussions for the local surgeon. The 'Role of Global Surgery' section argues that, while local institutional shortfalls are likely to be rigid, global surgery can alleviate part of the problem by training sets of local surgeons and enhancing their incentives and capacities to learn, innovate, and conduct research. Therefore, global surgery can circumscribe at least some of the challenges associated with limited organisational resources and help promote services such as spine surgery. The 'Conclusion' section summarises and concludes the chapter's arguments.

ORGANISATIONAL CHALLENGES IN DEVELOPING COUNTRIES

In the simplest terms, organisational efficiency refers to the ability to combine and use (i.e.

organise) resources efficiently, hence to make the most out of existing resources. This includes the organisation of material resources, such as (in a medical setting) from whom to buy medical equipment, how to distribute it across departments, how to market and expand the hospital's reach, and so on. It also includes the organisation of personnel resources, such as overseeing hiring and training and managing, facilitating, and supporting the work of doctors, nurses, administrators, and others. Because organisational efficiency is tied to the strength of the institutions that oversee material and personnel, it can also be referred to as institutional efficiency.

Therefore, whereas financial constraints imply there is a limited total amount of resources available (small pie), organisational constraints imply there is a limited ability, due to weak institutions, to manage these resources successfully (to make the most out of the existing pie). These are two related but distinct concepts. Greater resources (a bigger pie) may ease organisational constraints, but this will not happen if institutional quality remains poor and if there is a lack of streamlined and efficient bureaucracy to manage finances and personnel. Organisational inefficiency within an institution may also create organisational inefficiency between institutions, as it becomes more difficult to coordinate tasks and communicate with each other.

The difference is stark between advanced and developing countries both in the size of their resources and the strength of the institutions that manage these resources. In developed countries, resources are relatively abundant and institutions are strong, with streamlined bureaucracy and relatively transparent rules and chains of command. In developing countries, by contrast, resources are, by definition, limited, institutions are generally weak, bureaucracy is more haphazard, and rules are less transparent [1]. This also makes coordination between different institutions difficult, slow, and potentially chaotic [2]. For these reasons, it is more difficult, in developing countries, to set expectations and plan forward in almost all settings (not just the healthcare sector). Therefore, when we talk about 'resource-limited' countries, it signifies that there are limitations on both financial and organisational resources.

In developed countries, because institutions are relatively strong and bureaucracy is streamlined, it is easy to overlook the problems that could arise organisationally, and the distinction between themselves and developing countries has been understood, at least historically and in popular discourse, in terms of the extent of financial resources (as exemplified by the prevalent language of 'rich' versus 'poor' countries). The fact that development requires much more than just having more resources is exemplified by the vastly different outcomes of resource-rich developing economies. For example, in 2019, the top two oil-rich countries in West Africa – Angola and Nigeria – had a combined average gross domestic product (GDP) per capita of $3,000 while the top two oil-rich countries in the Persian Gulf – Saudi Arabia and the United Arab Emirates – had a combined average GDP per capita of about $30,000. Similarly, many countries receive aid and financial assistance from the West, but this aid is not equally successful across the board in promoting development, owing in part to institutional differences that influence how the funds are utilised [3].

Because global surgery programs are predominantly developed and organised by healthcare institutions and surgeons from the United States and Europe, the viewpoints of global surgery are largely informed by this perspective. Financial or quasi-financial assistance via donations or short-term volunteer missions are the primary concern of a majority of programs; see for example Gutnik et al. [4] on estimated financial contributions and Shrime et al. [5] on short-term surgical missions. (Volunteer missions are quasi-financial because they are equivalent to providing funding for those surgeries, with the funding source being the international surgeons who forgo their standard fees.)

Financial and quasi-financial assistance certainly alleviate short-term supply problems but cannot, on their own, address long-term problems. Providing funds for equipment and other purchases is of limited helpfulness if the domestic workforce is unable to utilise these resources effectively. Similarly, volunteering to conduct surgeries offers a short-term service that cannot be sustained nor replicated if local surgeons do not eventually learn how to provide this service themselves. In turn, as will be discussed in the 'Learning and the Local Surgeon' section, improving the ability of medical personnel to utilise resources effectively and to learn best practices is highly demanding on organisations. Therefore, the effectiveness of global surgery's financial assistance to developing countries is tied to complementary organisational improvements that allow local healthcare providers to learn and adapt some of those fundamental skills brought by global surgeons.

Of course, global surgery and the contributions of international surgeons cannot and would not be able to fix a developing country's healthcare system. Institutions are historically rooted and difficult to change except in the very long term, and, even then, institutional change is the outcome of the interaction of domestic political and economic factors [6]. In fact, part of the appeal of limited programs such as donations or volunteer surgeries is that they are doable and pragmatic in their goal of offering short-term relief. Nonetheless, while global surgery cannot be expected to change a country's institutions, there are ways it can use its resources to allow local surgeons to work around some of these organisational problems that are likely to persist in the long run.

In particular, global surgery – through its administrative bodies and networks of surgeons – can work with local institutions to offer space, skilled surgeons, and logistical support to train sets of local doctors on global best practices; in turn, as suggested above, this also supports the efficacy of financial and quasi-financial assistance to developing countries. The next section addresses more closely the concept of learning and innovation in developing countries, using EOS surgical training as an example. It will elaborate why training is not an automatic outcome of greater funding and needs to be organised and supported strategically, thereby paving the way for a discussion of the role of global surgery in this area.

LEARNING AND THE LOCAL SURGEON

THE LEARNING PROCESS

To set the stage for a discussion on the training of local surgeons, a useful starting point is the distinction between information and knowledge. Per economists who study how people learn in different settings, *information* describes a set of 'blueprints' that can be easily codified and freely transferred to a person who reads them [7]. For example, a simple set of instructions for putting together a child's toy constitutes information in that the full instructions can be written out, and the person who reads it will, with little effort, understand how to carry out the instructions perfectly.

By contrast, *knowledge* may incorporate components that are tacit, or hidden, because they are difficult to codify because of complexity and context specificity; acquiring this knowledge involves solving problems that are 'ill-structured', for which no automatic solution is available [8, 9]. As a result, knowledge cannot be fully transferred to another person through a manual or a blueprint, and the recipient must actively exert effort to uncover the tacit components and solve the relevant problem. For example, suppose the problem is how to design a large building. One cannot learn how to become an architect only by reading books because designing buildings is highly complex and depends on terrain, weather, building materials, zoning laws, etc. Extensive hands-on experience is necessary to fully acquire that knowledge. This is the reason architects must not only complete schooling in which they read books (codifiable information) but also apply themselves in internships and other projects before they are licensed. In the United States, for example, one must complete a 3-year internship before being licensed.

How and where does the 'uncovering' of the tacit components of knowledge take place? Because much of the tacitness is due to context specificity, the uncovering largely takes place through trial and error on the job itself. Attempting to solve the problem in a controlled setting, such as an architecture internships with supervision, enables people to figure out what works and what does not in the target context and to use that experience to gradually improve their ability to deal with the problem at hand. In that way, the knowledge-acquisition process involves (among other things) solving problems for which no codified solution exists, largely through trial and error on the job. This type of learning process is aptly named 'learning by doing'.

The nature of the learning process implies that, in fields for which problems are highly complex, ill-structured, and context specific, a lot of hands-on experience is necessary, and simply transferring equipment and information is not enough for building local expertise. This is because information transfer is not the same as knowledge transfer. It is critical that the target personnel are afforded the opportunity to get involved directly through guided learning by doing. For this to be successful, it must involve appropriate mentoring, supervision, guidance, assessment, and feedback, and this must be planned on a time frame that is long enough to sufficiently enable learning from experience and from trial and error.

To sum, learning in highly complex fields is not only potentially financially costly but also highly organisationally demanding [10].

The Surgeon in Developing Countries

Surgical intervention is a prime example of a problem that is highly complex, ill-structured, and context specific. For this reason, surgeons must acquire extensive hands-on experience before they are qualified to operate on patients, through rotations, multiyear residency programs, and potentially further training. Paediatric spinal surgery, particularly the treatment of EOS, is especially challenging. It is continually evolving and requires training in addition to standard orthopaedic surgical training. It is also highly context specific, with the most appropriate procedure varying with the child's medical history, the equipment available locally, and experience necessary for making critical on-the-spot decisions during the surgery itself.

In line with the above discussion, this implies that building local capacity for the management of EOS requires a great deal of organisational resources and that developing countries are at a significant disadvantage in this regard. Building capacity requires experienced surgeons to act as mentors for learning by doing, as well as institutional support in the form of planning and organising the training; patient outreach; equipping the nursing and other auxiliary staff; setting clear expectations about surgical outcomes and quality; and structuring appropriate intake, follow-up, and accountability procedures. It also requires extensive and transparent coordination between the different relevant institutions of a country, including its healthcare ministry, medical schools, training hospitals, and other hospitals. These organisational facets are somewhat or extremely deficient in countries with limited resources. Added to the existing financial burden of procuring often expensive equipment, this paints a bleak picture for surgical capacity in those countries

What does this mean at the individual level, for prospective spinal or EOS surgeons in a developing country? First, they face significantly more hurdles toward intellectual and clinical development than their counterparts operating in a streamlined bureaucratic system in the United States or Europe. Lack of institutional support also means they have little incentive to enter this highly complex, time-consuming, and risky surgical field, particularly given the high incidence of postoperative complications and unclear ways to protect the surgeon from medical negligence claims. The availability of an untapped market for spine and EOS surgery may motivate doctors, offsetting some of the incentive problem, but here, too, surgeons may encounter a wary population and will need to exert effort to display credibility to build a reputation.

As a result, often only the very ambitious individuals are able to move forward and essentially train themselves. They have to bear much of the burden of finding mentors and scouring training opportunities, coordinating the requirements and opportunities of different healthcare organisations, reaching out to patients, and building a skilled auxiliary team, all while bearing significant risk on the financial and medical side. Instead of institutions fostering medical talent (as in the advanced economies) the result is medical talent arising despite institutional hurdles and inefficiencies. Of course, this means too few spine and EOS surgeons and lack of provision of an important service to spine patients in developing countries. At the turn of the twenty-first century, about 80% of all orthopaedic surgeons in the world resided in 26 advanced economies, and the concentration was likely even higher for orthopaedic spine specialists [11].

This discussion also highlights the complementarity between financial and organisational resources. Procuring the right equipment is a financial hurdle for many countries, but even with funding for the right equipment, lack of a skilled staff that knows how to operate this equipment makes the tools more or less useless. Moreover, unlike equipment for which acquisition is largely a financial and operational problem, the acquisition of a skilled staff is much more complex and organisationally demanding. The next section expands on how global surgeons can realistically help promote progress in this challenging and institutionally constrained context, with continued focus on spinal and EOS surgery.

THE ROLE OF GLOBAL SURGERY

LONG-TERM TRAINING PROGRAMS

The most important healthcare resource in any country is the knowledge and skill of its medical staff, but, as discussed above, the nature of the problem of improving surgical training in countries with limited resources is twofold. First, training personnel to solve complex, ill-structured, and context-specific problems, such as spine and EOS surgery, is not only costly equipment-wise, but also highly organisationally demanding. Second, healthcare institutions that would usually be responsible for such training, including teaching hospitals, are usually organisationally weak (to varying extents) in countries with limited resources. They may have limited capability or experience in planning and coordinating who can train medical students and local surgeons, where and how often this training will take place, how it can be funded in the long term, what auxiliary staff is needed, and the set of outcomes/metrics expected and accounted for at the end, among other things. This creates an unfortunate situation in which the regions that need significant improvements in surgical outcomes remain the most in need, even as they occasionally receive financial or quasi-financial assistance from global health organisations.

Laying out the root of the problem clearly is important for thinking about solutions. It is hardly controversial to suggest that the nature of the learning process itself – and the fact that it is highly organisationally demanding – cannot be changed. Even though there are ongoing advancements in virtual reality (VR) surgical intervention, it is unclear how quickly these advancements will become mainstream in surgical training institutions. Moreover, even if or once VR training becomes widespread, effective use of it to train doctors in developing countries would still require significant organisational effort, albeit in a different capacity.

Therefore, the way forward is to somehow overcome the organisational weakness in countries with limited resources so that training, especially for highly complex surgeries, can be accommodated. While it is almost impossible for global surgery to make drastic changes to a country's domestic institutions, it can support existing arrangements, or offer new ones, for meeting certain realistic training goals.

What would such an involvement of global surgery look like? Though the exact program would be context specific, the main function of global surgery (specifically, the training or education committees of its associations) would be to coordinate between international surgeons, local healthcare systems, and local surgeons:

- **International surgeons.** Global surgery associations can draw systematically on the thousands of members they have and, without too much difficulty, elicit the enthusiastic participation of a sizable number of spinal and EOS surgeons for volunteer training missions. The participating surgeons would be highly experienced in training and mentoring and would be comfortable committing to a program that involves consistent travel (for example, once every 3 months) for a number of years to a specific country or region. They would also be financially comfortable doing this on a volunteer basis but with the understanding that their flights and basic accommodations are provided for. Follow-up and consistency over a sufficiently long time frame is key to generating learning results, for the reasons listed above, and is the primary differentiator between a program like

this and the existing popular short-term missions.

- **Local healthcare systems.** Global surgery associations can reach out to various contacts in each potential country of choice to see if there is agreement and enthusiasm among key local actors, such as health ministers and heads of training hospitals, about the desirability of an externally organised multiyear spine/EOS training program. After narrowing down a list of host countries, the difficult but important job is to negotiate key logistics such as where these training programs would take place, how often, what the appropriate metrics who be and how regularly they would be assessed (this is crucial), who would provide the equipment and/or cover the cost of hosting the international surgeons. Ironing out the details is context specific, but it might be important to ask that the local healthcare system bear part of the financial cost if possible. This increases the stakes of the program succeeding and provides an incentive for local administrators to manage and monitor progress closely.

- **Local surgeons.** Though local surgeons' main points of contact will be their own local healthcare administrators and the (visiting) international surgeons, it is beneficial for the global surgery logistics team to also establish some direct contact. Before training, a first step would be to ask surgeons from that country who are involved in global surgery networks what they think the major needs and challenges are of surgeons in their community and their view of the relationship between surgeons and local healthcare institutions. Once the training program is underway, it is important to receive and incorporate feedback from the group of surgeons being trained about the efficacy of training, the areas they need more focus on, and how the training is translating into results in their own local surgical practice.

This type of work would involve some financial costs (though not prohibitive because much of it would be done on a volunteer basis by the relevant committees), but, more importantly, it is highly organisationally demanding. Effectively, the institutions and networks of global surgery would be using their power and resources to ease some of the organisational burden on the healthcare system of the country in question, thereby facilitating the achievement of certain important targets. In a sense, this is parallel to financial assistance (in which funds ease the budget constraints of poor countries) and, as argued above, equally important but more often neglected.

Logistically and strategically, it is very important that long-term does not mean infinite or having a vague end date. Though some flexibility may be necessary as the programs get underway, it is imperative to have an end date in mind at the outset (such as 2 or 3 years). It is also necessary to have a protocol from the beginning specifying what the final goals are and how to assess progress in terms of these goals at regular intervals. This will increase transparency, help avoid complacency in the program, and encourage international surgeons to volunteer their time and effort, knowing that there is a specific desired outcome and end date in mind.

COLLABORATION OVER HIERARCHY

It is clear from the above discussion that global surgery institutes and networks would not (and cannot) supplant local healthcare institutions but, rather, would collaborate with them to ease some of the underlying constraints and facilitate the achievement of concrete targets. The organisational burden, though in part borne by the international institute owing to its resources, would be shared by the local organisations (such as health ministries and training hospitals), and two-way communication would be essential to continually assess and improve the training programs.

In parallel, the relationship of the international surgeon to the local surgeon should reflect a collaboration rather than a top-down chain of command. International surgeons are there to offer a resource (experience in highly complex surgeries) to ease the learning constraints on local surgeons. Though there is some power dynamic inherent in the mentor-mentee relationship, it is critical to be aware of this and mitigate the hierarchical dynamic to the extent possible.

Fostering a collaborative, versus a hierarchical, approach between the international and local surgeon is important not only because it can aid the working relationship but also because it is imperative for the success of the learning process. As discussed in the 'Learning and the Local Surgeon' section, learning often involves components that are context specific and that must be uncovered with experience and trial and error on the job. This includes how to adapt existing technologies or techniques to best fit the local environment, which is not something that can be known ex ante and is uncovered actively as the technology is being used in the target context. In fact, while developing countries often innovate by producing new technologies at the frontier of science, people in developing countries also innovate when they adapt existing technologies to best fit a complex local context.

With surgical intervention, while international surgeons brings their skills and experience in global best practices, local surgeons bring their intimate familiarity with the local context and a superior ability to gauge how to best adapt these standard practices to that context. For example, the surgeon being trained may figure out, with experience, how to create moderate adjustments in technique that utilise fewer expensive surgical materials, improving the accessibility of this surgery in an environment with limited financial resources (see Ahmad et al. [12] and the innovation of the four-rib construct for EOS treatment as an example). For this reason, the optimal learning process would combine insight from and feedback between both the international and local surgeon.

From the international surgeons, such a collaborative approach would require a dose of humility and an understanding of their role in perspective, including what they do not know and what they rely on the local surgeon for help with. It requires that international surgeons are cognisant of and work proactively to overcome the cgo problems embedded in volunteer missions (for a discussion of this problem, see Ahmad [13]). They should be comfortable acting as temporarily senior colleagues who are training surgeons in less developed countries to eventually become their peers. There needs to be an active effort to elevate local surgeons to the status of a peer, and to not view them as a perennial mentee, because that is the point and hallmark of successful training.

From the local surgeons, though in the long run it is in their best interest to form an active part of the surgical intervention and acquire the skill, there may be strong initial reluctance to get involved and potentially be held accountable for the outcomes of complex and risky surgeries. A clear understanding for these surgeons about what constitutes a medical error in these surgeries is helpful as is a measured and gradual approach in which local surgeons become more involved over successive training sessions. A protocol of expected outcomes and frequent assessment of performance would also incentivise local surgeons to exert effort and improve their performance confidence through successive rounds of feedback.

DATA COLLECTION

Data supports learning, progress, and innovation in all scientific fields, and surgery is no exception. The collection of data on the outcomes of different surgical techniques is at the heart of understanding what constitutes best practices. In addition, data on the distribution and correlation of different variables – for example, relating to patient characteristics, medical history, and ex post complications – would help surgeons better gauge the local context in which they are operating and innovate accordingly.

Unfortunately, the collection of aggregate medical data in developing countries is difficult [14], which is unsurprising given that it requires both financial and organisational resources. Global surgery cannot suddenly overturn or fix these problems; however, it can facilitate the collection of surgical data on the individual level by the local doctors it trains. Therefore, though macroanalysis of medical outcomes based on large data sets or experimental trials would remain elusive, more micro data sets, building on individual surgeon's experiences, can be encouraged, leading as well to potential research and publication outlets for these surgeons.

Accordingly, training programs provide a valuable venue to not only teach surgical best practices, but also to demonstrate data collection practices to the surgeons in training. The good news is that with surgery, data collection involves the somewhat time-consuming but not too complicated task of documenting key variables relating to patient characteristics and medical history preoperatively, and key surgical outcomes and complications ex post. Here, too, the sustainability of the training program makes a difference: because training would be organised on a relatively long-term basis with numerous follow-ups for each patient, the local surgeon would be able to use the follow-ups to apply the data collection skills learned in training.

In addition to training, global surgery may also be able to aid the microcollection of surgical data by creating the templates of relevant questions the local doctors would ask, and the observations they would document in the process. These templates can be standardised or somewhat differentiated by region. Such an endeavour would not require a great deal of financial resources, but it would be important to digitise this template, to disseminate it through various local networks, and potentially organise target training sessions for surgeons on the use and long-term adoption of such templates.

CONCLUSION

Healthcare systems in developing countries grapple with limited financial and organisational resources. Whereas the financial constraints are common knowledge, the organisational constraints these countries' institutions face are less well understood; these relate to the ability to utilise existing material and human resources effectively and to coordinate among different institutions to achieve shared objectives. Organisational constraints impede, among other things, effective training of the surgical cadre, especially on highly complex interventions such as spine and EOS surgery. This limits the ability of local surgeons to learn best practices and to refine existing techniques to best fit their local environment and keeps these interventions out of reach for much of the population.

Global surgery, with its organisational resources and network of skilled surgeons, can help partially offset these problems in target surgical fields by organising long-term training programs, fostering collaboration between international and local surgeons, and facilitating the collection of clinical data at the local level. Such programs would likely be more organisationally demanding than financially burdensome and would go much further in facilitating improvements to surgical care and access in developing countries than only financial assistance and/or short-term volunteer surgical missions.

REFERENCES

1. Rodrik D, Subramanian A, Trebbi F. Institutions rule: The primacy of institutions over integration and geography in economic development 2004. *IMF Working Papers*. 2002;WP/02/189.
2. Bardhan P. Understanding underdevelopment: Challenges for institutional economics from the point of view of poor countries. *Journal of Institutional and Theoretical Economics*. 2000;156(1):216–235.
3. Banerjee A, Duflo E. *Poor Economics: A Radical Rethinking of the Way to Fight Global Poverty*. New York, NY: PublicAffairs; 2011.
4. Gutnik L, Yamey G, Riviello R, et al. Financial contributions to global surgery: An analysis of 160 international charitable organizations. *Springerplus*. 2017;5(1):1558.
5. Shrime M, Sleemi A, Ravilla T. Charitable platforms in global surgery: A systematic review of their effectiveness, cost-effectiveness, sustainability, and role training. *World Journal of Surgery*. 2015;39(1):10–20.
6. Khan M. Political settlements and the governance of growth-enhancing institutions; Unpublished https://eprints.soas.ac.uk/9968/1/Political_Settlements_internet.pdf [Accessed April 7 2020].
7. Nelson R, Winter S. *An Evolutionary Theory of Economic Change*. Cambridge, UK: Harvard University Press; 1982.
8. Dahlman C, Westphal L. The meaning of technological mastery in relation to transfer of technology. *The Annals of the American Academy of Political and Social Science*. 1981;458(1):12–26.
9. Dosi G, Freeman C, Nelson R, et al. *Technical Change and Economic Theory*. Pisa, Italy: Laboratory of Economics and Management (LEM). Sant'Anna School of Advanced Studies; 1988.
10. Khan M. Technology policies and learning with imperfect governance. In: Stiglitz JE, Lin JY (eds). *The Industrial Policy Revolution I*. London, UK: Palgrave Macmillan; 2013:79–115.
11. Dormans J, Fisher R, Pill S. Orthopaedics in the developing world: Present and future concerns. *Journal of the American Academy of Orthopedic Surgeons*. 2001;9(5):289–296.
12. Ahmad A, Aker L, Hanbali Y, et al. Growth-friendly implants with rib clawing hooks as proximal anchors in early onset scoliosis. *Global Spine Journal*. May 2019;10(4):370–374.
13. Ahmad A. What's important: Recognizing local power in global surgery. *Journal of Bone and Joint Surgery. American Volume*. 2019;101(21):1974–1975.
14. Bram J, Warwick-Clark B, Obeysekare E, Mehta K. Utilization and monetization of healthcare data in developing countries. *Big Data*. 2015;3(2):59–66.

3a Blended Learning in Training Paediatric Deformity Surgeons

Emre Acaroglu and Alpaslan Senkoylu

CONTENTS

INTRODUCTION

Arguably the most important novelty in the twenty-first century has been the development and recognition of a new generation of internet (the so-called Web 2.0), which enabled ordinary people to communicate and produce and share content through it. Education is probably one of the most affected fields, as it has embraced these changes and the new paradigms being developed along with them. This chapter will provide a summary of the applications of education via the internet, defined as 'online learning' (OL) and its advantages and disadvantages.

WHAT IS ONLINE LEARNING?

OL is a form of e-learning that primarily uses the internet as the learning environment. In this regard, not all e-learning types are online, as learning through any electronic media, such as television, cassette players, CDs, may also be considered e-learning but not OL. OL provides several distinct advantages over the more traditional educational contexts, such as the traditional schools, and as may be expected, some disadvantages as well. Firstly, the advantages include [1, 2, 3]:

- It affords flexibility to the learners in using their time. In this regard, OL does not necessarily have to be synchronous, i.e. the learner does not have to attend the learning activity as it happens but, rather, at any time that is convenient. This is a contrast to the mandated synchronousness of schools.
- It allows and promotes users to use a wide range of educational resources.
- It is easy to update.
- It provides learners with a deeper and more prolonged exposure to the course materials. Learners are free to visit any content available in the learning management system (LMS) and interact with their instructors and peers at any time during their learning.
- It creates an economy of scale in that, once the LMS is developed and populated with content, expansion of the learning materials/courses can be realised with marginal costs. This quality makes OL particularly suitable for learning in underdeveloped areas of the world.

In this regard, a transition to making OL one of the primary educational contexts may also allow educators to be able to change the current predominant educational paradigm in schools. That is, instead of conceiving of learning as teachers instructing students to think and behave in certain ways, OL may allow education to adapt into more state-of-the-art conceptions of learning and teaching such as:

- Learning as a conscious process, fueled by personal interests and directed toward changing as a person [4], and
- Teaching as bringing about conceptual understanding and intellectual development in students [5].

As can be seen, these conceptions exclude the idea of unidirectional information flow and, instead, embrace the notion of the learner and teacher combining efforts to create new meanings that may be used in life. OL provides an excellent medium for such a conception of education.

On the other hand, its main disadvantage appears to be the inability to provide adequate learning on manual and technical skills as compared to cognitive skills. Basically, it is a great tool for cognitive learning but not necessarily so for technical learning. Learners still need to be embedded in learning environments, such as medical schools or residency programmes, to be able to train them on technical skills.

WHAT IS BLENDED LEARNING (BL)?

Blended learning (BL) is a term that refers to a blend of OL and face-to-face (F2F) learning. As mentioned above, OL offers exceptional opportunities for cognitive learning, such as memorising the anatomical parts of the human body or understanding the conceptual basis of the treatment for paediatric deformity, but it falls short in providing learners with guided practise inserting pedicle screws. So, BL is a mix of an OL component, in which the learner works on cognitive abilities, and a practical F2F component, in which the technical skills are practised.

BL not only translates theory into practise [6], but also enables adaptive and collaborative learning and transforms the teacher's role from transmitting knowledge to facilitating learning. Medicine has been reported as a suitable discipline for BL [7, 8]. Studies indicate that medical students reported that they were satisfied with e-learning [9, 10], but they did not think of it as a strategy to replace traditional teacher-centred education. Another advantage of OL for clinical medical disciplines is that training can be done at any time and be tailored to the individual's learning needs [11]. BL provides flexibility in teaching and learning processes using adult learning principles [8] and potentially eliminates problems of crowded classrooms with little real teacher-learner interaction [9]. The integration of technology into educational methods enables flexible, learner-centred learning, as well as asynchronous communication and collaboration, while providing interaction between the student and the instructor [10].

BL is highly dependent on content as well as context, and interdisciplinary transitions are controversial; therefore, there is no guarantee that a successful BL application in one field will be equally successful in another domain. BL requires the use of computers and the internet, but it should not be forgotten that the focus is not technology. The educator should first determine how best to teach the subject and then decide how to integrate technology into instruction [10]. OL environments are characterised by the autonomy of the learner; therefore, self-regulation is a critical factor for students. To support this prediction, researchers demonstrate self-regulated learning as a predictor of academic achievement for technology-mediated learning environments [12]. In 2003, the American Society for Training and Development identified BL as one of the top ten areas of development and advancement in the information industry [13].

BL aims to improve the development of quality educational activities on vertical and horizontal planes using different tools. It facilitates learning under the learning strategy in the horizontal plane, maintains a deep analysis of learning on a vertical plane, and provides a better understanding of the educational material [14].

BL is also on the rise in subspecialty medical education [3, 7, 9, 10, 15, 16]. A study on BL found that allowing students to participate in a course before it began and after it had completed increased student satisfaction of BL as student age increased [16]. The BL technique used for training in maxillofacial surgery demonstrated that participants preferred the OL programme over the traditional alternative and were very satisfied [17]. BL has been shown to be effective in reducing obstetric anal sphincter injuries in a programme attended by doctors and midwives [18]. In family planning education, it has been reported that participation in BL education results in the highest gains of acquiring information when compared to OL alone [19]. In another study, it was shown that this method is valuable in terms of cost for spine surgeons with limited time because of intensive work [20].

HOW BL COULD BE APPLIED TO THE TRAINING OF DEFORMITY SURGEONS

In regard to the specific area of paediatric spinal deformity, we recently conducted a study to investigate the efficacy of BL as a learning/teaching tool [21]. This study will be summarised here briefly to provide an example of how BL may be used in deformity surgery training.

To construct the course in our study, the topics to be covered and faculty members to cover these topics were decided first. Then, two or three learning outcomes (LO) for each topic were generated with the assistance and supervision of the medical educator members of the team. The team then developed a modified needs assessment (NA) questionnaire and a quiz. The NA survey served as the self-assessment of needs, whereas the quiz provided a more objective measure of the baseline at the beginning of the course and at several other points during the course.

The NA was based on the LO, and participants were to mark three of the questions on an analogue scale from zero to 10 with 0.5 increments, in which zero indicated 'none' and 10 indicated 'perfect'. Students were asked:

1. How do you rate your current level on this LO?
2. How do you rate your desired level on this LO?
3. How do you rate the likelihood of using your learning on this LO in your practice?

For the quiz, faculty members were assigned to specific topics and instructed to prepare two questions (multiple choice or open book) per the LO relevant to that topic. These questions were then pooled and canvassed on a blueprint table based on the LO and difficulty (attained by the faculty member). Based on this blueprint, a quiz was constructed consisting of ten questions (two per four topics, one per two topics), six of which were classified as difficult. Of the ten, eight questions were multiple choice and two allowed students to use their notes.

An LMS was used as the educational framework for the online part of the course. An open invitation was emailed to a group of spine surgeons, orthopaedic surgeons, and neurosurgeons inviting participants to register for the course, which included the mandatory NA and quiz to be taken for completion. Twenty-nine participants who took the quiz and filled the NA form were admitted to the course and formed the population of this study. Thirteen of them (Group A) completed both online and F2F parts, whereas 16 of them (Group B) attended only the online part.

ONLINE PART

The online portion of this course took 3 weeks. Within this 3-week period, participants had access to the course content online, which included PowerPoint presentations with or without voice-over recordings, video lectures, operation videos, supplementary text, and scientific articles related to the topics presented. Moreover, participants were also encouraged to participate in a discussion forum, which was specifically created for this course and facilitated by the faculty members. After allowing the participants some time to study the learning objects for the specified week and topics, faculty members asked the participants open-ended questions or gave small practical assignments, such as classifying scoliosis cases and sharing with the group, in the class discussion forum. Every topic of the course is designed in such a way that, upon completion, a set of LOs is satisfied. These LO were listed at the beginning of each topic so that participants knew what to expect from that section. Participants and the faculty were monitored for their active participation in this part of the course by two mechanisms. Firstly, faculty members were presented with information on the login times of the participants (and other faculty members) so that they were aware of the amount of participation by individuals; and secondly, by a discussion forum facilitated by faculty that encouraged and promoted peer discussion amongst the group of learners. One week after completion of online portion of the course, participants were asked to complete the quiz and the NA again before proceeding with the F2F portion of the course.

FACE TO FACE PART

Attending the online part of the course was a prerequisite for the F2F portion. Amongst those eligible, 13 attended this part and were divided into three groups, each of which was supervised by a faculty member who was there to facilitate and maintain the discussions. The F2F part consisted only of case discussions, one case per topic, one hour per case. This hour was divided into parts consisting of:

- Presentation of the case (by faculty) and questions: 10 mins.
- Discussion of the case within groups: 15 mins.
- Discussion of the case and each groups' solutions: 20 mins.
- Case solution (by faculty) and discussion of the solution: 10 mins.
- Reflection: 5 mins.

During the discussions, participants were able to exchange their ideas regarding the cases with each other and learn about the experiences of their peers and faculty to arrive at conclusions as to what to do regarding each particular case. After the discussions, each group nominated a spokesman to communicate the decisions of that the particular group to other groups. After these discussions were over, the faculty member who had presented the case presented his/her solution as well, which the participants also discussed. At the end, participants were asked to prepare a question or 2–3 tweets on what they had learned during the case discussion as a means of reflection. At the end of the day, after all cases were presented and discussed, participants were

asked to take the same quiz and NA before the course was adjourned (Table 3a.1).

Participants were also asked to complete the quiz and NA three months after the course had ended, but as only three participants responded to the invitation, those results were not included in the analysis. Results of quiz scores at different time points (i.e., enrolment, end of online portion, end of F2F portion) were analysed.

Although the learning analytics data on login times was too scattered to provide concrete conclusions, in general, the active participants who had spent more time on the OL portion of the course and engaged in the discussion forum who went on to participate in the F2F part. The faculty and participants used the discussion forum for 18 separate discussion threads (12 by participants and six by faculty) which generated 34 replies. Faculty members were active in these forums, the last entry to 16/18 chains were by faculty members.

For the analysis of efficacy in learning, quiz scores of the participants were compared. Group A was composed of participants who attended both online and F2F parts, and Group B consists of those who attended only the online part. Basically, participants in Group A took the quiz three times (before and after online and after F2F), whereas participants in Group B completed the quiz twice (before and after online). The precourse quiz scores for both

TABLE 3A.1
A Summary of the Concept and Programme of a BL Course

Item	Timeline
Needs Assessment for Planning Events	Prior to the induction of an education programme
Once Planned	
Assignment of Faculty, Development of LOs, and Programme	2–3 months prior
Prepare/Curate content and Upload	1–2 months prior
Perform Needs Assessment, Start an Online Part	3–6 weeks prior
Start F2F Part	

TABLE 3A.2
Median Quiz Scores of Participants at Time Points

[Median (min–max)]	Group A	Group B	P Value
Before Online Part (1)	5.4 (0.0–9.2)	5.4 (0.0–7.9)	>0.05
After Online Part (2)	6.8 (4.2–9.6)*	6.8 (5.1–9.3) *	>0.05
After F2F Part (3)	7.9 (6.8–8.9)**	N/A	N/A
P Value	*0.014 **0.023	0.014	

*Represents statistical significance of **After Online Part (2)** when compared to **Before Online Part (1)**.
Represents statistical significance of **After F2F Part (3) when compared to **After Online Part (2)**.

groups are quite similar, with a *p* value of 0.368 (Table 3a.2). Both groups improved their scores in the prelearning quiz significantly (*p* = 0.014). Further improvement can be seen for Group A at the end of F2F learning session (*p* = 0.023).

In summary, this study demonstrated that BL may be used very effectively in training surgeons on deformity surgery. It may be useful to recognise that, although skills training was not a part of this study, the F2F component could easily have been designed to incorporate training on models, recorded or live surgeries, or even virtual or augmented reality tools to provide skills training as well.

FUTURE OF EDUCATION IN PAEDIATRIC SPINAL DEFORMITY SURGERY

The pace of technological change is accelerating so fast, which is bringing about many emerging opportunities in healthcare and medical education. New technologies such as machine learning, artificial intelligence, and simulations, including virtual and augmented reality, have been utilised at different levels of medical education. Conventional teaching methods are becoming automated, and these newer techniques are increasing patient safety. They also allow for efficient skill assessment by chunking complex tasks into small components that can be easily evaluated via artificial intelligence or machine learning [22, 23].

Minimally invasive spine surgery is one of the first application areas of the simulation-based teaching because of its steep learning curve and cost. Different kinds of procedures, including percutaneous endoscopic discectomy, vertebroplasty, percutaneous pedicle screw fixation, and tumor ablation can be practised by using virtual, augmented, or mixed reality [24].

Simulators may also allow trainees to acquire key competencies in a secure environment, important in a subspecialty such as paediatric spine deformity in which technical mistakes can cause devastating complications [25]. In addition to surgical skills, BL can also assist in teaching preoperative planning and decision-making in paediatric spine deformity education. A combination of OL and simulators should permit distance education for key competencies of complex surgical procedures. This is a promising educational method, especially for the junior surgeons from underdeveloped countries who have financial difficulties obtaining standard paediatric deformity education.

However, the aforementioned emerging technologies have some drawbacks, including cost and not providing an optimal tactile sensation during practise. No doubt, they need optimisation for common use.

CONCLUSION

BL is a feasible and effective tool for paediatric spinal deformity education if applied in a specific format. While it calls for relatively low cost, BL can facilitate the training of the junior deformity surgeons from underdeveloped countries. Combining BL with newer technologies such as simulators, which still require optimisation, will provide an even more robust educational tool for this subspecialty.

REFERENCES

1. Herbert C, Velan GM, Pryor WM, et al. A model for the use of blended learning in large group teaching sessions. *BMC Medical Education.* 2017;17(1):197.
2. Lewin LO, Singh M, Bateman BL, et al. Blended learning B. Improving education in primary care: Development of an online curriculum using the blended learning model. *BMC Medical Education.* 2009;9:33.
3. Facharzt NM, Abos KIK, Algaidi S, et al. Blended learning as an effective teaching and learning strategy in clinical medicine: A comparative cross-sectional university-based study. *Journal of Taibah University Medical Sciences.* 2013;8(1):12–17.
4. Van Rossum E, Taylor IP. The relationship between conceptions of learning and good teaching: A scheme of cognitive development. Paper presented at the *Annual Meeting of the American Educational Research Association,* Washington, DC; April 1987.
5. Kember D. A reconceptualisation of the research into university academics' conceptions of teaching. *Learning and Instruction.* 1997;7(3):255–275.
6. Keifenheim KE, Velten-Schurian K, Fahse B, et al. A change would do you good: Training medical students in motivational interviewing using a blended-learning approach – A pilot evaluation. *Patient Education and Counseling.* 2019;102(4):663–9.
7. Lewin LO, Singh M, Bateman BL, et al. Improving education in primary care: Development of an online curriculum using the blended learning model. *BMC Medical Education.* 2009;9(33):33.
8. Gray K, Tobin J. Introducing an online community into a clinical education setting: A pilot study of student and staff engagement and outcomes using blended learning. *BMC Medical Education.* 2010;10:6.
9. Rowe Michael, Frantz Jose, Bozalek Vivienne. The role of blended learning in the clinical education of healthcare students: A systematic review. *Medical Teacher.* 2012;34(4):e216–e221.
10. Kassab Salah Eldin, Al-Shafei Ahmad I, Salem Abdel Halim, et al. Relationships between the quality of blended learning experience, self-regulated learning, and academic achievement of medical students: A path analysis. *Advances in Medical Education and Practice.* 2015;6:27–34.
11. Fachartz NM, Abos KIK, Algaidi S, et al. Blended learning in in clinical medicine: A comparative cross-sectional university-based study. *Journal of Taibah University Medical Sciences.* 2013;8(1):12–17.
12. Duque G, Demontiero O, Whereat S, et al. Evaluation of a blended learning model in geriatric medicine: A successful learning experience for medical students. *Australasian Journal on Ageing.* 2013;32(2):103–109.
13. Karamizadeh Z, Zarifsanayei N, Faghihi AA, et al. The study of effectiveness of blended learning approach for medical training courses. *Iranian Red Crescent Medical Journal.* 2012;14(1):41–44.
14. Luo L, Cheng X, Wang S, et al. Blended learning with moodle in medical statistics: An assessment of knowledge, attitudes and practices relating to e-learning. *BMC Medical Education.* 2017;17(1):170.
15. Protsiv M, Rosales-Klintz S, Bwanga F, et al. Blended learning across universities in a South–North–South collaboration: A case study. *Health Research Policy and Systems.* 2016;14(1):67.
16. Bock A, Modabber A, Kniha K, et al. Blended learning modules for lectures on oral and maxillofacial surgery. *British Journal of Oral and Maxillofacial Surgery.* 2018;56(10): 956–61.
17. Ali-Masri HS, Fosse E, Fosse E, et al. Impact of electronic and blended learning programs for manual perineal support on incidence of obstetric anal sphincter injuries: A prospective interventional study. *BMC Medical Education.* 2018;18(1):258.
18. Munro V, Morello A, Oster C, et al. E-learning for self-management support: Introducing blended learning for graduate students – A cohort study. *BMC Medical Education.* 2018;18(1):219.
19. Limaye RJ, Ahmed N, Ohkubo S, et al. Blended learning on family planning policy requirements: Key findings and implications for health professionals. *BMJ Sexual and Reproductive Health.* 2018;44(2):109–113.
20. Gunzburg R, Szpalski M, Lamartina C. Postgraduate education in spine surgery: The blended online learning concept. *European Spine Journal.* 2018;27(9):2059–2061.
21. Senkoylu A, Senkoylu B, Budakoglu I, et al. Blended learning is a feasible and effective tool for basic paediatric spinal deformity training. *Global Spine Journal.* 2020;1–5. doi: 10.1177/2192568220916502

22. Mirchi N, Bisonette V, Yilmaz R, et al. The virtual operative assistant: An explainable artificial assistance for simulation-based training in surgery and medicine. *PLOS ONE*. 2020. doi: 10.1371/journal.pone.0229596

23. Schwartz AW, Yilmaz R, Mirchi N, et al. Machine learning identification of surgical and operative factors associated with surgical expertise in virtual reality simulation. *JAMA Network Open*. 2019;2(8):e198263.

24. Lohre R, Wang J, Lewandrowski KU, et al. Virtual reality in spinal endocopy: A paradigm shift in education to support spine surgeons. *Journal of Spine Surgery*. 2020;6(suppl-1):S208–23.

25. Senkoylu A, Daldal I, Cetinkaya M. 3D printing and spine surgery. *Journal of Orthopaedic Surgery*. Jan–Apr 2020; 28(2): 2309499020927081, doi: 10.1177/2309499020927081.

3b Evidence-Based Medicine in Low- and Middle-Income Countries

Patrick Thornley, Devin Peterson and Mohit Bhandari

CONTENTS

INTRODUCTION TO EVIDENCE-BASED MEDICINE AND EVIDENCE-BASED SURGERY

The evidence-based movement in medicine began in the early 1990s as a response to a call from the medical community to understand how best to utilise published evidence to advance patient care [1]. The initial doctrines of evidence-based medicine (EBM) sought to teach clinicians the role of critical appraisal and to develop a hierarchy of evidence on which to base such appraisals. EBM progressed from the initial goal of educating clinicians in critical appraisal of the medical literature to increasingly stressing the role of incorporating patient values through shared decision-making. The first decade of this movement demonstrated that efforts to teach EBM to medical trainees would likely fail, as few clinicians would neither have the skills nor possess the time to conduct sophisticated analysis of the evidence relevant to their practise [2]. This process is further complicated by the explosion of information from publications, with estimates of greater than 6 million academic journal articles being published in more than 22,000 journals each year [3]. By the mid-2000s, EBM had evolved to form the essential background of young clinician training to consistently stress the importance of critical appraisal of the medical literature, while further improving the practise of medicine by developing methods and techniques to create systematic reviews and guidelines to inform clinical practise [1–3]. EBM has further contributed to a sophisticated hierarchy of evidence, emphasising the need for the best evidence and systematic summaries to guide patient care with the requirement of considering patient values in important clinical decision-making [1, 3].

Surgeons are often criticised for falling behind their medicine colleagues in incorporating EBM and utilising higher quality evidence [4]. Unlike EBM in nonoperative practise, evidence-based surgical practise is hampered by inherent problems and obstacles by virtue of the ethics of some surgical trials. This difficulty has led to a slower adoption and advancement of EBM within surgery. Nevertheless, much progress has been seen in the advancement of EBM in surgery, and orthopaedic surgery has been at the forefront of progressing this movement over the past quarter century.

Often lost in this movement, has been the contributions and standardisation of EBM in low- and middle-income countries (LMICs).

LMICs are herein defined by the 2015 World Bank definition: low-income economies are those with a gross national income (GNI) per capita of US$1,025, lower middle-income economies with a GNI per capita from US$1,026 to US$4,035 and upper middle-income economies with a GNI per capita from US$4,036 to US$12,475 [5]. While non-LMICs have seen dramatic increases in the quality and sheer volume of disseminated evidence during the EBM movement, there has not been equitable development among LMICs.

Developing the research capacity of LMICs has repeatedly been shown to be a key way for international health research to effect sustained benefit in these countries [6]. As a means to highlight this discrepancy, Kelaher et al. [6] sought to quantify the contributions of LMICs' researchers from 1990 to 2013, conducting studies on randomised controlled trials (RCTs) on HIV/AIDS, malaria, and tuberculosis. While an absolute increased number of publications was shown throughout the study period, there was only a modest increase in LMIC first authorship against a much larger increase in first authorship from non-LMIC authors [6]. Similarly, Sinha et al. analysed a total of 669 Cochrane systematic reviews, noting a low proportion of Cochrane authors from LMICs [7]. The authors subsequently conclude that capacity-building in systematic reviews and good quality, primary research throughout LMICs is warranted and necessary. Certainly, adoption of more inclusive policies to transfer research control to clinical researchers in LMICs is an important component of the engagement of healthcare providers in LMICs in the EBM movement [8].

EVIDENCE-BASED MEDICINE IN LOW- AND MIDDLE-INCOME COUNTRIES: A FOCUS ON THE ORTHOPAEDIC LITERATURE

Given the nature of the difficulties with establishing large banks of data, there remains significant uncertainty surrounding incidence/prevalence, aetiology, management and prognosis of many conditions among patients in LMICs. Such uncertainty reduces our ability to appropriately intervene in an effective manner

for these patients and highlights the importance of conducting research to guide clinical care in countries in which cultural and resource differences are profoundly discrepant from those of high-income nations. Certainly, it is important to establish the evidence base on which barriers and facilitators to health information exchange exist in LMICs [8, 9]. A key principle of EBM, and one of the most important strategies to get effective interventions into routine clinical practise, is to develop and implement evidence-based clinical practise guidelines [10]. It is increasingly recognised that for guideline implementation strategies to be effective, it is important to understand why some guidelines are ineffective. It is important to develop guidelines with an understanding that, within different cultures and resource settings, context-specific barriers may exist to limit the effect of changes in treatments [10].

Understanding the inherent difficulties with creating EBM models of care in LMICs is important when critically appraising the best method to treat patients in LMICs. Recent efforts to apply increased attention to pragmatic trials is a response to address contextually sensitive and important clinical care decisions in multiple routine care settings with interventions compared with the existing standard of care [9, 11]. Improvement of health outcomes will require timely delivery of interventions that are not only effective but feasible to implement in LMICs [11]. Regrettably many clinical care decision-making guidelines within surgery continue to draw upon low-level evidence. Global efforts are needed to support pragmatic research trials to complement current evidence-based guidelines [10, 11].

As a starting point for EBM in orthopaedic surgical care, efforts within LMICs have been made to quantify and understand the burden of musculoskeletal conditions. Joshipura et al. [12] attempted to identify the surgical burden of musculoskeletal conditions in LMICs. This first-of-its-kind publication highlights the uncertainty of establishing a global burden of musculoskeletal conditions within LMICs given the paucity of credible and vetted databanks [12]. The authors concluded that LMICs account for more than 70% of the world population, however, they account for only a quarter of the volume of major surgery. In contrast, only 15% of the global population in high-income countries accounts for approximately 60% of musculoskeletal surgeries; a staggering figure [12]. While it is indeed difficult to establish a true numerical burden of musculoskeletal conditions within LMICs, the aggregate number of patients globally within LMICs who may benefit from enhanced nonoperative or surgical intervention is undoubtedly continuing to increase.

Much recent work in orthopaedic surgery evidence in LMICs has highlighted attempts to establish an understanding of not only the current burden of pathology faced by clinicians but also to understand their current treatment practises. Curran et al. [13] conducted a survey of 413 surgeons from 83 countries, 53 of which were low to LMICs to understand current paediatric femur fracture management [13]. Unsurprisingly, decreasing socioeconomic status was associated with increased rates of nonoperative treatment. From low and LMICs respondents 63%–65% of all paediatric femur fractures, regardless of age and fracture type, were routinely treated with bed rest and traction. The authors concluded that future studies should investigate the value of treatment options in resource-limited settings, a recurring theme in all surgical literature involving LMICs [13].

While orthopaedic trauma literature has largely been a prime focus among emerging EBM publications focussing on LMICs, little is known about common paediatric pathologies and their management in these countries. Owen et al. [14] attempted to provide some global perspective to clubfoot management in LMICs. Clubfoot occurs in an estimated incidence of 1.24/1000 live births, affecting upwards of 174,000 children born annually, with approximately 90% of these children born in LMICs [14]. Untreated, clubfoot has lifelong impairment, deformity, and long-term consequences on overall health and function. With a primarily nonsurgical approach adopted globally after the popularisation of the Ponseti serial casting method, Owen et al. [14] reported on the difficulties of incorporating such a care practise to LMICs. A cross-sectional survey of clinicians treating clubfoot was conducted with respondents from 55 countries comprising an estimated coverage of nations with up to 79% of predicted clubfoot cases. Compiled responses revealed low coverage for these patients with less than 15% of children born with clubfoot in LMICs receiving treatment [14]. Importantly, however, the authors noted that responses indicate increased coverage since 2005 when Ponseti treatment became more widely known and accepted. The importance of early intervention to prevent or diminish lifelong deformity and functional impairment in these patients cannot be overstated. With an understanding of the difficulties of quantifying the burden of orthopaedic pathology in LMICs and trying to establish an understanding of the type of care being provided, we can now begin to better understand the difficulties with approaching evidence-based spine care in LMICs with a focus on the paediatric spine.

EVIDENCE-BASED MEDICINE IN SPINE SURGERY IN LOW- AND MIDDLE-INCOME COUNTRIES

In the resource-limited setting, decisions for healthcare interventions need to consider increased patient volume and demands, as well as infrastructure and budgetary limitations that may render higher cost interventions that are impractical in a given setting. Guidelines, such as those outlined by the 2016 International Scientific Society on Scoliosis Orthopaedic and Rehabilitation Treatment (SOSORT), on conservative management of scoliosis during growth are critical to the care of patients in LMICs [15]. These guidelines serve as expert opinion regarding which patients can be managed conservatively and which are predicted to fail with conservative management. The prevalence of both EOS and adolescent idiopathic scoliosis (AIS) changes according to latitude and varies from 0.93% to 12% of the paediatric population; however, only 0.1% to 0.3% of AIS cases will require surgical correction [15]. Thus, the importance, both for the patient and budget, of appropriately identifying and intervening upon the remaining population who may only require conservative management during growth is clear.

The recurring theme in assessing the available evidence to inform best paediatric spinal deformity management is that it is sparse and of low quality. Low-grade evidence in the form of

Level 4 case reports and retrospective Level 3 cohort studies form the bulk of the best available management decisions. With such uncertainty, there is a need for a degree of synthesis nuanced with expert opinion and consensus agreements to standardise practises and identify areas of uncertainty. With such low-quality available evidence in the paediatric spinal deformity literature, and even worse evidence for EOS, it is no surprise that there is a paucity of paediatric spinal deformity evidence from LMICs.

It is important to first highlight the efforts currently being made to address and impact spinal care in LMICs, which, until very recently, has largely focussed on adult spine patients. A discussion will then follow regarding paediatric spine research that is available from LMICs.

Spinal disorders are increasingly being recognised as a major cause of disability, morbidity, and economic hardship in LMICs [16]. While the available evidence is sparse, it is expected that the burden of spinal disorders among the adult and young adult populations in LMICs is just as, if not more, significant than in high-income countries [16–18]. To be able to respond to this predicted growing burden of disability, inability to work, and associated economic hardships, intervention must be effective in LMICs as has been discussed above. Guidelines need to be readily and culturally adaptable, evidence-based, financially sustainable, easily accessible and neither ineffective, harmful, nor wasteful. In response to this, World Spine Care (WSC) was established in 2008 with the mission to 'improve lives in underserved communities by providing sustainable, integrated and evidence-based spine care … a world in which everyone has access to the highest quality spine care possible' [16–18]. Sixty-eight leading spine clinicians from 24 countries, representing all aspects of allied, primary, and specialist-level spine care were involved in developing guidelines for this project [16–18]. The mandate of this programme reflects admirable goals that, hopefully in the future, can be applied to paediatric spine care in LMICs. The tenants of the programme include a low-cost and efficient model of care, ability to be taught to providers with varying levels of education/training, evidence-based; and transferrable applicability to any existing healthcare system in LMICs. As part of the Global Spine Care Initiative (GSCI) through the World Spine Care group, the global burden of spinal pathology was better elicited [17]. An example of this is a study showing the prevalence of low back pain increased in adult women, particularly those with less education; psychological factors, such as depression/anxiety; and increased alcohol consumption [17]. They concluded that a call to action to devote increased resources to address the gaps in medically underserved areas in LMICs for patients with chronic low back pain is imperative [17]. As part of the GSCI publication series, Cedraschi et al. [19] published a narrative review of 29 cohort, cross-sectional, qualitative, and mixed-methods studies investigating adults with low back pain. The authors concluded that few studies evaluate the psychological and social factors associated with back pain in LMICs thus limiting the adaptation of such recommendations to this population. Furthermore, the authors stressed that instruments need to be developed for people with low literacy in medically underserved areas in LMICs, especially where psychological and social factors are poorly understood and difficult to address [19].

From the GSCI review, the primary doctrines of their intervention protocols were established with a strong emphasis on prevention of first-presentation and prevention of worsening spinal conditions regardless of pathology. Through WSC, spinal programmes have been initiated in the Dominican Republic, India, and Ghana and are supported by government agencies, local, and international university volunteers and are integrated into existing healthcare systems [5]. One of the first Level 4 evidence studies of spine patients within an LMIC population resulted from this project. The authors provided a case report outlining the demographics and pathology type of patients presenting to the WSC clinics in the Dominican Republic for care and further highlight the issues that researchers face when attempting to conduct research and ethics board reviews within LMICs [5].

EVIDENCE-BASED MEDICINE IN PAEDIATRIC SPINE CARE IN LOW- AND MIDDLE-INCOME COUNTRIES

The overt prevalence of low-quality data makes the utilisation of evidence-based decision-making on scoliosis history, available treatment options, and outcome projections difficult [20]. Currently, much of EBM in paediatric spinal deformity management is employed in conjunction with patient's values and individual clinician expertise. Negrini et al. [21] demonstrated through their Cochrane review that brace treatment in AIS does not change patient quality of life, with low-grade evidence supporting brace treatment preventing deformity progression [21]. As better evidence continues to evolve supporting brace treatment for AIS management, the impetus to disseminate and optimise this practise globally and to LMICs is emphasised.

At the time of publication of this chapter, only a few research studies, all primarily case reports or retrospective cohort studies, on the LMICs paediatric spinal deformity population exist. Of the available evidence-based publications on paediatric spine deformity in LMICs, most studies focus on outreach groups and their associated surgical results.

Verma et al. [22] provided insights into the discriminate validity of the Scoliosis Research Society Questionnaire (SRS-22r) in Ghana between adolescents with and without AIS and compared these with matched cohorts in the United States. In Ghana, 84 healthy, mean age of 13 years (healthy-G), and 61 AIS patients of a mean age of 15 years (AIS-G) were included. Comparatively, from New York City, 450 healthy adolescents (healthy-US) of a mean age 16 years, and 302 patients with AIS (AIS-US) and a mean age of 15 years were included. When controlling for curve magnitude, a significant difference between all four study groups was found in all domains and total score (P<0.01). AIS-G showed significantly lower scores in activity, image, pain, and mental health domains (P<0.01), reaching the minimum clinically important difference for these domains. AIS-G patients initially presented with a larger curve magnitude compared to the American cohort (67° vs. 52°), likely a representation of resource access in Ghana for conservative management. Overall Ghanaian adolescents with AIS had significantly worse health-related quality of life compared to their AIS American counterparts [22].

When conservative management efforts are either not indicated or fail in the paediatric spinal deformity population, surgical correction is recommended. Poor access to appropriate resources for children with spinal deformity in LMICs over represents the number of patients who would benefit from surgical correction to minimise adulthood dysfunction and morbidity. Furthermore, scoliosis correction surgery is expensive and highly specialised.

The Scoliosis Research Society Global Outreach Mission Programs (SRS-GOP) are medical missions endorsed by the Scoliosis Research Society (SRS) with the goal of providing spinal deformity care for children in LMICs [23]. Boachei-Adjei O et al. [24] provided the largest comprehensive review of major perioperative complications from an SRS global outreach programme site from 1998 to 2015. Overall, a total of 427 patients were included in the study with 60% females of an average age of 15 at the time of surgery. Forty-seven percent of surgical indications were AIS. The overall complication rate within the study was 19.9% with a 2.3% rate of permanent neurological deficit. Furthermore, three-column osteotomies were identified as an independent risk factor for postoperative complication as was surgical treatment of curves greater than 100° [24].

Halo-gravity traction also has promise for reducing the severity of preoperative deformity in paediatric spinal deformity, potentially lowering morbidity during surgical intervention (Figure 3b.1). Nemani et al. [25] reported a single-centre retrospective cohort study on the use of a modified halo-gravity traction protocol for patients with severe spinal deformities in Ghana. The authors' rationale for undertaking the study was to assess the amount of possible correction that could be obtained with halo-gravity traction before surgical intervention to minimise the number of three-column osteotomies they would be required to perform to decrease the associated operative risks. A total of 29 patients underwent halo-gravity traction beginning at 20% of body weight and increasing 10% weekly until 50% of total body weight. The average time for traction was 107 days with an average 131° to 90° preoperative curve correction (31% curve correction), ultimately achieving an average postoperative curve of 57° (56% overall correction). They found halo-gravity traction to be highly effective, with few complications,

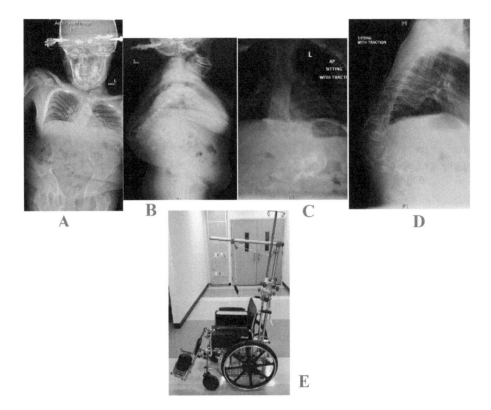

FIGURE 3B.1   A and B – pretraction images of a 12-year old patient with early onset spinal deformity caused by neurofibromatosis. C and D – traction film after multiple weeks of halo-gravity traction used prior to definitive surgery. E – simple traction setup using a hospital wheelchair, traction equipment used for femur fractures, a fish scale, and other products purchased at a local hardware store.

and indicated that it may reduce the number of three-column osteotomies required at time of surgery [25].

Despite 20 approved SRS surgical outreach sites, reported studies from these sites are extremely limited. Fletcher et al. [23] reported on spinal deformity surgical correction in a low-income country, Ecuador. In the Ecuador Spine Deformity Program project, 28 of 38 children (74%), with an average age of 14 at the time of surgery, and 18 at follow-ups were available for review. The mean total score on the SRS 22r was 4.3, with a mean percentage major curve correction of 57%, no infections and only two revision surgeries were required for pseudarthrosis and delayed paraplegia, both of which were resolved. It was concluded that the Ecuador Spine Deformity Program demonstrated that the SRS global outreach programme goals of self-sufficient spine centres to provide care to children in LMICs is possible [23].

The Fletcher [23] study also demonstrated some of the barriers and challenges with implementing successful paediatric spinal deformity surgery programmes in LMICs. A cooperative effort is required between the country receiving care and the volunteers attending from higher income nations until the programme gains self-sufficiency. Higher income nations need to help coordinate clinical scheduling and plan for provision of the necessary supplies, nursing, anaesthesia, surgical skill, neurologic monitoring, and appropriate postoperative intensive care [23].

CONCLUSION

Paediatric spinal deformity is a highly prevalent pathology in LMICs. Access to appropriate and timely care is imperative in preventing progression to a surgical pathology in many instances within this population. Furthermore, creating a healthcare delivery model for paediatric spine

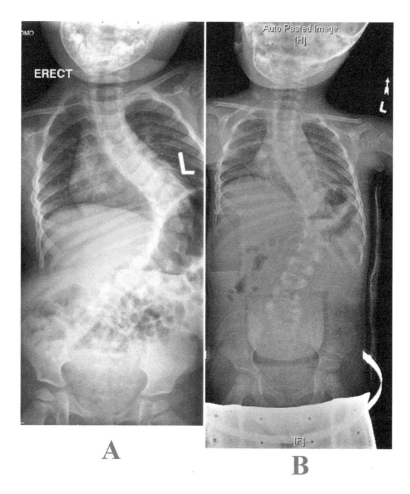

FIGURE 3B.2   A – precasting of a 31-month-old with EOS. B – Postcasting under general anaesthesia

deformity in LMICs is fraught with many barriers, including resource limitations, expertise limitations, and difficult generalisability of published findings on this population when the bulk of the literature comes from the data of higher income nations.

Recent interest has centred on the optimisation of bracing therapy and other conservative management strategies (Figure 3b.2) for paediatric scoliosis. With this impetus, care of these complex patients in LMICs has a higher likelihood of being implemented. This will require collaboration with experts from higher income nations who are willing and able to help teach and develop sustainable programmes to deliver this care in LMICs. Furthermore, it will also be important to create large databanks on the outcomes of these patients. Only through this collaborative approach, emphasising and supporting

not only quality provision of resource-conscious care to these patients but also emphasising the importance of further evidence generation, will we be able to optimise global paediatric spinal deformity care for all children.

REFERENCES

1. Djulbegovic B, Guyatt G. Progress in evidence-based medicine: A quarter century on. *Lancet.* 2017;390(10092):415–423.
2. Guyatt G, Meade M, Jaeschke R, et al. Practitioners of evidence based care. Not all clinicians need to appraise evidence from scratch but all need some skills. *BMJ.* 2000;320(7240):954–955.
3. Djulbegovic B, Elqayam S, Dale W. Rational decision making in medicine: Implications for overuse and underuse. *J Eval Clin Pract.* 2018;24(3):655–665.

4. Evidence MA. 0based surgery: The obstacles and solutions. *Int J Surg*. 2005;18:159–162.

5. Brady O, Nordin M, Hondraw M, et al. Global forum: Spine research and training in underserved, low and middle-income, culturally unique communities: The world spine care charity research program's challenges and facilitators. *J Bone Joint Surg Am*. 2016;98(24):e110:1–9.

6. Kelaher M, Ng L, Knight K, et al. Equity in global health research in the new millennium: Trends in first-authorship for randomized controlled trials among low- and middle-income country researchers 1990–2013. *Int J Epidemiol*. 2016;45(6):2174–2183.

7. Sinha A, Ovelman C, Pradhan A. Profile of published Cochrane systematic reviews in child health From low- and middle-income countries. *Indian Pediatr*. 2019;56(1):45–48.

8. Akhlaq A, Sheikh A, Pagliari C. Barriers and facilitators to health information exchange in low- and middle-income country settings: A systematic review protocol. *J Innov Health Inform*. 2015;22(2):284–292.

9. Hunt A, Saenz C, Littler K. The global forum on bioethics in research meeting, "ethics of alternative clinical trial designs and methods in low- and middle-income country research": Emerging themes and outputs. *Trials*. 2019;20(Suppl 2):701.

10. Stokes T, Shaw E, Camosso-Stefinovic J, et al. Barriers and enablers to guideline implementation strategies to improve obstetric care practice in low- and middle-income countries: A systematic review of qualitative evidence. *Implement Sci*. 2016;11(1):144.

11. English M, Karumbi J, Maina M, et al. The need for pragmatic clinical trials in low and middle income settings – Taking essential neonatal interventions delivered as part of inpatient care as an illustrative example. *BMC Med*. 2016;14:5.

12. Joshipura M, Gosselin R. Surgical burden of musculoskeletal conditions in low- and middle-income countries. *World J Surg*. 2020;Apr;44(4):1026–1032.

13. Curran P, Albright P, Ibrahim J, et al. Practice patterns for management of pediatric femur fractures in low- and middle-income countries. *J Pediatr Orthop*. 2020;May 12;40(5):251-8..

14. Owen R, Capper B, Lavy C. Clubfoot treatment in 2015: A global perspective. *BMJ Glob Health*. 2018;3(4):e000852.

15. Negrini S, Donzelli S, Aulisa A. SOSORT guidelines: Orthopaedic and rehabilitation treatment of idiopathic scoliosis during growth. *Scoliosis Spinal Disord*. 2016;13:3.

16. Haldeman S, Nordin M, Chou R, et al. The global spine care initiative: World spine care executive summary on reducing spine-related disability in low- and middle-income communities. *Eur Spine J*. 2018;27(Suppl 6):776–785.

17. Hurwitz E, Randhawa K, Torres P, et al. The global spine care initiative: A systematic review of individual and community-based burden of spinal disorders in rural populations in low- and middle-income communities. *Eur Spine J*. 2018;27(Suppl 6):802–815.

18. Green B, Johnson C, Haldeman S, et al. The global spine care initiative: Public health and prevention interventions for common spine disorders in low- and middle-income communities. *Eur Spine J*. 2018;27(Suppl 6):838–850.

19. Cedraschi C, Nordin M, Haldeman S, et al. The global spine care initiative: A narrative review of psychological and social issues in back pain in low- and middle-income communities. *Eur Spine J*. 2018;6:828–837.

20. Oetgen M. Current use of evidence-based medicine in pediatric spine surgery. *Orthop Clin North Am*. 2018;49(2):191–194.

21. Negrini S, Minozzi S, Bettany-Saltikov J, et al. Braces for idiopathic scoliosis in adolescents. *Cochrane Database Syst Rev*. 2015;6:CD006850.

22. Verma K, Lonner B, Toombs C, et al. International utilization of the SRS-22 instrument to assess outcomes in adolescent idiopathic scoliosis: What can we learn from a medical outreach group in Ghana? *J Pediatr Orthop*. 2014;34(5):503–508.

23. Fletcher A, Schwend R. The Ecuador Pediatric Spine Deformity Surgery Program. An SRS-GOP site, 2008–2016. *Spine Deform*. 2019;7(2):220–227.

24. Boachie-Adjei O, Yagi M, Nemani V, et al. Incidence and risk factors for major surgical complications in patients with complex spinal deformity: A report from an SRS GOP site. *Spine Deform*. 2015;3(1):57–64.

25. Nemani V, Kim H, Bjerke-Kroll B, et al. Preoperative halo-gravity traction for severe spinal deformities at an SRS-GOP site in West Africa: Protocols, complications, and results. *Spine*. 2015;40(3):153–161.

4 Normal and Abnormal Development and Growth of Spine and Thoracic Cage

Federico Canavese, François Bonnel, and Alain Dimeglio

CONTENTS

GROWTH HOLDS THE BASICS

Spinal growth is a mixture of hierarchy, synchronisation, and harmony among more than 130 growth plates; the slightest error can lead to a complex malformation. Growth starts around the third month of intrauterine life and ends during the second decade of life. It is a dynamic process, although it does not progress linearly, with periods of acceleration followed by periods of deceleration [1–4]. In particular, three periods can be identified: between birth and 5 years of age; between 5 and 10 years of age, and between age 10 and skeletal maturity.

The anterior and posterior part of each vertebra, as well as cervical, thoracic, and lumbar spine regions, grow at a different rate. In particular, the thoracic region, the posterior components of the thoracic spine, grow at a faster pace than their anterior counterparts, while the opposite occurs in the lumbar spine. This allows the spinal column to progressively change morphology and modify its relationships with the spinal cord [1, 2].

Standing height is not the best parameter to evaluate spinal growth because it does not directly measure the length of the spinal column. The best parameter to assess spinal growth is the sitting height; the spine represents about 60% of the sitting height, while the head and pelvis represent the remaining 40% (20% each). In children with progressive scoliosis, there is a decrease of longitudinal growth and a loss of the normal proportionality of trunk growth, and this phenomenon is highlighted by the loss of sitting height. The loss of sitting height is related to the severity of the deformity [1–4].

Idiopathic scoliosis is a progressive disorder that negatively affects spinal growth as asymmetrical forces act on the growth plates of the vertebral column [1], the younger the child is, the higher the risk is of progression. Timely control and correction of the spinal deformity are needed to restore the harmony and the hierarchy of growth between the different growth plates. If action is delayed, the abnormal growth and the subsequent anatomical modifications will lead to a progressive and irreversible clinical picture [2, 5]. Puberty is a turning point in all children with scoliosis, as it increases the risk of progression [3, 4].

Importantly, spine and thoracic cage growth are closely related, although their growth is not synchronous. In particular, Dimeglio et al., Canavese et al., and Charles et al. reported that that thoracic parameters should always be related to growth parameters, such as weight and sitting height, rather than age, because of possible height variations within one age section [1, 2, 6, 7].

WEIGHT

Careful weight assessment is an important part of the orthopaedic evaluation. Weight is another useful parameter for assessing growth, as most children with severe progressive scoliosis exhibit a deficit in weight [1, 2, 5–7]. The weight increases by twentyfold between birth (about 3 kg and 32% of final weight) and skeletal maturity; it is about 20 kg, 30 kg, and 60 kg at age

5, 10, and 16, respectively. As a rule of thumb, weight usually doubles during pubertal growth spurt.

CERVICAL SPINE (C1–C7) GROWTH

At birth, the cervical spine (C1–C7) measures 3.7 cm; it will double in length by age 6 and will gain an additional 3.5 cm during the pubertal growth spurt to reach the adult length of about 13 cm; it represents 22% of the C1–S1 segment and about 16% of the sitting height [1, 2, 6, 7].

MEDULLAR CANAL

The diameter of the cervical spinal canal varies with location, typically decreasing in width from C1 to C7 or from C1 to C3, then widening slightly. The average width of the cervical canal is 13.2 mm, and the average anteroposterior depth is 7.7 mm [1, 2, 6, 7]. Therefore, the transverse and sagittal diameters of the cervical canal are important because the room available for the spinal cord can vary significantly within the cervical spine. In the adult, at C3, the normal transverse diameter is 27 mm, and the average sagittal diameter is approximately 19 mm [1, 2, 6, 7].

THORACIC SPINE (T1–12) GROWTH

The growth of the thoracic spine (T1–T12) is characterised by a rapid phase from birth to 5 years of age (+7.3 cm), a slower phase from 5 to 10 years of age (+3.8 cm), and rapid growth through puberty (+6.5 cm–7 cm) [1, 2, 6, 7]. The thoracic spine measures about 11 cm at birth and will reach a final length of about 28 cm in boys and 26 cm in girls.

The T1–12 segment represents 30% of the sitting height, and a single thoracic vertebra and its disc represents 2.5% of the sitting height. A T1–T12 segment of at least 18 to 22 cm is necessary to avoid respiratory compromise as it corresponds to about 70% of expected T1–T12 length [1, 2, 5, 6].

MEDULLAR CANAL

The thoracic spinal canal is narrower than both the lumbar and the cervical canal. The fifth finger may be introduced into this canal at age 5, when it has attained 95% of its final size [5]. The average transverse and anteroposterior diameter at T7 is about 15 mm.

LUMBAR SPINE (L1–L5) GROWTH

The growth of the lumbar spine (L1–L5) is characterised by a rapid phase from birth to 5 years of age (+3 cm), a slower phase from 5 to 10 years of age (+2 cm), and rapid growth through puberty (+3 cm). The lumbar spine measures about 7 cm at birth, and will reach a final length of about 16 cm in boys and 15.5 cm in girls; at age 10, the lumbar spine has reached 90% of its final height but only 60% of its final volume [1, 2, 6, 7].

The lumbar spine represents 18% of the sitting height, and a single lumbar vertebra and its disc account for 3.5% of the sitting height [1, 2, 6, 7].

MEDULLAR CANAL

The medullar canal in the lumbar spine is wider than that of the thoracic spine. The forefinger can be introduced. At birth, the spinal cord ends at L3, and at maturity, it ends between L1 and L2.

SPINE AND THORACIC CAGE GROWTH FROM BIRTH TO 5 YEARS OF AGE

Between birth (35 cm) and age 5 (62 cm), there is a significant increase in the sitting height (+27 cm–30 cm) and the gain in spinal height is the same as the gain between age 5 and skeletal maturity; moreover, during the first two years of life, sitting height will increase by 63% (22 out of 35 cm) [2, 5]. During this period, the spine is mostly cartilaginous as only 30%–40% is ossified and thus vulnerable to the changes induced by a progressive spinal deformity.

Growth of the spine cannot be dissociated from the thoracic cage growth, as these two entities are closely interrelated. The thoracic cage has a perimeter of about 32 cm at birth (36% of its final length and 98% of the sitting height). By age 5, thoracic perimeter will reach 63% of its final size [1, 2, 5].

Severe infantile scoliosis leads to progressive deformity of the thoracic cage. Over time, a mainly orthopaedic disorder shifts toward a systemic paediatric disease characterised by severe spine distortion and cardiopulmonary impairment; a multidisciplinary approach is required for patients in this population. Severe, progressive infantile spine deformities are characterised by a cascade of growth disorders that amplify each other, like a *domino effect*: abnormal growth of the spine leads to abnormal growth of the thorax, which leads to abnormal growth of the cardiopulmonary system. The goal of treatment is to break this vicious cycle by restoring thoracic motion and provide enough space for the lungs and heart (referred to as the *parasol effect*).

In this respect, an offensive strategy is essential to protect lung development and growth. Canavese et al. [6–10] have experimentally proven that an early spinal arthrodesis can have negative effects on the development of the thoracic cage and of the lungs. Karol et al. [8] have confirmed clinically the negative consequences of early spine fusion in children with early onset spinal deformity. In particular, a spinal arthrodesis of the thoracic spine performed early in life can have negative repercussions on the heart, lungs, respiratory muscles, nervous system, and endocrine system [9–13]. There is an interaction between the organic components of the spine, the thoracic cage, and the intrathoracic and some extrathoracic organs. Fusion causes respiratory insufficiency and adds loss of pulmonary function to the spinal deformity [8–13]. It has been shown that, to develop significant modifications of cardiorespiratory status, a deformed spine and significantly reduced spinal height must be present simultaneously. The simultaneous presence of a short spine and deformity alter plastic properties of the thoracic cage [6, 7, 9, 11, 13]. Xun et al. [14] suggested that, when correcting severe scoliosis, the surgeon should not only straighten the spine, but also preserve the kinematics of the spinal column and thoracic cage, with the diaphragm perpendicular to the spine to restore its function as a respiratory piston. At skeletal maturity, the goal is to have a vital capacity of at least 50%, a weight of at least 40 kg, and a thoracic spine length of at least 18 cm–22 cm [2, 6–8, 14].

The thoracic volume has reached only 6% and 30% of its definitive size at birth and at age 5, respectively.

SPINE AND THORACIC CAGE GROWTH BETWEEN 5 AND 10 YEARS OF AGE

Between 5 and 10 years of age, the annual growth rate of the spine slows down; it is a deceleration period. In particular, the gain in sitting height is about 2.5 cm/year, while the T1–S1 spine segment will gain about 1.1 cm–1.2 cm/year and the annual weight increase is of about 2.5 kg/year [1, 2, 5]. During this period, the thoracic perimeter increases by 10 cm (from 56 cm to 66 cm) with an annual growth rate of about 2 cm/year; however, this increase is lower compared to the first 5 years of life [7].

RIB-VERTEBRAL-STERNAL-COMPLEX (RVSC)

The thoracic cage is part of the rib-vertebral-sternal-complex (RVSC). Severe scoliosis (Figure 4.1) can adversely affect thorax development by changing its shape and reducing its normal motility. The RVSC, which fits the thoracic cavity three-dimensionally (3D), tends to constitute an elastic structural model similar to a cube in shape [10, 11]. However, in the presence of scoliosis, it becomes flat and rigid and

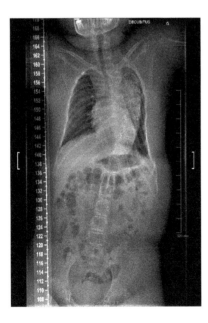

FIGURE 4.1 9-year-old boy with infantile scoliosis and distortion of thoracic cage growth.

turns elliptical, thus preventing the lungs from expanding [10, 11, 14]. At birth, the difference between thoracic depth and width is minimal, and the ratio of thoracic depth/thoracic width is very close to 1. Conversely, at skeletal maturity, the thoracic depth/thoracic width ratio is lower than 1, as width has grown more than depth. For this reason, the overall thoracic cage shape evolves from ovoid at birth to elliptical at skeletal maturity. At skeletal maturity, thoracic depth and width represent about 20% and 30% of sitting height, respectively [1, 2, 6, 7, 10, 11].

LUNG GROWTH

Lung growth is a process involving different pulmonary structures growing at different paces. At birth, the newborn has the same number of conducting airways as an adult. From infancy to adulthood, the tracheal caliber increases two- to threefold, while alveolar (peripheral areas containing alveoli) and acinar regions (peripheral area containing pulmonary capillaries) undergo substantial postnatal growth and development. At the end of lung development, the total number of alveoli has increased sixfold, and alveolar-capillary surface has increased by more than tenfold. A progressive spinal deformity, inducing distortion of the thoracic cage, can compromise lung development and growth, as up to 85% of alveoli develop after birth. In particular, during the first 7 years of life, there is an increase in the number of alveoli (alveolar multiplication), while after that period, there is an increase in the alveolar size (alveolar growth), and the overall number of alveoli does not change anymore [2, 6, 7, 15].

The thoracic volume will reach 50% of its definitive size by age 10, while the normal number of alveoli increase from 20 million at birth to 300 million at age 7; during this period, 60% of the spine has ossified. Therefore, the crucial time frame for both spine and thoracic cage growth occurs during the first 5–7 years of life and it coincides with lung development. Reduction of spine growth and subsequent alterations of thoracic cage size and function during the period of alveolar multiplication can cause progressive postnatal pulmonary hypoplasia (Figure 4.2) [2, 6, 7]. Gollogly et al. [16] reported that lung parenchyma volume is a function of age. Lung parenchyma volume is about 400 cc at birth, 900 cc at age 5, 1500 cc at age 10, and about 4000 cc at skeletal maturity [16]. Recent studies reported normal values of 3D thoracic growth from childhood to adult ages, while others found that mild to moderate scoliosis do not affect thoracic width, depth, and volume at any stage of growth [1, 2, 6, 7, 14, 15, 17, 19, 20].

SPINE AND THORACIC CAGE GROWTH DURING THE PUBERTAL GROWTH SPURT

Puberty is a turning point in children with idiopathic scoliosis, as the pubertal growth spurt increases the risk of deformity progression. During puberty, standing height increases by approximately 1.4 cm–1.5 cm/year, and a new period of acceleration of the spine growth is observed [2–4, 19, 20]. Duval Beaupere et al. [22] have demonstrated that, during the pubertal growth spurt, scoliosis will worsen substantially in most cases. Charles et al. have shown that if curve magnitude reaches 30° at the beginning of puberty, the need for surgery is very close to 100%; on the other hand, the need for surgery is about 20% if the curve magnitude at the beginning of puberty is 20° [21–25].

A prefect knowledge of the different stages of puberty is essential to provide a rationale, and well balanced, treatment strategy. However, the chronological age is a poor indicator of remaining growth and bone age should be used whenever possible [26–29].

Puberty starts at 11 years of bone age in girls and at 13 years of bone age in boys. The onset of puberty is characterised by a dramatic increase in stature, a significant change in the proportions of the upper and lower body segments, a modification of the overall morphology of the body, the first appearance of pubic hair, the budding of the nipples, and testicular growth (secondary sexual characteristics) [1–4, 22–25]. The secondary sexual characteristics generally develop in harmony with bone age, but there are discrepancies in about 10%–20% of cases [1–4].

The first physical sign of puberty in boys is testicular growth. In 70% of cases, it occurs 3.5 years before attaining adult height. At onset of puberty, boys have approximately 13 years of bone age, the Risser sign is 0, the triradiate cartilage is still open and have 13% of remaining growth (22.5 cm; 12.5 cm in sitting height and 10 cm in subischial length). At this age, girls have well-developed secondary sexual characteristics, and their rate of growth is already decelerating.

In more than 90% of girls, the first physical sign of puberty is breast budding; menarche occurs at Risser I, about 2 years after breast budding, and final height is usually achieved 2.5–3 years after menarche [1–4, 22–25]. At the onset of puberty, girls have approximately 11 years of bone age, the Risser sign is 0, the triradiate cartilage is still open and have 12% of remaining growth (20.5 cm; 11.5 cm in sitting height and 9 cm in subischial length). After menarche, girls will gain the final 5% of their standing height, about 3 cm–5 cm [1–4, 22–25].

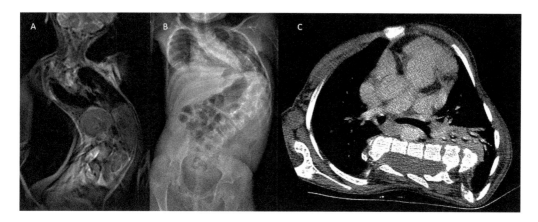

FIGURE 4.2 9-year-old girl with untreated early onset scoliosis. MRI (A), radiographs (B), and transverse CT scan (C) show severe alteration of spine/thoracic cage relationship.

During the pubertal growth spurt, growth is far more noticeable in the trunk than in the lower limbs; in particular, during puberty, two-thirds of growth is at the level of the trunk (sitting height) and one-third at the level of the lower extremity (subischial length) [1, 2]. Charles et al. and Canavese et al. found that the anterior-posterior thoracic diameter at the level of the xiphoid process, the thoracic width, and the thoracic perimeter correspond to 20%, 30%, and almost 100% of sitting height, respectively [6, 19, 20].

The peak growth velocity occurs between 13 and 15 years of bone age in boys and between 11 and 13 years of bone age in girls. After this period, there is a substantial decrease in the annual growth rate, with growth in the the lower limbs stopping rapidly; the remaining growth is about 5.5 cm (1.5 cm in the lower limbs) [1–4].

PUBERTAL DIAGRAM

By plotting the gain in sitting and standing height every 6 months, the pubertal diagram, which represents the pubertal growth spurt, can be obtained. Within the pubertal diagram, two very distinct periods can be identified: 1) the acceleration phase or 'ascending side of the pubertal growth spurt', between 11 and 13 years of bone age in girls and 13 and 15 years of bone age in boys and 2) the deceleration phase or 'descending side of the puberty', between 13 and 15 years of bone age in girls and between 15 and 17 years of bone age in boys; this phase is characterised by a significant deceleration of growth. During the ascending side, the gain in sitting height is approximately 8.5 m in boys and 7.7 cm in girls; on the other hand, the gain is about 5 cm for boys and 4.5 cm for girls during the descending side [3, 4, 21, 27]. Whatever the population or the ethnicity, the chronology of puberty is always the same: an acceleration phase (ascending side) followed by a deceleration phase (descending side).

The spine surgeon must be aware of the following radiographic parameters.

- Elbow closure (13 and 15 years of bone age in girls and boys, respectively) and fusion of the distal phalanx of the hand split the pubertal growth spurt into two parts: ascending and descending side.

- Triradiate cartilage closes during the ascending phase at 12 and 14 years of bone age in girls and boys, respectively.
- Risser sign appears during the descending phase. Risser I appears at 13.5 and 15.5 years of bone age in girls and boys, respectively.
- The peak height velocity it is not a point in the curve, as it takes place during the first 2 years of puberty (ascending side).
- During puberty, the peak of growth results from a combination of three smaller peaks (micropeaks); the first peak involves the lower limbs, the second peak involves the trunk, and the third peak involves the thorax.

Risser 0 makes up two-thirds of the ascending phase of puberty, and it can be divided into two parts: 1) Risser 0-triradiate cartilage open (11–12 and 13–14 years of bone age in girls and boys, respectively) and 2) Risser 0-triradiate cartilage closed (12–13 and 14–15 years of bone age in girls and boys, respectively).

When plotting all these data on the pubertal diagram, four distinct zones (Figure 4.3) can be identified: two in the ascending side and two in the descending side [2 ,21, 26, 29]:

- *Zone 1:* Risser 0, triradiate cartilage open (ascending side).
- *Zone 2:* Risser 0, triradiate cartilage closed (ascending side).
- *Zone 3:* Risser I-II, greater trochanter open (descending side).
- *Zone 4:* Risser III-V, greater trochanter closed (descending side).

To evaluate the potential for progression of a spinal curvature, it is important to evaluate the behaviour of the curve during the ascending side of the pubertal diagram, when the risk of progression is significantly higher [21–25].

BONE AGE

It is essential to evaluate the bone age, as only 50% of the population has a bone age in concordance with the chronological age. There are many options to assess bone age, but the

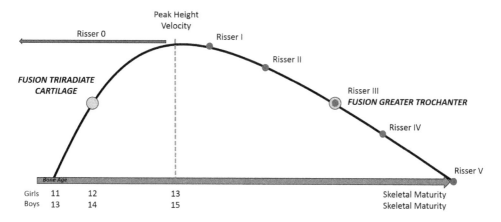

FIGURE 4.3 Pubertal diagram.

simplified olecranon method should be preferred during the ascending phase of puberty, as it is more precise than the Greulich and Pyle atlas. On the descending phase, the Risser sign is helpful although not precise enough when complex decisions must be taken; during this period, methods involving the hand are more detailed, although a good correlation has been proved between hand and iliac crest radiographs [19, 20, 22, 25, 26, 28, 30].

Despite all useful information bone age can provide, it must always be balanced with secondary sexual characteristics, annual growth rate and, in girls, the onset of menarche. Sometimes Risser V (complete ossification of the iliac apophysis) never appears and is, therefore, difficult to decide whether a specific treatment can be stopped, as clinical signs are also important. If there is no more increase in sitting height, a treatment can be stopped. Usually, 2–2.5 years after the onset of menarche, the trunk stops growing [1 ,2, 5].

Parents frequently ask how much a spinal fusion for scoliosis will decrease the final height of their child. To determine the answer to this question, the surgeon needs to know the remaining sitting height and the contribution to it made by the vertebrae that will be fused. After a bone age of 13 years in girls, when there are only 4 cm of remaining growth in sitting height, and after a bone age of 15 years in boys, when there are only 5 cm of remaining growth in sitting height, there is little need for concern about final height [1–4, 6, 7, 22–25].

THE CRANKSHAFT PHENOMENON

The crankshaft phenomenon was described by Dubousset in 1973 [30] and Dubousset et al. in 1989 [31]. It occurs when there is a solid posterior arthrodesis with sufficient anterior growth remaining to produce a rotation of the spine and trunk with progression of the curve [29, 30]. To control a scoliotic curve, all growth plates involved in the deformity should be neutralised at once. This fundamental concept is at the heart of the crankshaft phenomenon; therefore, the surgeon must consider the state of skeletal maturity and the amount of growth remaining in the portion of the spine that is to be fused [30, 31].

The younger the patient, the higher the risk of crankshaft phenomenon. During the pubertal growth spurt, the risk still persists. Sanders et al. [32] have demonstrated that the risk of crankshaft phenomenon is lower when the triradiate cartilage is closed; however, triradiate cartilage closes 1 year after the onset of puberty when the remaining sitting height is about 8 cm–9 cm in both boys and girls [1, 2, 5, 21, 27, 29]. Full screws constructs can reduce the risk of crankshafting, although the risk cannot completely be eliminated. Sanders et al. [33] performed a retrospective study of posterior spinal instrumentation with fusion in 43 patients with idiopathic scoliosis, who were at Risser 0 at the time of surgery. The triradiate cartilage was open in 23 patients and closed in 20. The crankshaft effect was observed in 10 of the 23 patients (43.5%)

with open triradiate cartilage, and in one patient (5%) with a closed triradiate cartilage.

The crankshaft phenomenon should not only be merely considered as worsening of the Cobb angle, as it carries several other negative effect, including aggravation of the spinal imbalance, deterioration of the thoracic deformity, and aggravation of the deformity above and below the instrumented segments [30, 31].

THE 'SCOLIOTIC RISK'

When dealing with patients with idiopathic scoliosis, the basic question is 'what is the scoliotic risk for the patient?' As a rule of thumb, the younger the child, the higher the scoliotic risk. A scoliosis of 20° does not have the same risk of deterioration at 5, 10 or 15 years of age. Several papers have been published on the surgical risk of scoliosis, and, by merging all published data together, a relatively simple approximation can potentially be used in daily practise [18, 24].

The scoliotic risk for a 20° curve should be multiplied by 5 at 5 years of age (20 × 5 = 100% risk of progression), by 4 at 10 years of age (20 × 4 = 80% risk of progression), by 3 at the beginning of puberty (20 × 3 = 60% risk of progression) and by 2 at the peak of pubertal growth spurt (Risser I; 20 × 2 = 40% risk of progression).

At Risser II, the risk of progression of a 20° curve drops to 20%, although more severe deformities (30°–40°) carry a higher risk of progression (30%) [21, 27].

However, the risk of progression for curves measuring 10°, 20°, or 30° for patients on the descending side of puberty is different, as the strategy of management essentially depends upon the topography of the curve. In particular, lumbar deformity should never be underestimated because of the potential for poor outcome during adulthood. A curve increasing by 10° during the first 2 years of puberty carries a high risk of requiring surgical treatment.

WHAT WILL BE THE FINAL DEFICIT OF THE TRUNK AFTER POSTERIOR SPINE INSTRUMENTED FUSION?

The deficit in trunk height induced by a posterior spine fusion can be easily assessed by a) evaluating the sitting height; b) evaluating the remaining sitting height; c) considering each single thoracic and lumbar vertebra will cause a 2.5% and 3.5% deficit is sitting height, respectively; d) adjusting these values to the age of the patient; and e) applying the following algorithm as some authors have suggested: 0.07 mm/vertebra/year of remaining growth). The overall loss of sitting height will be compensated by the correction of the deformity [1–4].

CONCLUSIONS

PERFECT KNOWLEDGE OF NORMAL GROWTH PARAMETERS IS MANDATORY

Only perfect knowledge of normal growth parameters allows a better understanding of both normal and abnormal spine and thoracic cage growth. Measurement of sitting height gives an indirect estimate of spinal growth, and it is certainly instructive to monitor sitting height rather than standing height.

ANTICIPATION IS THE BEST STRATEGY

There is a reciprocal interaction between spine, thoracic cage, and cardiorespiratory system. Progressive spinal deformities and early spinal arthrodesis can alter spinal and thoracic cage growth by altering both shape function. As the spinal deformity progresses, a *domino effect* causes modification to the size and shape of the thoracic cage. If action is delayed or not taken, the abnormal growth and the subsequent anatomical modifications of both spine and thoracic cage will lead to a progressive, evolutive, and irreversible clinical picture.

ESSENTIAL KEY POINTS TO KEEP IN MIND WHEN DEALING WITH PAEDIATRIC SPINAL DEFORMITIES

- The growing spine is a complex phenomenon characterised by the interaction among more than 130 growth plates.
- Repeated clinical measurements allow identification and treatment of anticipated progressive deformities.
- Sitting height is more precise than standing height.

- Bone age is more precise than chronological age.
- Careful weight assessment is an important part of the orthopaedic evaluation, as weight doubles during pubertal growth spurt.
- Ask yourself: a) What is the sitting height? b) What about remaining sitting height? c) What is the bone age? d) Is the patient on the ascending or descending side of puberty?
- Most spinal deformity arises within the T1–S1 segment (strategic segment).
- The T1–S1 segment makes up about 49% of the sitting height at skeletal maturity.
- The T1–T12 segment represents about 30% of the sitting height (at maturity).
- The L1–L5 segment represents about 19% of the sitting height (at skeletal maturity).
- Spine and thoracic cage growth are closely interrelated.
- About half of trunk growth occurs during the first 5 years of life.
- As the spinal deformity progresses, a 'domino effect' causes modification to the size and shape of the thoracic cage.
- The crankshaft phenomenon is at the heart of paediatric spinal pathology.
- The timing of spinal arthrodesis should be decided after accounting for all growth parameters.

Ethical statement: The authors are accountable for all aspects of the work in ensuring that questions related to the accuracy or integrity of any part of the work are appropriately investigated and resolved.

Conflict of interest: None declared.

REFERENCES

1. Dimeglio A, Bonnel F. *Le rachis en croissance*. Paris, France: Springer Verlag; 1990.
2. Dimeglio A, Canavese F. The growing spine: How spinal deformities influence normal spine and thoracic cage growth. *Eur Spine J.* 2012;21(1):64–70.
3. Dimeglio A, Canavese F, Charles YP. Growth and adolescent idiopathic scoliosis: When and how much? *J Pediatr Orthop.* 2012;31(1) (Suppl.):S28–S36.
4. Dimeglio A, Canavese F. Progression or not progression? How to deal with adolescent idiopathic scoliosis during puberty. *J Child Orthop.* 2013;7(1):43–9.
5. Dimeglio A. Growth of the spine before age 5 years. *J Pediatr Orthop B.* 1993;1(2):102–7.
6. Canavese F, Dimeglio A, Bonnel F, et al. Thoracic cage volume and dimension assessment by optoelectronic molding in normal children and adolescents during growth. *Surg Radiol Anat.* 2019;41(3):287–96.
7. Canavese F, Dimeglio A. Normal and abnormal spine and thoracic cage development. *World J Orthop.* 2013;4(4):167–74.
8. Karol L, Johston C, Mladenov K, et al. Pulmonary function following early thoracic fusion in non neuromuscular scoliosis. *J Bone Joint Surg Am.* 2008;90(6):1272–81.
9. Canavese F, Dimeglio A, Volpatti D, et al. Dorsal arthrodesis of thoracic spine and effects on thorax growth in prepubertal New Zealand white rabbits. *Spine.* 2007;32(16):E443–50.
10. Canavese F, Dimeglio A, D'Amato C, et al. Dorsal arthrodesis in prepubertal New Zealand White rabbits followed to skeletal maturity: Effect on thoracic dimensions, spine growth and neural elements. *Indian J Orthop.* 2010;44(1):14–22.
11. Canavese F, Dimeglio A, Granier M, et al. Arthrodesis of the first six dorsal vertebrae in prepubertal New Zealand White rabbits and thoracic growth to skeletal maturity: The role of the "Rib-Vertebral-Sternal complex". *Minerva Ortop Traumatol.* 2007;58:369–78.
12. Canavese F, Dimeglio A, Granier M, et al. Influence de l'arthrodèse vertébrale sélective T1-T6 sur la croissance thoracique: Étude expérimentale chez des lapins New Zealand White prépubertaires. *Rev Chir Orthop Reparatrice Appar Mot.* 2008;94(5):490–7.
13. Canavese F, Dimeglio A, Stebel M, et al. Thoracic cage plasticity in prepubertal New Zealand white rabbits submitted to T1-T12 dorsal arthrodesis: Computed tomography evaluation, echocardiographic assessment and cardio-pulmonary measurements. *Eur Spine J.* 2013;22(5):1101–12.
14. Xun FX, Canavese F, Xu H, et al. Dynamic three-dimensional reconstruction of thoracic cage and abdomen in children and adolescents with scoliosis: Preliminary results of optical reflective motion analysis assessment. *J Pediatr Orthop.* 2020;40(4):196–202.
15. Canavese F, Samba A, Dimeglio A, et al. Serial elongation-derotation-flexion casting for children with early-onset scoliosis. *World J Orthop.* 2015;6(11):935–43.

16. Gollogly S, Smith JT, White SK, et al. The volume of lung parenchyma as a function of age: A review of 1050 normal CT scans of the chest with three-dimensional volumetric reconstruction of the pulmonary system. *Spine.* 2004;29(18):2061–7.

17. Canavese F, Kaelin A. Adolescent idiopathic scoliosis: Indications and efficacy of non-operative treatment. *Indian J Orthop.* 2011;45(1):7–14.

18. Canavese F, Botnari A, Dimeglio A et al. Serial elongation, derotation and flexion (EDF) casting under general anesthesia and neuromuscular blocking drugs improve outcome in patients with juvenile scoliosis: Preliminary results. *Eur Spine J.* 2016;25(2):487–94.

19. Charles YP, Marcoul A, Schaeffer M, et al. Three-dimensional and volumetric thoracic growth in children with moderate idiopathic scoliosis compared with normal. *J Pediatr Orthop B.* 2017;26(3):227–32.

20. Charles YP, Canavese F, Dimeglio A. Curve progression risk in a mixed series of braced and non-braced patients with idiopathic scoliosis related to skeletal maturity assessment on the olecranon. *J Pediatr Orthop B.* 2017;26(3):240–4.

21. Charles YP, Daures JP, De Rosa V, et al. Progression risk of juvenile idiopathic scoliosis during pubertal growth. *Spine.* 2006;31(17):1933–42.

22. Duval-Beaupère G, Dubousset J, Queneau P. Pour une théorie unique de l'évolution des scolioses. *Presse Med.* 1970;78(25):1141.

23. Duval-Beaupère G, Combes J. Segments supérieur et inférieur au cours de la croissance physiologique des filles: Étude longitudinale de la croissance de 54 filles. *Arch Fr Pediatr.* 1971;28(10):1057.

24. Duval-Beaupère G. Les repères de maturation dans la surveillance des scolioses. *Rev Chir Orthop.* 1970;56(1):59.

25. Duval-Beaupère G. Croissance résiduelle de la taille et des segments après la première menstruation chez la fille. *Rev Chir Orthop.* 1976;62(5):501.

26. Canavese F, Charles YP, Dimeglio A. Skeletal age assessment from elbow radiographs. Review of the literature. *Chir Organ Mov.* 2008;92(1):1–6.

27. Charles YP, Dimeglio A, Canavese F, et al. Skeletal age assessment from the olecranon for idiopathic scoliosis at Risser grade 0. *J Bone Joint Surg Am.* 2007;89(12):2737–44.

28. Diméglio A, Charles YP, Daures JP, et al. Accuracy of the Sauvegrain method in determining skeletal age during puberty. *J Bone Joint Surg Am.* 2005;87(8):1689–96.

29. Canavese F, Charles YP, Dimeglio A, et al. A comparison of the simplified olecranon and digital methods of assessment of skeletal maturity during the pubertal growth spurt. *Bone Joint J.* 2014;96(11):1556–60.

30. Dubousset J. *Recidive d'une scoliose lombaire et d'un basin oblique après fusion precoce: Le phénomène du Villebrequin. Proceeding Group Etude de la Scoliose.* Paris, France; 1973.

31. Dubousset J, Herring JA, Shufflebarger HL. The crankshaft phenomenon. *J Pediatr Orthop.* 1989;9(5):541.

32. Sanders JO, Khoury JG, Kishan S, et al. Predicting scoliosis progression from skeletal maturity: A simplified classification during adolescence. *J Bone Joint Surg Am.* 2008;90(3):540–53.

33. Sanders JO, Herring JA, Browne RH. Posterior arthrodesis and instrumentation in the immature (Risser-grade-0) spine in idiopathic scoliosis. *J Bone Joint Surg Am.* 1995;77(1):39–45.

5 Pulmonary Evaluation and Management of Early-Onset Scoliosis

Laura Ellington, Mary Crocker, and Gregory Redding

CONTENTS

Early onset scoliosis (EOS), which begins before 10 years of age, impairs breathing to variable degrees during childhood. Severe EOS can be lethal due to cardiopulmonary failure with or without pulmonary hypertension; however, other children with EOS have minor spine and thoracic deformities and are as active as their peers. While there is an interest in using structural features of scoliosis, such as the coronal curve magnitude (also known as the Cobb angle), as a proxy for impairments in respiratory function, most studies have found weak correlations at best between Cobb angle and spirometry, sleep quality, or exercise tolerance [1–3]. This chapter addresses the breathing disorders associated with EOS, the ways to evaluate them (both quantitatively and qualitatively), and the role of medical providers in managing children with EOS in resource-limited settings (RLS).

PULMONARY MANIFESTATIONS OF EOS

EOS is often classified by aetiology, but diagnosis and strategies for care depend on the age at presentation [4]. *Congenital* scoliosis results from primary malformations of the vertebrae, usually due to hemivertebrae or failure of segmentation, producing a bar of fused bone. In the newborn period, congenital scoliosis, with or without abnormal ribs, can lead to immediate respiratory distress, requiring supportive care, such as oxygen, enteral tube feedings, and mechanical ventilation to survive. However, congenital scoliosis can present late in childhood if there is an isolated hemivertebra or two hemivertebrae that are balanced (one on either side of the spine) thereby producing a relatively straight back. *Neuromuscular* scoliosis results from conditions producing muscle weakness or spasticity, such as cerebral palsy. Progressive scoliosis occurs with progressive neuromuscular weakness [5]. This can begin early in life, such as spinal muscular atrophy Type I, or during adolescence; however, neuromuscular weakness can also compromise respiratory function before scoliosis begins [6]. *Syndromic* scoliosis is usually part of a multi-organ condition often due to a genetic disorder. Syndromic EOS is often associated with multi-organ disease, such as VACTERL syndrome, in which the vertebral abnormalities are overshadowed by other congenital abnormalities that require more immediate intervention. *Thoracogenic* scoliosis develops after cardiac or thoracic surgery, such as congenital diaphragmatic hernia or rib resection early in life. Finally, *idiopathic* EOS includes infantile (0–3 years of age) and juvenile (4–10 years of age) scoliosis, based on the age at first detection [7]. In older infants and toddlers, a spine deformity may be the first indication of EOS rather than respiratory features. However, poor nutritional status, i.e. low weight for length and failure to thrive, may be the presenting problem, as tachypnoea with feeding and limited oral intake often go unnoticed. This may be additionally challenging to diagnose in RLS where additional factors, including low socioeconomic status, contribute to malnutrition. In older children, EOS can produce fatigability and dyspnoea with exercise and may limit activities during play or sports. As children adapt to the increased work of breathing, they often opt for a more sedentary lifestyle. Consequently, patients may not report dyspnoea because they choose not to exert themselves. Alternatively, children present with respiratory distress associated with an acute lower respiratory tract infection or with prolonged symptoms during and after the infection.

PATHOPHYSIOLOGY OF EOS

Several pathophysiologic processes coexist in children with EOS. Spine and chest wall deformities lead to malalignment of the vertebral body, ribs, and sternum. This malalignment may be rigid initially, as with congenital scoliosis, or become more rigid over time due to prolonged joint immobility, as occurs with neuromuscular weakness. Surgical implantation of rigid devices and spine fusion also lead to loss of spine and thoracic flexibility, producing additional stiffness [8]. Increased chest wall rigidity leads to greater respiratory work to maintain chest wall excursion with breathing. With severe deformities, the chest wall moves minimally, and excursion occurs with paradoxical abdominal motion. Patients minimise respiratory work by changing their breathing pattern. Minute ventilation is maintained by breathing more shallowly but faster.

In addition, the intercostal muscles become less effective as ribs become immobile and patients rely increasingly on the diaphragm to generate force during inspiration. Inspiratory force, such as maximal inspiratory pressure, is diminished in many children with EOS, even in the absence of underlying neuromuscular weakness disorders [9]. Inspiratory muscle weakness directly correlates with reduced vital capacity in older children with EOS. This is likely due to rotation and tethering of the diaphragm to deformed skeletal structures in EOS. It is unclear if reduced movement with contraction results in atrophy of certain muscles, such as the intercostal muscles. Poor nutritional status also results in respiratory muscle weakness and fatigability. The combination of a stiffer chest wall and weaker respiratory muscles predisposes children to hypercapnia, particularly during respiratory infections and during sleep.

The chest wall deformity also leads to reduced lung volumes and local distortion of lung shape, as illustrated in Figure 5.1. Loss of lung volume regionally or generally leads, in turn, to reduced lung compliance, contributing to respiratory system stiffness. Loss of lung volume also predisposes patients with EOS to recurrent hypoxaemia during sleep when pauses in breathing occur [3]. This occurs because some airways are narrowed with reduced functional residual capacity (FRC) and close with relaxation of thoracic muscles during rapid eye movement (REM) sleep. These are called hypopnoeic hypopxaemic episodes during sleep and differ from obstructive apnoeas that are more prolonged and due to upper airway obstruction or collapse. In children with large tonsils and adenoids, obstructive sleep apnoea and recurrent hypoponeic hypoxemic events can coexist and disturb sleep quality.

PULMONARY EVALUATION OF CHILDREN WITH EOS

On physical exam, a posterior rib hump is present with or without changes in the anterior chest. One shoulder is often higher than the other. Posteriorly, the scapula may protrude more on one side than the other. Isolated rib prominence may be present due to abnormal rib alignment, and large gaps between the ribs can often be palpated. Pectus deformities, such as pectus excavatum or pectus carinatum, may coexist with spine deformities. Pectus excavatum,

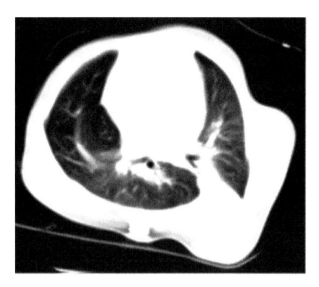

FIGURE 5.1 Computerised tomogram of the chest and spine in a transverse cut demonstrating differences in left and right lung size and shape.

especially in the presence of thoracic lordosis, leads to reduced chest wall depth, known as pectus gracilus, and often compression of large airways, producing fixed airway obstruction [10, 11]. This is illustrated in Figure 5.2, which demonstrates the limited chest wall depth related to the thoracic lordosis and pectus gracilus. The pulmonary arteries and even the esophagus can also be compressed with loss of chest wall depth.

Inspection will also reveal that children use their abdominal muscles to exhale more forcefully at rest; however, this is not a prolonged exhalation but a short push with every breath. This likely reflects abnormal diaphragmatic position and an attempt by the child to reposition the diaphragm during exhalation to its most effective position higher in the chest to initiate the next breath. Abnormal findings on auscultation include unilaterally reduced breath sounds or bilaterally reduced breath sounds despite maximal inspiratory efforts. Breath sounds may be asymmetric due to asymmetric restrictive constraint of the ribs on one side or reduced diaphragm function and excursion on one side. Alternatively, breath sounds may be louder than normal on a more functional side due to mainstem or lobar bronchial compression by the spine and mediastinal organs. Rales, rhonchi, and wheezes are not common in EOS in the absence of underlying lung or airway disease

and should raise questions about concurrent primary pulmonary disease.

The physical examination in young children who are able to run should include an examination after running to hear breath sounds with deeper breathing and to count the respiratory rate. This manoeuver will produce breath sounds that were diminished at rest and also demonstrate exercise-related tachypnoea, which is the earliest manifestation of restrictive chest wall disease.

In addition, the examination should survey for cardiac disease, neuromuscular weakness or spasticity, and nutritional state. The abdomen should be examined to assess subdiaphragmatic reasons for restrictive lung disease, such as hepatosplenomegaly and distension due to air swallowing and/or constipation. The abdomen should also be examined for pelvic obliquity, associated with thoracolumbar scoliosis, as this elevates one iliac crest to abut, enclose, or intrude beneath the ribs unilaterally. This is assessed by placing your fingers between the iliac crest and lower ribs and palpating the distance between them.

An examination of the hypopharynx is important in children with EOS who snore, thrash in bed, and or sweat when asleep. Upper airway obstruction due to tonsil and adenoid hypertrophy is more likely to produce hypoxaemia during sleep when lung volumes are

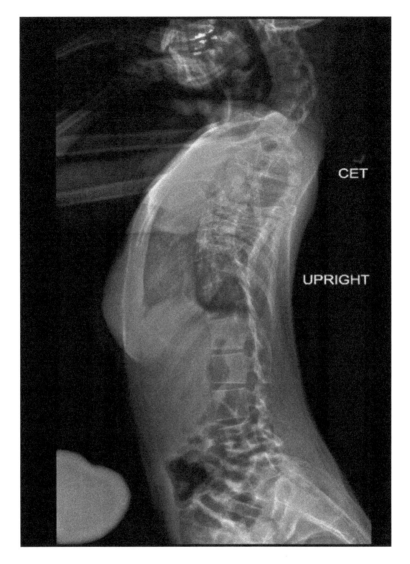

FIGURE 5.2 Sagittal view of the spine in a child with thoracic lordosis, producing a reduced chest wall depth, contributing to lower lung volumes and restrictive lung disease.

reduced due to scoliosis. Nutritional status can be assessed using weight for age, weight velocity on appropriate growth curves, or weight for length using arm span instead of length in children with significant spine curvature.

Unfortunately, apart from respiratory rate and weight, these features are not quantitative. Nonetheless, these findings are important to note in estimating degree of restrictive or obstructive lung disease due to spine and thoracic deformity over time. Presence of breath sound asymmetry, abdominal expiratory push, tachypnoea at rest, pelvic obliquity, and poor nutritional status

represent different pathophysiologic features of EOS, but together, they indicate more severe respiratory disease.

DIAGNOSTIC TESTS

The spine radiograph and spirometer are necessary to understand the spine deformity and its respiratory consequences for an individual. Pulse oximetry is useful at night more than during wakefulness, as sleep related oxyhemoglobin desaturation is more common than hypoxaemia when awake. In children with severe spine and rib deformities, an assessment of hypercapnia using blood gas and serum bicarbonate levels identifies high-risk patients in chronic respiratory failure. Lung function testing is most useful to rule out primary lung disease, such as asthma, and then, after the pulmonary disease has been treated, as an objective measure of the spine and chest wall impact on breathing.

The spine radiographs should include anterior-posterior and lateral views (coronal and sagittal views, respectively) in order to better assess the thorax and diaphragmatic contours. One reason for these films is to rule out aetiologies for poor pulmonary status due to conditions other than scoliosis. Abnormalities, such as lobar or whole lung atelectasis, occur during acute respiratory illnesses in children with EOS due to localised restriction of lung expansion. Recurrent pneumonias and aspiration events may lead to airway damage and even regional bronchiectasis. Scoliosis after repair of a congenital diaphragmatic hernia repair is particularly problematic as restrictive changes result from the hypoplastic lung(s) and/or the spine deformity. Herniation of the lung is often identified when ribs are absent or abnormally spaced.

In addition, special attention should be focussed on the contour of the diaphragm. The diaphragm is attached posteriorly at the first to the third lumbar vertebrae, to the pericardium in the chest, and to the xiphoid process anteriorly. Distortions in the relationships of these insertion points of the central tendon can lead to tethering of the crural portion of the diaphragm. In addition, the diaphragm is attached at the lower ribs as it descends to become the coastal region, apposed by the surface of the abdomen; therefore, deformation of the lower ribs can further distort, rotate, or tether the diaphragm, reducing its mobility. A flattened diaphragm and one in which the pleural sulcus is absent reflects a diaphragm with decreased excursion. Diaphragmatic flattening illustrated in Figure 5.3 is associated with kyphosis.

Central airway compression by the spine posteriorly and mediastinal structures anteriorly is not readily apparent from a chest radiograph, but the presence of thoracic lordosis, especially in the presence of a pectus excavatum, should alert the clinician to this cause for unilateral obstructive lung disease [10]. It can be further confirmed by CT scan of the chest or flexible bronchoscopy if these tests are available.

Spirometry is simple to conduct but needs to be practised and mastered by the child in order to be interpretable. This is particularly true for children ≤6 years of age. Emphasis on the

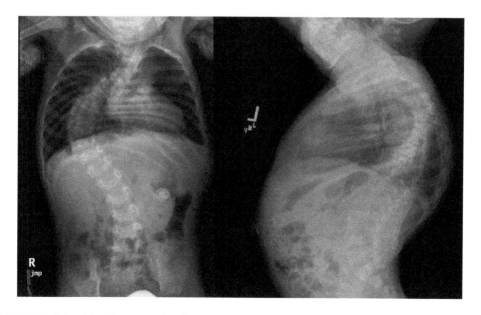

FIGURE 5.3 Spine films demonstrating flattened diaphragms in a child with kyphoscoliosis in the anterior-posterior and lateral images.

complete deep inspiration before the expiratory manoeuver is particularly important, as it is difficult for children to inhale to total lung capacity unless they are coached to do so. Most children with EOS have restrictive features on spirometry with a reduced FVC as a percent of normal. A forced expiratory manoeuver will help to identify underlying obstructive disease. Although this occurs in only 10%–30% of patients with EOS, it should be further investigated if present on more than one spirometric test [12]. In our study of children with EOS who demonstrated obstructive lung disease by spirometry, a third of those tested before and after a bronchodilator trial had reversible airway obstruction, i.e. asthma, compared to two-thirds with irreversible obstruction, likely due to airway compression or airway traction [13].

Vital capacity is usually normalised for height to compare to children of different ages without scoliosis who are normal. However, children with significant scoliosis are shorter than predicted because of the spine curvature, therefore, arm span should always be used as a surrogate for height in children with scoliosis. Ulnar length can also be measured as there are formulas for ulnar length to height relationships that allow for this measure to be used as a surrogate for predicted height as well. In different parts of the world, there are different prediction equations based on ethnicity.

Serial measures of vital capacity in absolute terms and as a % of predicted value are particularly important. They can identify progressive loss of lung function as the spine deformity worsens, and this can assist the spine surgeon in deciding when to intervene. Spirometry is also useful to measure the pulmonary consequences of different spine surgical (and nonsurgical) strategies. In one long-term study, lung function declined by 25% despite treatment with spine distraction devices over a 6-year period [14]. Serial spirometric assessments should be continued after all surgical treatment is completed, as lung function can improve, decline, or stay the same after spine fusion. Spirometry has also been measured when children with EOS transition to adult care. In some series, there is progressive loss of lung function, particularly when the vital capacity is <70% after spine fusion in childhood or adolescence [15].

OTHER DIAGNOSTIC TESTS

In children with underlying neuromuscular weakness, the vital capacity does not discriminate between the impact of scoliosis and of respiratory muscle weakness. To do this requires a more direct assessment of inspiratory and expiratory muscle strength. Respiratory muscle strength can be assessed using maximum inspiratory (MIP) and expiratory pressures (MEP) measured with a manometer connected to a closed system with no change in airflow [16]. This can be done at the mouth, or alternatively at the nose, to measure maximum sniff pressures, which some patients find more intuitive to do. The MIP is measured after a complete exhalation, known as the Mueller manoeuver, when the patient has exhaled to residual volume. It can also be performed at functional residual capacity, but the normal values differ at different lung volumes. MIP is age and gender dependent, as boys can generate greater pressures than girls, and adolescents have stronger respiratory muscles than preadolescent children [17].

MEP can also be measured as an indication of abdominal muscle strength required to cough. It can be reduced more when neuromuscular weakness is present. Maximum expiratory pressure is measured after a patient inhales as much as possible and then exhales against a closed system. MEP may be reduced when a patient's total lung capacity is reduced, such as in scoliosis. MEP is also gender and age dependent. Reduced maximum expiratory pressure may indicate a reduced ability to cough, although the exact value at which cough is impaired is not clear.

There are multiple other tests that can complement thoracic imaging and spirometry if available. Exercise testing using a treadmill or stationary bicycle will demonstrate a limited ability to perform external work, a reduced maximum oxygen consumption despite an expected elevated heart rate, and often deconditioning [1]. The 6-minute walk test has also been used in children with EOS, and the distance walked is often reduced. This test, like the formal cardiopulmonary exercise test, is not specific to lung function limitations, as it is also affected by strength, cardiac status, balance, and developmental status. Neither test has been used to make decisions regarding surgery and cannot be used as a surrogate for lung function alone, as correlates between exercise-derived data and spirometric data are poor until pulmonary limitations are severe.

Sleep-related breathing disorders have also been identified in children with EOS. These occur most often during REM sleep and are associated with hypoxaemia and hypercapnia. The Apneoa-Hypopnoea Index is abnormal in the majority of children who undergo formal polysomnography. Among children who have been studied overnight with polysomnography, more than half required noninvasive positive ventilation or supplemental oxygen [18]. Sleep quality is also abnormal in the majority of children tested, and this may affect growth velocity, intellectual development, and daytime behaviour. Sleep-related disorders in this population include risks described in normal children, such as tonsil and adenoidal hypertrophy, obesity, and midface hypoplasia. In centers that do not have paediatric sleep facilities, examination of the hypopharynx for enlarged tonsil should prompt earlier consideration of tonsil and adenoid removal. In lieu of a formal polysomnogram, overnight assessments of hypoxaemia with a pulse oximeter would be a reasonable screening procedure. Polycythaemia has been reported in up to 28% of children with EOS, likely reflecting nighttime hypoxaemia during sleep [19]. This finding should prompt some investigation of breathing during sleep. Nap studies have been reported in children with EOS but are normal in many cases, probably because children do not often enter REM sleep during naps [20]. Improvements in sleep quality and nighttime hypoxaemia have been described in children with EOS undergoing serial sleep studies; however, the impact of spine surgery to treat EOS on breathing during sleep is not known

IMPLICATIONS OF LUNG FUNCTION TESTING IN CHILDREN WITH EOS

There is no data as yet that any surgical procedure to correct or improve EOS leads to improvement in lung functions [2, 21]. There is data that absolute volumes in litres increase as children grow, even after growth-friendly devices are inserted to reduce the Cobb angle and increase vertebral length; however, when corrected for assumed height using arm span or ulnar length to calculate expected normal height, predicted FVC declines over time with ongoing somatic growth [22, 23]. In other words, lung growth in functional terms does not keep pace with somatic growth, probably because of thoracic cage constraints. In patients with EOS followed for 25 years after spine fusion, lung function tended to remain the same as a % of predicted values if preoperative values were >80% (reflecting minimal lung function impairment initially) [15]. However, for children with more severe pulmonary impairment, further decline in adulthood should be anticipated.

The advances in development of expandable growing titanium distraction devices, which can be increased in length noninvasively, has revolutionised orthopaedic management of severe early spine deformities. Advances in spinal growth modulators, such as vertebral tethers, hold promise of alternative surgical treatment strategies for selected populations in the future. This has produced a new population of children who are growing up with chronic restrictive lung disease often with prospects for further deterioration in adulthood. This population will require long-term pulmonary assessment and treatment to mitigate the long-term impact of spine deformities that have been surgically corrected.

PULMONARY MANAGEMENT OF EOS

There are three epochs of care that require a pulmonary assessment. The first is when a child initially presents for spine care. The medical evaluation must focus on any preexisting comorbid conditions that could complicate the functional consequences of the scoliosis. Malnutrition, anaemia, and other pulmonary conditions should be addressed before a pulmonary assessment related primarily to scoliosis can be made. At that point, the lung functions preoperatively are the major determinant of lung functions throughout adulthood regardless of surgical therapy. This assessment may also impact how quickly a surgical or nonsurgical treatment (such as a brace) should be initiated.

The second epoch of assessment and care occurs during the preoperative and postoperative period for each procedure, but especially for initial insertion of growing rods or spine fusion. The preoperative assessment should determine the level of lung function and, therefore, risk of postoperative complications. In patients with adolescent idiopathic scoliosis, a FVC<40% triples the risk of postoperative pulmonary problems [24]. There is no threshold value established for younger patients with EOS. We believe that pulmonary hypertension and hypercarbia preoperatively carry a higher pulmonary complication risk following any spine surgery in children with EOS. Finally, children should be actively gaining weight for the period before surgery to improve wound-healing postoperatively. Postoperatively, children with restrictive chest wall disease may benefit from airway clearance treatments if their cough seems compromised, nutritional supplementation to avoid weight loss in the perioperative period, and adequate pain control.

Finally, at least 3 months after the final surgical procedure, such as spine fusion, lung functions should be measured to identify the best spirometric values to be expected thereafter. There is little data on children who have undergone prefusion growing rod treatment to prognosticate about degree of decline in adulthood. Danielsson [15] reported that 25 after spine fusion for EOS, adults who experienced further pulmonary decline in adulthood where those with a preoperative value of <70% for FVC. Such individuals merit serial pulmonary assessments as they age.

CONCLUSION

Decisions to treat EOS in young children are based on both structural and functional assessments. Children may be too marginal to tolerate surgery if their deformity is severe and their lung function is severely compromised. This is a case-by-case decision ideally made by an interdisciplinary team. Children with EOS may not have the diagnostic modalities to assess lung structure and function objectively in RLS. Fortunately, important information may be gained through history, physical examination, and growth trends alone that should assist with decisions regarding surgical treatment and long-term care.

REFERENCES

1. Jeans KA, Johnston CE, Stevens WR, et al. Exercise tolerance in children with early onset scoliosis: Growing rod treatment "graduates". *Spine Deform.* 2016;4(6):413–9.
2. Mayer OH, Redding G. Early changes in pulmonary function after vertical expandable prosthetic titanium rib insertion in children with thoracic insufficiency syndrome. *J Pediatr Orthop.* 2009;29(1):35–8.
3. Striegl A, Chen ML, Kifle Y, et al. Sleep-disordered breathing in children with thoracic insufficiency syndrome. *Pediatr Pulmonol.* 2010;45(5):469–74.
4. Willams BA, Matsumoto H, McCalla DJ, et al. Development and initial validation of the classification of early-onset scoliosis (C-EOS). *J Bone Joint Surg Am.* 2014;96(16):1359–67.
5. Mayer OH. Scoliosis and the impact in neuromuscular disease. *Paediatr Respir Rev.* 2015;16(1):35–42.
6. LoMauro A, Romei M, Gandossini S, et al. Evolution of respiratory function in Duchenne muscular dystrophy from childhood to adulthood. *Eur Respir J.* 2018;51(2):1701418.
7. James JI. Idiopathic scoliosis; the prognosis, diagnosis, and operative indications related to curve patterns and the age at onset. *J Bone Joint Surg Br.* 1954;36-B(1):36–49.
8. Motoyama EK, Deeney VF, Fine GF, et al. Effects of lung function of multiple expansion thoracoplasty in children with thoracic insufficiency syndrome: A longitudinal study. *Spine.* 2006;31(3):284–90.
9. Redding G, Mayer OH, White K, et al. Maximal respiratory muscle strength and vital capacity in children with early onset scoliosis. *Spine.* 2017;42(23):1799–804.
10. Borowitz D, Armstrong D, Cerny F. Relief of central airways obstruction following spinal release in a patient with idiopathic scoliosis. *Pediatr Pulmonol.* 2001;31(1):86–8.
11. Redding GJ, Kuo W, Swanson JO, et al. Upper thoracic shape in children with pectus excavatum: Impact on lung function. *Pediatr Pulmonol.* 2013;48(8):817–23.
12. McPhail GL, Boesch RP, Wood RE, et al. Obstructive lung disease is common in patients with syndromic and congenital scoliosis: A Preliminary Study. *J Pediatr Orthop.* 2013;33(8):781–5.
13. Redding GJ, Hurn H, White KK, et al. Persistence and progression of airway obstruction in children with early onset scoliosis. *J Pediatr Orthop.* 2020;Apr 3;40(4):190–195.
14. Dede O, Motoyama EK, Yang CI, et al. Pulmonary and radiographic outcomes of

VEPTR (vertical expandable prosthetic titanium rib) treatment in early-onset scoliosis. *JBJSAM*. 2014;96(15):1295–302.

15. Danielsson AJ, Ekerljung L, Hallerman KL. Pulmonary function in middle-aged patients with idiopathic scoliosis with onset before the age of 10 years. *Spine Deform*. 2015;3(5):451–61.

16. Fauroux B, Aubertin G. Measurement of maximal pressures and the sniff manoeuvre in children. *Paediatr Respir Rev*. 2007;8(1):90–3.

17. Fauroux B. Respiratory muscle testing in children. *Paediatr Respir Rev*. 2003;4(3):243–9.

18. MacKintosh EW, Ho M, White KK, et al. Referral indications and prevalence of sleep abnormalities in children with early onset scoliosis. *Spine Deform*. 2020;Feb 18:1–8.

19. Caubet JF, Emans JB, Smith JT, et al. Increased hemoglobin levels in patients with early onset scoliosis: Prevalence and effect of a treatment with vertical expandable prosthetic titanium rib (VEPTR). *Spine*. 2009;34(23):2534–6.

20. Yuan N, Skaggs DL, Davidson Ward SL, et al. Preoperative polysomnograms and infant pulmonary function tests do not predict prolonged postoperative mechanical ventilation in children following scoliosis repair. *Pediatr Pulmonol*. 2004;38(3):256–60.

21. Gadepalli SK, Hirschl RB, Tsai WC, et al. Vertical expandable prosthetic titanium rib device insertion: Does it improve pulmonary function? *J Pediatr Surg*. 2011;46(1):77–80.

22. Gauld LM, Kappers J, Carlin JB, et al. Prediction of childhood pulmonary function using ulna length. *Am J Respir Crit Care Med*. 2003;168(7):804–9.

23. Torres LA, Martinez FE, Manco JC. Correlation between standing height, sitting height, and arm span as an index of pulmonary function in 6–10-year-old children. *Pediatr Pulmonol*. 2003;36(3):202–8.

24. Zhang JG, Wang W, Qiu GX, et al. The role of preoperative pulmonary function tests in the surgical treatment of scoliosis. *Spine*. 2005;30(2):218–21.

6 Conservative Management of Early-Onset Scoliosis

Muhammad Tariq Sohail and Shahid Ali

CONTENTS

INTRODUCTION

Early-onset scoliosis (EOS) is defined as a spinal deformity occurring before the age of ten years [1] (see Figure 6.1). (EOS) is a complex and heterogeneous condition of significant diversity with respect to etiology, natural history, and management [2]. If left untreated or if surgery is performed too early, it can result in increased mortality and cardiopulmonary compromise [3, 4] The complexity and heterogeneous nature of EOS establishes the importance of understanding the growth of the spine and the etiology of EOS.

GROWTH OF SPINE

Truncal height will increase by 350% and weight twentyfold from birth to adulthood [8–11]. In addition to two-dimensional (2D) growth, volumetric growth occurs. At birth, the volume of the thorax is 6.7% of the final volume, and the volume of lumbar vertebrae will be multiplied by 6 from the age of 5 to skeletal maturity (Figure 6.2) [5].

Ossification of the vertebral bodies starts at the third month of intrauterine life. Three primary ossification centres are present within each vertebra, except for C1, C2, and the sacrum. Ossification first appears in the lower thoracic and upper lumbar spine and radiates from there in both cranial and caudal directions [6].

The skeleton has two rapid growth periods: from birth to 5 years and during puberty [7]. At birth, the standing height of the neonate is about 30% of the final height. The spine makes up to 60% of the sitting height, whereas the head represents 20%, and the pelvis the remaining 20% [7]. The length of the spine will nearly triple between birth and adulthood. The T1–S1 segment measures about 19 cm at birth, 28 cm at the age of 5 and 45 cm at skeletal maturity (Figure 6.2). This segment represents 49% of the sitting height and 64% of the length of the spine. During the first 5 years of life, its rate of growth is >2 cm per year, 0.9 cm between the ages of 5 and 10 years and 1.8 cm during puberty [6]. The thoracic spine (T1–T12) is about 11 cm long at birth, 18 cm at 5 years of age, and 22 cm at 10 years of age, and will reach a length of 28 cm in boys and 26 cm in girls at maturity [7].

The length of the thoracic spine is critical for normal lung development. The final length of the thoracic spine is closely related to the lung volume obtained at skeletal maturity [8]. If the

69

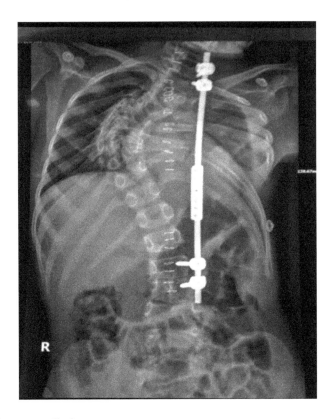

FIGURE 6.1   Early-onset scoliosis.

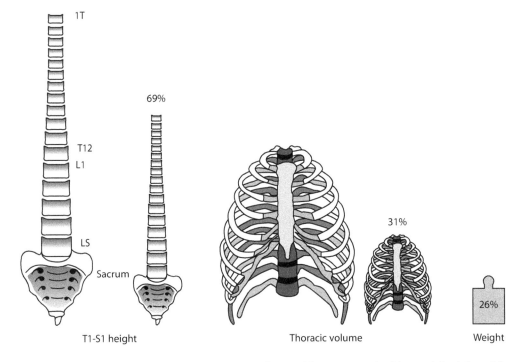

FIGURE 6.2   Relative size of thorax and spine in a 5-year-old as compared with an adult. Adapted from Helenius, I.J. (2011) 'Normal and abnormal growth of spine', with permission from Springer.

T1–T12 segment reaches the length of 18 cm (normal value at the age of 5 years) at maturity, a lung volume (vital capacity) of approximately 45% of normal is achieved, which is compatible with survival [5]. However, the T1–T12 segment should achieve the length of 22 cm (normal length at the age of 10 years) to obtain normal lung volume at maturity [8].

To address this heterogeneous and complex condition, a uniformly accepted classification has been proposed (Figure 6.3) [1]. This includes age, etiology (congenital, neuromuscular, syndromic, and idiopathic), major curve, kyphosis, and progression modifier.

Age-related classification by SRS (Scoliosis research society) differentiating scoliosis according to its age of onset and radiological classification:

- infantile (0–3 years; IIS)
- juvenile (3–10 years; JIS)
- adolescent (10–18 years; AIS)
- adult (>18 years)

Primary degenerative or 'de novo' scoliosis has to be differentiated

Age-related classification by Dickson:

- early onset (0–5 years)
- late onset (after 5 years of age)

The rationale behind this classification is that growth of the spine in the juvenile (ages 3–10 years) is rather steady and that the pulmonary maturity reached after 5 years of age exhibits fewer cardiopulmonary risks

Etiology-related classification:

Etiologies are listed in prioritised order from highest to lowest. When etiology is mixed and/or unclear, etiologic assignment should be made starting from the top of the list.

- **Congenital/Structural**: Curves developing because of a structural abnormality or asymmetry of the spine and/or thoracic cavity, e.g. hemivertebrae (Figure 6.4), fused ribs, post thoracotomy, thoracogonic, iatrogenic (postthoracotomy), tumor (pre- or postresection), amniotic band syndrome, hemihypertrophy, neurofibromatosis (NF) (dysplastic type), congenital diaphragmatic hernia, congenital heart defect, Proteus syndrome, Jeune's syndrome, Congenital chest wall deformity, Jarcho-Lovin syndrome, spondylothoracic dysplasia, spondylocostal dysplasia, and VATER/VACTERL.

- **Neuromuscular**: Curves without congenital or structural abnormalities in which the deformation is primarily attributable to a neuromuscular abnormality of high or low tone (Figure 6.5) e.g. flaccid spinal cord injury, spinal muscular atrophy, muscular dystrophy, spina bifida, low tone cerebral palsy (CP), Freidrich's ataxia, familial dysautonomia, syringomyelia, Charcot-Marie-Tooth disease, CHARGE syndrome, spastic CP, spastic spinal cord injury, and Rett syndrome.

- **Syndromic**: Syndromes with known or possible association with scoliosis that

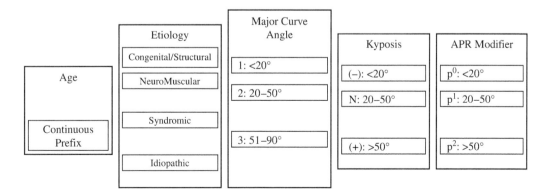

FIGURE 6.3 Classification of early-onset scoliosis (C-EOS)

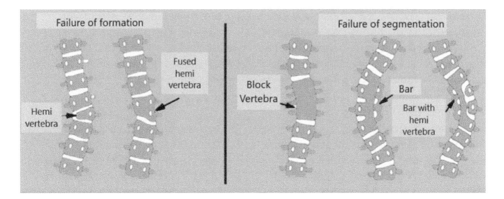

FIGURE 6.4   Congenital – Vertebrae develop incorrectly *in utero*. There is either failure of formation, failure of segmentation, or a combination of both. It is sometimes associated with cardiac and renal abnormalities. Evaluation may include studies of heart and kidneys.

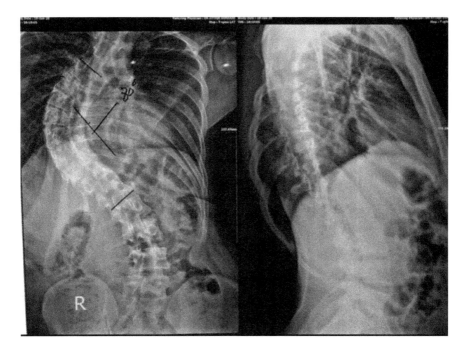

FIGURE 6.5   Neuromuscular – children with neuromuscular disorders, including spinal muscular atrophy, cerebral palsy, spina bifida and brain or spinal cord injury.

are not primarily related to congenital/ structural or neuromuscular etiology, e.g. spinal dysraphism, Ehlers-Danlos syndrome (and other connective tissue disorders), Prader-Willi syndrome, Marfan syndrome, achondroplasia, arthrogryposis, diastrophic dysplasia, Ellis Van Creveld syndrome, NF, osteogenesis imperfecta, spondyloepiphyseal dysplasia. Down's syndrome, Goldenhar syndrome, Klippel Feil syndrome.

- **Idiopathic**: No clear causal agent (can include children with a significant comorbidity that has no defined association with scoliosis).

All radiographic assessments should be posteroanterior and performed in the most gravity dependent position possible for the patient (i.e. standing preferred to sitting preferred to supine) **Major Curve**: Measurement of major spinal curve in the most gravity dependent position.

Kyphosis: Maximum measurable kyphosis between any two levels

Annual Progression Ratio (APR) Modifier (optional): Progression calculations should be made with two separate clinical evaluations at times t_1 and t_2 that are spaced a minimum of 6 months apart:

APR (Major Curve @ t_2) − (Major Curve @ t_1) × 12 months/[t_2_t_1]

INDICATIONS FOR INTERVENTIONS

EOS can be treated with serial casting, bracing, or surgery. Casting is indicated for progressive infantile scoliosis (diagnosed before the age of 3) [9], while surgery is typically recommended when the Cobb angle progresses beyond 50° for patients for whom conservative management has failed and progression has been documented [10–12]. Progressive and nonprogressive infantile scoliosis are typically differentiated mainly by using the rib-vertebra angle difference (RVAD) [12]. A RVAD of 20° or more is typical of progressive infantile scoliosis, while most resolving curves show a RVAD <20°. A definitive hallmark of progressive infantile scoliosis is the apical rib head in Phase 2. In this stage, the shadow of the head of the rib overlaps the corresponding vertebral body [9].

NONSURGICAL

Because of the high complication rate associated with surgical management of EOS and increasing evidence of successful treatment with early serial casting, nonsurgical management is becoming more common. Serial casting for infantile scoliosis may result in complete correction in some patients, but it also plays an important role in delaying the need for surgery in most patients. Nonsurgical treatment of progressive EOS includes bracing, casting, and halo-gravity traction (HGT) [13]. Mehta [9], recommended repeat radiographs after 3 months to evaluate the Cobb angle and RVAD in the setting of resolving or questionable spinal curves. At 3 months after the initial radiographs, the Cobb angle and RVAD of resolving curves had decreased in size [9].

BRACING

Although bracing is efficacious for adolescent idiopathic scoliosis [14], no studies have examined its efficacy for EOS. Nevertheless, it remains the most common nonsurgical treatment for EOS. However, successful management with this method has varied [15]. Brace fit is often difficult in young patients. Infants and toddlers typically have large abdomens, making a proper pelvic mould difficult, and their inability to hold still can make the lumbar and thoracic corrective moulding challenging. Young children also have more pliable ribs than adolescents, and braces using a three-point bend on the apical ribs can deform the chest wall by pushing the ribs toward the spine. Furthermore, the habitus in young children is typically more cylindrical in shape than in adolescents. This is compounded by the need to make the brace sufficiently flexible for donning and doffing. An experienced orthotist and a dedicated family that is educated in the principals of brace wear are required for proper bracing in young patients because each time the brace is worn, it must be put on in an ideal position. Proper bracing should focus on the rotation and three-dimensional (3D) deformity to maximise chest wall corrections rather than simply the Cobb angle. Although bracing is convenient because the brace can be removed for bathing and other activities, being removable precludes it from being a continuous corrective force. Moreover, because a brace functions predominantly to stabilise a deformity rather than reverse it, bracing is less likely than casting to permanently correct a deformity in a patient with EOS. Nevertheless, bracing plays an important role in delaying the need for surgery. With improved understanding of EOS pathophysiology and mechanics, more effective braces may be developed.

CASTING

Sayer [16] initially described casting for correction of scoliosis in 1877, but the early history of casting to treat scoliosis was really confined to correcting curves preoperatively and maintaining the correction postoperatively using the turnbuckle cast for uninstrumented fusions developed by Hibbs et al. [17]. Turnbuckle casting did not permit walking, and Risser [18] later developed 'localiser casting', which used a frame with a head halter and pelvic traction and 'localisers' that pushed on the curve for correction. Cotrel and Morel [19] further developed Risser's technique by identifying the key factors of traction, derotation, and bending with an ambulatory cast. They called the technique EDF casting for 'elongation (traction), derotation, and flexion (bending)' and suggested that serial EDF casting could correct infantile scoliosis. However, with the introduction of effective spinal instrumentation by Harrington [20], casting became a less popular method of managing adolescent scoliosis, and knowledge of the EDF casting technique persisted in only a few centres. Mehta [21] and Sanders et al. [22] reported on their experience using serial EDF casting for infantile scoliosis. Since the publication of these encouraging reports, there has been resurgent interest in serial EDF casting, particularly because of the challenges associated with growing instrumentation. EDF casting has now been successfully used in numerous centres. Compared with bracing, casting allows for improved fit and a constant corrective force. Patients with very large spinal curves may benefit from precast HGT, with the goal of delaying surgical intervention.

The EDF cast is applied with the child positioned on a table with a head halter and pelvic traction. The table must provide support for the child while ensuring that the thorax, shoulders, and pelvis are free for cast application and manipulation. Sufficient traction is applied to narrow the thorax and allow the spine to be manipulated. The table must allow secure positioning of the patient with head and pelvic traction, allowing full access to the torso, shoulder girdle, and pelvis (Figure 6.6) [22].

Manipulation rather than traction is the primary means of correction because traction will be removed after casting, and the patient's spine will recoil unless the cast includes the occiput and mandible. This recoil must be anticipated, or the cast may ride up. A silver-impregnated undergarment can be helpful in preventing cast irritation. Silver nanoparticles do, however, have the capacity to penetrate the skin, particularly when it is damaged, although the clinical effects of this are unknown [23]. Patients must be intubated during the cast moulding because thoracic pressure can make ventilation temporarily difficult.

Peak airway pressures can double during the procedure, and the anaesthesiologist should be prepared for this possibility. Peak airway pressures return to baseline after windows are cut in the cast [24]. For curves with an apex superior to T8, the shoulders are included in the cast, and high thoracic curves may require an occipital-mandibular extension. When the apex of the curve is at or inferior to T8, casting below the shoulders is an option. A mirror slanted under the table is useful for visualising rib prominence, the posterior cast, and the moulds. As the plaster is applied, it is important to obtain a good mould over the iliac crests because the pelvis is the foundation of the cast. A well-moulded and snug cast is less likely to rub and cause pressure sores than a cast that is excessively padded, poorly moulded, or loose. Plaster is preferred because it is very mouldable and expands slightly when setting, unlike fibreglass, which contracts.

The cast must not push the ribs toward the spine because that would narrow the space available for the lungs. Rather, the posteriorly rotated ribs are rotated anteriorly to create a more normal chest configuration, with counter rotation applied through the pelvic mould and upper torso (Figure 6.7) [22]. For a typical lower-left thoracic curve, the pelvis is carefully moulded and stabilised while the left posterior thorax is rotated anteriorly, and the right anterior thorax is rotated posteriorly and stabilised against the left pectoral girdle.

Two windows are made to improve the patient's respiratory capacity while preventing the lower ribs from rotating. An anterior window is made over the chest and abdomen to relieve the pressure on the chest and allow for abdominal distention and breathing because younger children are diaphragmatic (i.e., belly) breathers (Figure 6.8). A posterior window is made on the concave side of the cast, allowing the depressed, concave ribs and spine to move posteriorly (Figure 6.8).

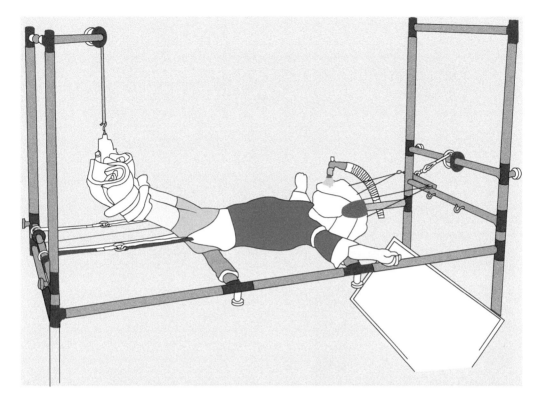

FIGURE 6.6 Illustration (A) and photograph (B) demonstrating patient positioning for elongation-derotation-flexion casting. The patient is positioned on a table with a head halter and pelvic traction. A mirror placed under the table can be used to visualise rib prominence as well as the posterior cast and the moulds.

For casts under the shoulders, the superior trim line is at the manubrium. This is not as important for casts that include the shoulders, as long as the upper thorax is casted. The lower trim should hold the pelvis securely while allowing the hips to flex >90°. Lack of hip flexion can cause the cast to ride up when the patient is sitting, particularly in car seats that require significant hip flexion.

Proper casting corrects the curve by rotating and shifting it toward the midline without pushing the ribs toward the spine. If the cast is pushing the ribs toward the spine and narrowing the convex side of the chest, we recommend removing the cast and either reapplying or abandoning it. Casts are changed every 2 to 4 months based on the child's growth. In select patients, typically those with supine curves of <20° or those with casts that are maintaining correction, we often use fibreglass with a waterproof liner and padding that allows patients to bathe and get into a swimming pool.

Casting is considered complete when the curve has resolved or the cast is obviously failing. We advise families that 1 year of casting is generally considered the minimum period of treatment. We consider a curve resolved when it measures ≤10° on standing radiographs after the cast is removed. In children with curves that have resolved, we use bracing for 1 year after the cast has been discontinued. We recommend continuation of casting for unresolved curves until the growth velocity has decreased, typically at age 4 or 5 years, and then using a brace for unresolved curves. If the curve is progressing, particularly if it is approaching 70°, we discuss the use of growing instrumentation with the family. Further reasons to discontinue casting include the ribs being pushed toward the spine on the convexity or continued curve progression despite casting. Other medical conditions, such as severe asthma, can make cast wear intolerable for patients and families.

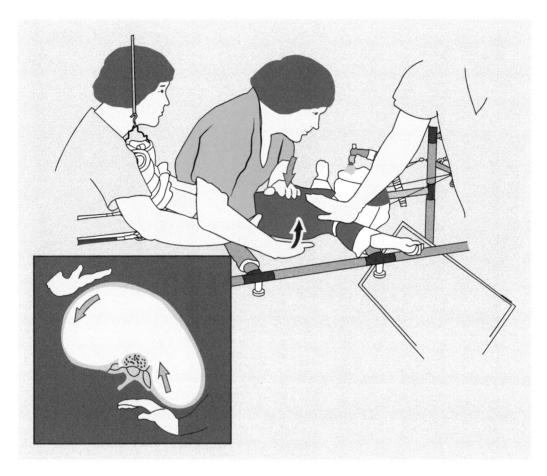

FIGURE 6.7 Illustration demonstrating the elongation-derotation-flexion casting technique. The posteriorly rotated ribs are rotated anteriorly (arrows) to create a more normal chest configuration, with counter rotation applied through the pelvic mould and upper torso. Inset, illustration demonstrating the location of force applied to the ribs. The goal is to derotate the spine toward normal.

COMPLICATIONS

Casting can cause skin breakdown although, in our experience, only minor skin irritation has occurred, and it has healed without further complications. The cast may need to be removed to manage other medical issues, such as viral respiratory illness, asthma exacerbation, and abdominal surgery, or if the cast becomes wet or soiled. The repeated use of anaesthetics for cast application may carry a risk of complications. In animal studies, neuron cell death associated with the repeated use of anaesthetics has been reported, but this has not been demonstrated in humans [25–27]. However, another study found that repeated use of anaesthetics

may be associated with learning delays in young children, although it is difficult to determine whether the delays are related to the etiologies that necessitate the repetitive use of anaesthetics [28].

There are several variable factors in casting, and the risk-benefit ratio for casting in certain patients is unclear. In patients with paralytic or neuromuscular scoliosis, such as those with spinal muscular atrophy or quadriplegic cerebral palsy, it is unclear whether the benefits of casting outweigh the risks of chest restriction in this population. Some patients with EOS have sleep apnoea, gastrostomy tubes, silent aspiration, and gastroesophageal reflux, which may be compounded by a cast. Furthermore, the

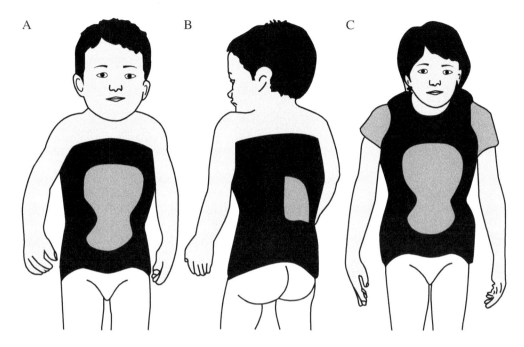

FIGURE 6.8 Photograph (A and C) of a child wearing an elongation-derotation-flexion cast, with an anterior window made to improve respiratory capacity. Photograph (B) posterior window on concave side allowing depressed, concave ribs and spine to move posteriorly.

psychological effect of casting in young children is unknown. Because the clinical presentation of these patients is highly variable, the goals and risks of casting must be balanced against the risks of early surgical management. Currently, many centres do not have the necessary equipment or education to successfully manage EOS with serial casting. Thus, it is rarely performed outside major academic centres [29].

RESULTS

In the landmark paper by Mehta [21], 136 children under the age of 4 with progressive infantile scoliosis (scoliosis diagnosed before the age of 3) were treated with casting. In 94 children with early referral (mean age 1 year 7 months) and with a mean Cobb angle of 32° (11°–65°), the scoliosis resolved by a mean age of 3.5 years. They needed no further treatment and went on to lead a normal life. In contrast, in 42 children with late referral (mean age 2.5 years) with a mean Cobb angle of 52° (23°–92°), casting could not reverse the deformity. In all, 15 of these children (36%) underwent spinal fusion.

CONCLUSION

It is very important to understand the disease etiology and its heterogeneity so that an appropriate management plan can be made. Conservative management is well established and produces very good outcomes if treatment is started at an appropriate age.

REFERENCES

1. Williams BA, Matsumoto H, McCalla DJ, et al. Development and initial validation of the classification of early-onset scoliosis (C-EOS). *J Bone Joint Surg Am.* 2014;96(16):1359–67.
2. Vitale MG, Trupia E. Classification of early-onset scoliosis. In: *The Growing Spine.* Springer; 2016:113–21.
3. Pehrsson K, Larsson S, Oden A, et al. Long-term follow-up of patients with untreated scoliosis. A study of mortality, causes of death, and symptoms. *Spine.* 1976;17(9):1091–6.
4. Karol LA, Johnston C, Mladenov K, et al. Pulmonary function following early thoracic fusion in non-neuromuscular scoliosis. *J Bone Joint Surg Am.* 2008;90(6):1272–81.
5. Helenius IJ. Treatment strategies for early-onset scoliosis. *EFORT Open Rev.* 2018;3(5):287–93.

6. Dimeglio A. Growth in pediatric orthopedics. In: Morrissy RT, Weinstein SL, eds. *Lovell and Winter's Pediatric Orthopaedics*. 6th ed. Philadelphia: Lippincott Williams & Wilkins; 2006:35–65.

7. Dimeglio A. Growth of the spine before age 5 years. *J Pediat Orthop B*. 1992;1(2):102–7.

8. Karol LA, Johnston C, Mladenov K, et al. Pulmonary function following early thoracic fusion in non-neuromuscular scoliosis. *JBJS*. 2008;90(6):1272–81.

9. Mehta M. The rib-vertebra angle in the early diagnosis between resolving and progressive infantile scoliosis. *J Bone Joint Surg Br*. 1972;54(2):230–43.

10. Akbarnia BA, Marks DS, Boachie-Adjei O, et al. Dual growing rod technique for the treatment of progressive early-onset scoliosis: A multicenter study. *Spine*. 1976;30(17 Suppl):46–57.

11. Akbarnia BA, Breakwell LM, Marks DS, et al. Dual growing rod technique followed for three to eleven years until final fusion: The effect of frequency of lengthening. *Spine*. 1976;33(9):984–90.

12. Akbarnia BA. Management themes in early onset scoliosis. *J Bone Joint Surg Am*. 2007;1:42–54.

13. Diedrich O, von Strempel A, Schloz M, et al. Long-term observation and management of resolving infantile idiopathic scoliosis a 25-year follow-up. *J Bone Joint Surg Br*. 2002;84(7):1030–5.

14. Weinstein SL, Dolan LA, Wright JG, et al. Effects of bracing in adolescents with idiopathic scoliosis. *N Engl J Med*. 2013;369(16):1512–21.

15. Emans JB. Orthotic management for infantile and juvenile scoliosis. In: *The Growing Spine*. Springer; 2011:365–81.

16. Sayre DLA. *Spinal Disease and Spinal Curvature, Their Treatment by Suspension and the Use of the Plaster of Paris Bandage, by Lewis A. Sayre*: Smith, Elder, and Company; 1877.

17. Hibbs RA, Risser JC, Ferguson AB. Scoliosis treated by the fusion operation an end-result study of three hundred and sixty cases. *JBJS*. 1931;13(1):91–104.

18. Risser JC. The application of body casts for the correction of scoliosis. *Instr Course Lect*. 1955;12:255–9.

19. Cotrel Y, Morel G. The elongation-derotation-flexion technic in the correction of scoliosis. *Rev Chir Orthop Reparatrice Appar Mot*. 1964;50:59–75.

20. Harrington PR. Treatment of scoliosis. Correction and internal fixation by spine instrumentation. *J Bone Joint Surg Am*. 1962:591–610.

21. Mehta MH. Growth as a corrective force in the early treatment of progressive infantile scoliosis. *J Bone Joint Surg Br*. 2005;87(9):1237–47.

22. Sanders JO, D'Astous J, Fitzgerald M, et al. Derotational casting for progressive infantile scoliosis. *J Pediatr Orthop*. 2009;29(6):581–7.

23. Larese FF, D'Agostin F, Crosera M, et al. Human skin penetration of silver nanoparticles through intact and damaged skin. *Toxicology*. 2009;255(1–2):33–7.

24. Jensen RD, Stasic AF, Kishan S, et al. Cardiorespiratory effects of derotational casting during anesthesia for children with early onset scoliosis. *Open J Anesthesiol*. 2014;2014:36–40.

25. Zhu C, Gao J, Karlsson N, et al. Isoflurane anesthesia induced persistent, progressive memory impairment, caused a loss of neural stem cells, and reduced neurogenesis in young, but not adult, rodents. *J Cereb Blood Flow Metab*. 2010;30(5):1017–30.

26. Ikonomidou C, Bosch F, Miksa M, et al. Blockade of NMDA receptors and apoptotic neurodegeneration in the developing brain. *Science*. 1999;283(5398):70–4.

27. Jevtovic-Todorovic V, Hartman RE, Izumi Y, et al. Early exposure to common anesthetic agents causes widespread neurodegeneration in the developing rat brain and persistent learning deficits. *J Neurosci*. 2003;23(3):876–82.

28. Wilder RT, Flick RP, Sprung J, et al. Early exposure to anesthesia and learning disabilities in a population-based birth cohort. *Anesthesiology*. 2009;110(4):796–804.

29. Fletcher ND, Larson AN, Richards BS, et al. Current treatment preferences for early onset scoliosis: A survey of POSNA members. *J Pediatr Orthop*. 2011;31(3):326–30.

7 Anaesthetic Management of Early-Onset Scoliosis

Damarla Haritha and Souvik Maitra

CONTENTS

INTRODUCTION

The vertebral column of human beings consists of natural bends along its course defined as curvatures. These can be either primary curvatures that are present since intrauterine development or secondary curves that develop after birth due to weight bearing. The primary curves are present in the thoracic and sacral regions, and the secondary curves in cervical and lumbar region develop as a result of head lifting and standing over course of time.

Scoliosis is the lateral and rotational deformity of the vertebral bodies, which causes the shift of the spines of vertebrae toward the concave side [1]. The bending of vertebral bodies toward one side leads to posterior shift of the ribcage on the convex side, forming a hump that deforms the chest wall. Moreover, there can be crowding of the ribs on the concave side and widening of the ribs on the convex side. With an overall incidence of 2%–3% in the general population, scoliosis poses a challenge to the anaesthesiologist as this chest wall deformity has serious consequences on the cardiorespiratory status of the patient [2].

CLASSIFICATION

The oldest and simple classification of scoliosis dates back to 1905, when Schulthess divided scoliosis based on the region of the abnormality as cervicothoracic, thoracic, thoracolumbar and lumbar [3]. But the classification given by the Terminology Committee of the Scoliosis Research Society (SRS) based on the aetiology is widely in use even at present (Table 7.1) [4].

TABLE 7.1

Classification of Scoliosis Based on Aetiology [4]

1. Congenital scoliosis	Associated with congenital abnormalities of the spinal cord and vertebrae such as spinal dysraphism, tethered cord, hemivertebrae, and rib anomalies
2. Idiopathic scoliosis a. Infantile (seen before 3 years of age) b. Juvenile (seen in 3–10 age group) c. Adolescent (seen after 10 years of age).	Most common type of scoliosis, adolescent variety being the most common of all. The aetiology is unknown, but various theories such as impaired ossification of the vertebrae and genetic component are suggested.
3. Associated with neuromuscular diseases	Seen in patients with cerebral palsy, poliomyelitis, Duchenne muscular dystrophy, and other myopathies
4. Associated with syndromes	Neurofibromatosis, Marfan syndrome, mucopolysaccharidoses, rheumatoid arthritis, and osteogenesis imperfecta.
5. Traumatic scoliosis	Associated with fractures, irradiation, burns, and surgery.
6. Neoplastic scoliosis	Associated with tumours of the vertebral column, nerve roots and spinal cord.

NOMENCLATURE AND GRADING OF SEVERITY

The scoliotic curves are generally named with the side facing the convexity as left-sided and right-sided curves. The left-sided curves are more frequently associated with congenital anomalies [2]. The most commonly used parameter for grading the severity is the Cobb angle [5]. It is measured by a plain radiograph of the spine, marking the most cephalic end of the curve and the caudal of the curve. A parallel line is drawn along the upper border of the most tilted upper vertebra and the lower border of the lower vertebra, and perpendiculars are dropped along these two parallel lines. The angle made by these two perpendicular lines is defined as the Cobb angle. A Cobb angle of less than 10° is considered normal. Curves less than 30° rarely progress over time, but the progression also depends on factors such as the age of onset of the deformity, the bone age, etc. A retrospective study by Yin et al. [6] reported that a Cobb angle >77° was associated with post-operative pulmonary complications. The main disadvantage of using Cobb angle is that it only quantifies the deformity in two-dimensions (2D) and does not give any information on the rotational deformity [7] and definition of end vertebra causes a source of error [8].

Systemic Effects of Scoliosis

1. **General Effects:** In a child with scoliosis, the typical presentation would be deformity of the back that manifests after the child starts walking [9]. The deformity can progress as the child grows, causing gross abnormality in the shape of the thorax and development of secondary curves in the other regions of the vertebral column. The child's functional capacity may be limited, including inability to play like the peers and frequent respiratory tract infections that can lead to frequent hospitalisations and malnourishment. In a child with syndromes such as neurofibromatosis, café au lait spots and axillary freckling is noticed, whereas tall stature and long limbs are noticed in a child with Marfan syndrome.

2. **Respiratory System:** The deformity of the chest wall leads to a restrictive kind of lung disease due to limitation of the movement of the rib cage upon inspiration and compression of the lung tissue; however mixed or obstructive lung disease may be present in 46% of the patients [10,11]. Altered respiratory mechanics and reduced lung volume leads to restrictive lung disease, and airway narrowing leads to obstructive lung diseases in some cases [12]. Total lung capacity (TLC) is reduced whereas residual volume (RV) usually remains within normal limit, hence RV/TLC ratio is increased [13]. The forced vital capacity (FVC)

and forced expiratory volume in the first-second (FEV1) both are reduced so that the ratio of FEV1 /FVC almost remains normal [14]. The reduction in the vital capacity represents the inability to cough and clear lung secretions effectively, leading to frequent lower respiratory tract infections [15]. The limitation of expansion of lung tissue leads to a decrease in respiratory compliance and, when combined with stretching of the intercostal muscles, leads to increase in work of breathing, resulting in decreased tidal volume and increased respiratory rate. The inspiratory capacity is maximally affected, while the functional residual capacity (FRC) is not that severely affected. In severe cases, as the curve progresses, an increase in residual volume may develop due to inadequate expiration as a result of muscle dysfunction.

The mechanical compression of the blood vessels in the lung and the ventilation perfusion mismatch in the lung causes chronic hypoxia, and it can lead to pulmonary hypertension and, ultimately, right ventricular dysfunction [16]. Diffusion limitation and alveolar hypoventilation can also contribute to hypoxaemia, especially in severe cases. With the deformity arising early in the life, there can be true pulmonary hypoplasia due to restriction of lung growth causing a decreased number of functional alveoli [13]. The alteration of lung volumes, frequent lower respiratory tract infections, and recurrent

aspirations due to bulbar dysfunction in patients with neuromuscular disease puts them at a more significant risk of respiratory complications in the perioperative period [17]. The severity of pulmonary compromise is generally found to correlate well with the Cobb angle in these patients and provide information on the postoperative risk stratification (Table 7.2) [18, 19].

3. **Cardiovascular System:** The hypoxia and pulmonary hypertension predisposes to right ventricular dysfunction. Diastolic dysfunction was also found to be associated with higher Cobb angle in thoracic scoliosis patients [20]. The increased work of breathing and hypoxia, coupled with baseline anaemia, which is often found in developing nations because of malnutrition, will cause resting tachycardia in these patients. Patients with idiopathic scoliosis have associated mitral valve prolapse and the congenital anomalies in patients with associated syndromes further complicate clinical management [21].

4. **Nervous System:** In a patient with syndromes, there can be gross mental retardation further leading to difficulty in communication and preoperative respiratory training. In a patient with congenital scoliosis, there can be spina bifida or meningomyelocele, leading to bladder and bowel involvement. Even in a child with idiopathic scoliosis, the progression of the deformity can cause compression of the nerve roots, causing

---

TABLE 7.2
Correlation of Cobb Angle and Respiratory System Involvement [3]

Cobb Angle	Suspected Involvement
1. >25°	Increased pulmonary artery pressures measured in echocardiography
2. >65°	Restrictive lung disease in pulmonary function tests (PFT)
3. >75°	Pulmonary hypertension on exercise
4. >100°	Symptomatic lung disease
5. >110°	Pulmonary hypertension at rest
6. >120°	Alveolar hypoventilation

reduction in sensation, parasthesia, and weakness of the lower limb.

5. **Musculoskeletal System:** In patients with congenital myopathies, there can be weakness of the muscles in general and bulbar involvement that leads to frequent aspirations, complicating the perioperative course. Duchenne muscular dystrophy is an X-linked recessive disorder caused by a defect in the gene coding 'dystrophin', a muscle protein [22]. The patient will be restricted to a wheelchair by 8–10 years of age, and the expected life span is 15–16 years. It is associated with cardiomyopathy and fatal arrhythmias. The corrective scoliosis surgery helps to improve nursing and quality of life in such patients and should be done at a lower Cobb angle to prevent progression of the curve and appearance of cardiomyopathy [23].

6. **Airway:** Difficulty in securing airway can be anticipated in patients with syndromes due to deformity of the face and upper airway. Distortion of the trachea and glottis can be seen in patients with deformities of the cervical spine [24]. Patients of Marfan syndrome can have a high arched palate, and patients with Duchenne muscular dystrophy can have hypertrophy of the tongue posing difficulty in securing airway [23].

PREOPERATIVE INVESTIGATIONS

Surgical treatment is indicated when the Cobb angle becomes more than 40° despite nonsurgical treatment [23]. It is indicated much earlier when the Cobb angle becomes more than 20° in a patient with Duchenne muscular dystrophy [23].

The severity of the patient's cardiorespiratory system involvement and other associated conditions must be assessed before the surgery. The various investigations necessary include:

1. **Blood investigations:** A hemogram is necessary to find out the baseline haemoglobin concentration of the patient and prepare the patient optimally for surgery. Room air arterial blood gas analysis is needed in patients with suspected respiratory failure or the room air plethysmography shows a peripheral saturation of less than 95%.

2. **Radiological investigations:** A chest x-ray will help in assessing the Cobb angle and any active infection of the lung. It is also an invaluable tool to assess for any distortion of the tracheobronchial tree, which can make positioning of the endotracheal tube difficult.

3. **Others:** An ECG will be helpful in suspected right ventricular failure due to pulmonary hypertension and shows right axis deviation, right ventricular hypertrophy indicated by R/S >1 in V_1 and right ventricular strain pattern with ST segment and T wave inversion in V_1 to V_3. Pulmonary function testing documents the baseline restriction of the lung volumes and helps to predict possible postoperative intensive care or mechanical ventilation requirements. 2D echocardiography may show the pulmonary hypertension due to chronic hypoxia but also rules out any congenital cardiac anomalies and establishes the ventricular function.

PREOPERATIVE OPTIMISATION

Reported incidence of postoperative complications after scoliosis surgery varies widely and largely depends upon the definition of complications used. In general, neuromuscular scoliosis is associated with the highest rate of complications followed by congenial scoliosis [25]. A large database review of more than 36,000 patients reported that 7.6% patients fulfiled the criteria of at least one in-hospital complication. Respiratory failure was the most common complication followed by reintubation and implant related complications [26]. Adequate optimisation of the patient will lead to uneventful surgery and early recovery of the patient. Ideally, the anaesthesiologist will assess the patient well in advance to identify other comorbidities, anomalies, syndromes, or any other cardiorespiratory disease, such as pneumonia, that should be treated before the surgery. In addition, the nutritional status of the patient should be built up by haematinics to improve the haemoglobin. Incentive spirometry and inspiratory muscle training might be useful in preventing postoperative pulmonary complications [27]. However, these modalities have not been specifically evaluated in patients undergoing scoliosis surgery for prevention of respiratory complications.

Identification of risk factors such as age, duration of surgery, a Cobb angle >77 associated with postoperative pulmonary complications (POPC) [28,29]. The various predictors for postoperative mechanical ventilation are mentioned in Table 7.3.

Adequate preoperative optimisation and preparation of the patients help to reduce complications and as does preparing well in advance for the postoperative care of the patient and optimal utilisation of resources.

INTRAOPERATIVE CONCERNS

The various intraoperative concerns for anaesthesiologists include prolonged surgery, blood loss, hypothermia, spinal cord monitoring, prone positioning, difficulty in access to the patient, etc. General anaesthesia, with or without neuraxial analgesia, is the anaesthetic technique of choice. Anaesthesia is induced intravenously with a fast-acting opioid, propofol and an intermediate-acting muscle relaxant such as atracurium or vecuronium. Appropriate assistance for difficult airways should be prepared in the operation theatre in anticipated cases and the use of succinylcholine should be avoided for patients with muscular disorders to prevent life-threatening hyperkalaemia and arrhythmias [30]. Apart from the American Society of Anaesthesiologists' standard monitoring such as ECG, noninvasive blood pressure, pulse oximetry, and capnography, additionally invasive blood pressure, central venous pressure, urine output, temperature, depth of anaesthesia monitoring (e.g. bispectral index), and spinal cord monitoring are usually required in major deformity correction cases. Placement of invasive lines such as central venous catheter can be difficult in patients with stiff deformity involving the cervical vertebra. It helps in monitoring the central venous pressure, though they are not reliable in prone position, and also for multiple drug infusions. Invasive arterial line is required for beat-to-beat blood pressure measurement and also for blood gas analysis. Maintenance of anaesthesia is usually performed by total intravenous anaesthesia (TIVA) technique by propofol infusion with a fast-acting opioid. Remifentanil is the opioid of choice for TIVA. Standard target-controlled infusion (TCI) models available include the Marsch and Schnider model for propofol and the Minto model for remifentanil [31]. The Marsch model requires the patient's total body weight to calculate the dose infused, whereas the Schnider model uses age, height, and lean body mass [32]. The plasma concentration of propofol for loss of consciousness in a patient that was not premedicated is 5–6mcg/mL and a concentration of 1–2 mcg/mL will awaken the patients from anaesthesia [32].

SPINAL CORD MONITORING

The anaesthesia technique as a whole revolves around spinal cord monitoring used in the intraoperative period to assess the integrity of the dorsal and ventral columns of the spinal cord. Previously, subjective tests such as the wake-up test and clonus test were used, but now, when

---

TABLE 7.3

Predictors of Postoperative Mechanical Ventilation

    a. Anterior spinal surgery [3]

    b. Preoperative FVC <50% predicted [3]

    c. Preoperative FEV1 <50% predicted [3]

    d. Maximum inspiratory pressure of less than 40 cm H_2O [3]

    e. Blood loss more than 30ml/kg [3]

    f. Pre-existing neuromuscular disorders, congenital heart disease, right ventricular failure [3]

    g. Cephalad location of the curve [3]

available at the facility, they have been replaced by more objective ways of measurement such as somatosensory-evoked potentials (SSEP) and motor-evoked potentials (MEP).

WAKE-UP TEST

The wake-up test includes waking up the patient during the surgery and observing the movement of lower limb fingers upon instruction. The patient must be counselled in the preoperative period itself and ensured that there will not be pain and he or she will not remember the procedure. The anaesthesiologist has to be notified at least 15 minutes before the wake-up test so that the muscle relaxant can be timed, inhalational agents discontinued, and haemodynamics ensured. The main disadvantages of this test included the inability to monitor at critical steps such as screw placement, the subjective nature of the test, and the risk of violent movements, disconnections of invasive lines, accidental extubation, etc. This has been replaced with more objective and sophisticated means of monitoring the integrity of columns of spinal cord such as evoked potentials. Evoked potentials are the discharges that are collected from a specific area after stimulating some other point.

SOMATOSENSORY EVOKED POTENTIAL

As the name suggests, this involves stimulating a peripheral nerve with surface electrodes and recording the evoked potentials from the sensory cortex through scalp electrodes. The process is continued throughout the surgery and the amplitude and latency of the wave form is compared with the baseline. The most common nerves used for monitoring are posterior tibial nerve, peroneal nerve, and median nerve. The decrease in amplitude of more than 50% and increase in latency by 10% is considered significant [3]. Various anaesthetic agents interfere in the recording of SSEP, and the anaesthesiologist must optimally maintain anaesthesia with other agents. The effect of anaesthetic agents on SSEP is represented in Table 7.4.

Muscle relaxants decrease the background noise in SSEP and helps in monitoring [23]. The other factors effecting SSEP include the

TABLE 7.4
Effect of Anaesthetic Agents on SSEP [23]

Anaesthetic Agent	Amplitude	Latency
Inhalational agents	Decrease	Increase
Nitrous oxide	Decrease	No effect
Propofol	No effect	No effect
Thiopentone	Decrease	Increase
Ketamine	Increase	No effect
Etomidate	Increase	No effect
Opioids	No effect	No effect
Dexmedetomidine	No effect	No effect

temperature, mean arterial blood pressure, PO_2, PCO_2, and haemoglobin concentration. The combination of opioid, muscle relaxant, and a sub MAC doses of inhalational agent or propofol infusion is considered optimal for SSEP monitoring [5]. The main advantage of SSEP is that there is no patient movement expected, the surgeon need not stop operating at critical steps; however, the inability to monitor motor tracts and the longer latency outweighs its benefits.

MOTOR EVOKED POTENTIALS

MEP is the compound muscle action potential (CMAP) recorded in various muscle groups after stimulating motor cortex through scalp electrodes. The muscle groups above the level of correction are considered the control group and are compared with the muscle groups below the level of correction and also with their corresponding baseline values. All anaesthetic agents that effect SSEP also effect MEP in a similar manner, but MEP are also affected with muscle relaxant [3]. A physiological and pharmacological steady state must be maintained during MEP monitoring [3]. A combination of a short-acting opioid and propofol total intravenous anaesthesia (TIVA) without muscle relaxant is considered optimal for MEP monitoring. The advantage with MEP monitoring is that it measures the integrity of motor tracts, and the latency is minimal [23]. The main disadvantage being movement of the patient every time the stimulus is given, leading to tongue lacerations, change in position of the patient causing compression of vital structures, such as the eyes, and damage to endotracheal tube. So, the position of the patient must be examined after each stimulus and a bite block has to be introduced before prone position to prevent injuries to tongue and damage to endotracheal tube.

PRONE POSITIONING

After intubation and the invasive lines have been secured, the patient must be positioned in the prone position for the surgery (Figure 7.1). The process of shifting a patient from supine to prone position is a complex procedure and requires knowledge of the appropriate technique. The equipment required for supporting the patient in the prone position must be in the operation theatre, and the anaesthesiologist is in charge of the head end of the patient, airway, invasive lines, and coordinating the shifting. The monitors and invasive lines are to be disconnected sequentially, the last being the circuit, and it must be reattached as soon as the patient is shifted. The position of the endotracheal tube must be checked again, and all the pressure points padded. Care should be ensured that there is no pressure on the eyes and the abdomen is free from compression and eyes must be padded (Figure 7.2). The compression of the abdomen can cause rise in intraabdominal pressure and thereby epidural pressure causing excessive bleeding during the surgery [33].

The position of the head and eyes should be checked every time the patient moves. Excessive abduction of the arms, flexion or extension of the neck should be avoided to avoid compression of the brachial plexus and compression of

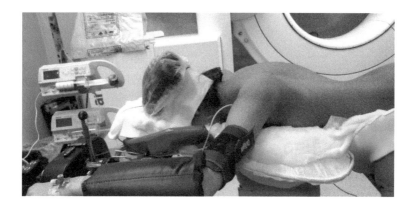

FIGURE 7.1 Optimum prone positioning for scoliosis surgery.

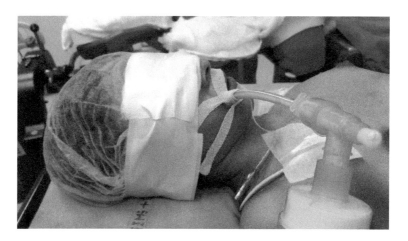

FIGURE 7.2 Eye protection by padding.

the jugular veins [33]. Severe haemodynamic consequences are not generally expected unless there is severe compression of the abdomen and there by inferior vena cava [33]. A slight head-up position prevents congestion of the conjunctiva in a prolonged surgery [33].

HYPOTHERMIA

Hypothermia is anticipated, as it is a prolonged surgery and most of the body is exposed for surgery. The measures to reduce hypothermia should start before the prone position itself. The fluids must be warmed and a forced air warmer can be used at the lower limbs to prevent hypothermia. The lack of access to the patient in a very small child makes this much more challenging, and children are more susceptible to hypothermia. Hypothermia prolongs the metabolism of anaesthetic agents and causes delayed awakening, effects intraoperative spinal cord monitoring, and causes platelet dysfunction and, thereby, excessive bleeding [34].

BLOOD CONSERVATION STRATEGIES

Blood loss is anticipated in the deformity correction, as it involves removal of the posterior elements of the vertebral column, which is a cancellous bone and very vascular. The 24-hour anticipated blood loss is about 200mL per segment operated [23]. The preoperative anaemia, limited ability to increase cardiac output in a stressful situation, and pulmonary hypertension in unison puts the patient at risk of haemodynamic compromise in case of bleeding. Therefore, blood loss should be anticipated and treated appropriately to prevent undue complications. The various blood conservation strategies that can be used and a brief explanation of their advantages and disadvantages are as follows.

1. **Nutrition and haematinics:** This technique requires assessment of the child well in advance of the surgery to build up the haemoglobin by starting on oral iron therapy. It is the most physiological way of increasing the haemoglobin of the child. Preoperative haematinics and erythropoietin have been shown to reduce perioperative transfusion requirements when combined with other interventions such as antifibrinolytics, cell salvage, and moderate hypotension [35,36]. The inability to utilise in case of acute haemorrhage and reduced compliance of oral iron in children are disadvantages for this method.

2. **Preoperative autologous donation (PAD):** A certain amount of blood is collected from the patient at regular intervals in the preoperative period and stored in the blood bank for later use. A reduction of allogeneic blood transfusion has been reported in patients who underwent preoperative autologous transfusion and has been studied along with other interventions such as antifibrinolytics and cell salvage [37,38]. This prevents use of allogenous blood in case of haemorrhage intraoperative haemorrhage, The main disadvantage is the difficulty in collecting blood from a small child in the preoperative period and its hemodynamic consequences.

3. **Acute normovolemic haemodilution (ANH):** This technique involves removing a calculated amount of blood from the patient immediately before the surgery and replacing the amount with crystalloids in a ratio of 3:1 or colloids in a ratio of 1:1. There is controversial evidence suggesting a reduction in allogenic blood transfusion with ANH alone [39,40,41]. This can cause haemodynamic disturbance during removal of blood and also reduce tolerability to intraoperative blood loss. ANH has also been shown to cause exponential reduction in the haemoglobin after bleeding but also lesser haemoglobin drop in the postoperative period after autotransfusion in patients undergoing scoliosis correction [39].

4. **Antifibrinolytic agents:** Infusion of antifibrinolytic agents such as tranexamic acid or epsilon amino caproic acid is postulated to decrease blood loss. Tranexamic acid has been studied extensively for reduction in transfusion requirements in not only

scoliosis correction but also in obstetrics, cardiac, neurosurgery, and urology [42]. The efficacy of tranexamic acid is postulated to be dose specific. Several dosing regimens such as high dose regimen (50mg/kg loading dose followed by 5mg/kg/hr) and low dose (10mg/kg followed by 1mg/kg) were compared with controversial results [43,44,45,46]. In most of the studies, the high dose regimen reduced blood loss and transfusion requirements more than low dose regimen [42]. Side effects, such as seizures and allergic reactions, limit the usage of high dose regimen. The optimal dose of tranexamic acid is yet to be determined [42].

5. **Infiltration of site with local anaesthetic and adrenaline**
6. **Preventing pressure over the abdomen to decrease epidural venous congestion**
7. **Hypotensive anaesthesia:** This method, also referred to as controlled hypotension, includes deliberate reduction of the mean arterial blood pressure with various anaesthetic drugs such as epidural, inhalational agents, intravenous infusions, and nonanaesthetic drugs including clonidine, nitroglycerine, nicardipine, esmolol, and labetalol. However, hypotension makes the patient more susceptible to haemodynamic instability in case of any sudden, severe haemorrhage and also puts the patient at risk of ischemic damage to various vital organ beds [46]. Throughout the literature, the goal mean arterial pressure to maintain the perfusion of spinal cord varies between 80mmHg to 90 mmHg without any strong evidence [47]. But selecting the same threshold for every patient goes against individual variability among the population and is not recommended [48]. The anaesthesiologist has to monitor invasive blood pressure and individualise the blood pressure goals according to the patient profile and intraoperative events.

8. **Cell Salvage:** This is a process of collecting the blood from the surgical field through a separate suction, removing the debris, washing the red blood cells and centrifuging them and mixing with an anticoagulant, such as heparin, and transfusing it to the patient. Avoiding exposure to allogenous blood and preventing waste are the advantages, but the requirement of a specialised apparatus, perfusionist, and concern with respect to red cell damage, oxygen carrying capability, hyperkalaemia, and coagulopathy due to heparin are the disadvantages.

SPINAL CORD PROTECTION

The anterior one third of the spinal cord is supplied by a single anterior spinal artery originating from vertebral artery and the posterior two third is supplied by two posterior spinal arteries originating from posterior inferior cerebellar artery [49]. Segmental arteries originating from the ascending cervical artery, posterior intercoastal arteries, and the lumbar arteries that join these spinal arteries form a plexus of vessels around the spinal cord. In the setting of hypoperfusion, the most prone area for ischaemia is the watershed zone at the T4 to T7 level, which is sparsely perfused [50]. The damage to the spinal cord depends on the length of the procedure, stretching of the nerve roots leading to reduced blood supply, systemic hypotension, direct contusion of the cord, blood loss, etc. This can be prevented by real-time monitoring of spinal cord perfusion with SSEP or MEP. As soon as any change in the evoked potentials is noted, the surgeon and anaesthesiologist should be alerted immediately. Any inhalational agent should be discontinued, and hypothermia, anaemia, and hypotension should be treated appropriately. Failure to improve the evoked potential should alert the surgeon to either remove the screw or decrease the traction. Treatment with methylprednisolone 30mg/kg bolus followed by 5.4 mg/kg infusion for 23 hours given within 8 hours of insult has been shown to improve neurological outcomes in patients with traumatic spinal cord injury but not specifically in scoliosis surgery [51].

ANALGESIA

Intraoperative dissection of bone and periosteum mandates appropriate analgesia in these patients. Multimodal analgesia regimens such as paracetamol, infusion of opioid, and dexmedetomidine are most widely practised. Nonsteroidal anti-inflammatory drugs (NSAIDS) are generally avoided in orthopaedic procedures, as there are concerns regarding delayed union and malunion. The prostaglandin pathway, which is inhibited by NSAIDS, is also responsible for expression of osteoprotegerin, a protein that helps in bone healing [52]. A meta-analysis concludes that there is strong evidence associating delayed union and malunion with NSAID exposure but it may be dependent even on dose and duration of exposure [52]. Intrathecal morphine administered by the surgeon at the end of surgery has been found to be associated with lower postoperative opioid consumption and improved pain control [53, 54]. However, a retrospective study reported that incidence of inadvertent dural tear was also increased without an increase in surgical site infection [55]. It should be remembered that, during intrathecal opioid administration, local anaesthetic has to be avoided to prevent interference in spinal cord monitoring.

The decision regarding extubation and the postoperative intensive care unit stay is made depending on the preoperative comorbidities, optimisation, degree of respiratory failure, intraoperative blood loss, haemodynamics and complications. There is a general trend toward extubation on table, which helps in early assessment of patient's motor and sensory response and recovery as a whole.

POSTOPERATIVE CONCERNS

The postoperative course is as important as preoperative optimisation in a patient with scoliosis because it takes time for the lung volumes and capacities to improve after surgery. There is a significant variation in the literature regarding this aspect. Various studies reported that the pulmonary function test (PFT) parameters improve after surgery [56, 57, 58, 59, 60], though few concluded that lung volumes decrease after surgery [61, 62], and a few reported that there is no change in the lung volumes after the correction [63, 64]. However, the surgical approach and the duration of evaluation after surgery will change the PFT parameters. Open anterior approach, requiring disruption of rib cage, injury to the respiratory muscles and pleural adhesions in the postoperative period, may prevent optimal change in lung volumes [65]. In the immediate postoperative period after posterior instrumentation, it studies have shown that the lung volumes actually decrease on Day 1, reach a plateau at Day 3, and reach baseline values 2 to 3 months after surgery [31]. This, along with the major fluid shifts, blood loss, and pain, makes the patient more at risk of postoperative pulmonary complications. The other anticipated complications are postoperative ileus due to prolonged infusion of opioids for analgesia, worsening of the neurological status, postoperative visual loss, nerve compression injuries due to intraoperative malpositioning and worsening of bulbar symptoms in a patient with previous history. Other rare complications such as pneumothorax, air embolism in prone position, and superior mesenteric artery syndrome due to compression of superior mesenteric artery between the third part of the duodenum and aorta during correction of severe deformities, and syndrome of inappropriate antidiuretic hormone release (SIADH) due to handling of the nerve tissue [23]. The postoperative care centres on chest physiotherapy, adequate analgesia, careful neurological monitoring, and early ambulation.

A patient with scoliosis posted for surgeries other than deformity correction also poses a significant challenge to the anaesthesiologist. The techniques of anaesthesia, spinal cord monitoring, analgesia, and preoperative assessment have evolved over time and led to a reduction in the complication rate and better outcomes for these patients. This is not only because of the advanced equipment available, but also thorough understanding of the physiology by both the surgeons and anaesthesiologists. The success of the surgery stems from teamwork and depends on communication between the members of the team.

CONCLUSION

Perioperative management of scoliosis patients undergoing deformity correction is always a challenge. Preoperative risk stratification, optimisation, and an anaesthetic protocol targeting optimum haemodynamics without hampering neurological monitoring is the key to the successful outcome in these patients.

REFERENCES

1. Horlocker TT, Wedel DJ. Anesthesia for orthopedic surgery, Chapter 40. In: *Clinical Anesthesia*, Barash PG, Cullen BF, Stoelting RK, eds. 5th edition. Lippincott Williams and Wilkins; Philadelphia, 2005.
2. Kynes MJ, Evans FM. Surgical correction of scoliosis, anaesthetic considerations. *ATOTW*. 10th July 2015;318.
3. Kulkarni AH, Ambareesha M. Scoliosis and anaesthetic considerations. *Indian J Anaesth*. 2007;51(6):486–95.
4. Goldstein LA, Waugh TR. Classification and terminology of scoliosis. *Clin Orthop*. 1973;93(93):10–22.
5. Cobb JR. Outline for the Study of Scoliosis. *Am Acad Orthop Surg Instr Course: Lect*. 1948;5:261–75.
6. Yin S, Tao H, Du H, et al. Postoperative pulmonary complications following posterior spinal instrumentation and fusion for congenital scoliosis. *PLOS ONE*. 2018;13(11):e0207657.
7. Kim H, Kim HS, Moon ES, et al. Scoliosis imaging: What radiologists should know. *RadioGraphics*. 2010;30(7):1823–42.
8. Gstoettner M, Sekyra K, Walochnik N, et al. Inter- and intraobserver reliability assessment of the Cobb angle: Manual versus digital measurement tools. *Eur Spine J*. 2007;16(10):1587–92.
9. Janicki JA, Alman B. Scoliosis: Review of diagnosis and treatment. *Paediatr Child Health*. 2007;12(9):771–6.
10. Farrell J, Garrido E. Effect of idiopathic thoracic scoliosis on the tracheobronchial tree. *BMJ Open Respir Res*. 2018;5(1):e000264.
11. Boyer J, Amin N, Taddonio R, et al. Evidence of airway obstruction in children with idiopathic scoliosis. *Chest*. 1996;109(6):1532–5.
12. Farrell J, Garrido E. Effect of idiopathic thoracic scoliosis on the tracheobronchial tree. *BMJ Open Respir Res*. 2018;5(1):1–8.
13. Tsiligiannis T, Grivas T. Pulmonary function in children with idiopathic scoliosis. *Scoliosis*. 2012;7(1):7.
14. Praud Jaen-Paul CE. *Chest Wall Function and Dysfunction. Kendig's Disorders of the Respiratory Tract in Children*. Edited by Chernick V, Boat TF, Wilmott RW, Bush A. Philadelphia: Saunders Elsevier; 2006:733–46.
15. Kozak OS, Eelco FMW. *Clinical Evaluation of Neuromuscular Respiratory Failure, Critical Care Medicine*. 3rd edition. 2008.
16. Li S, Yang J, Li Y, et al. Right ventricular function impaired in children and adolescents with severe idiopathic scoliosis. *Scoliosis*. 2013;8(1):1.
17. Matsumoto M, Miyagi M, Saito W, et al. Perioperative complications in posterior spinal fusion surgery for neuromuscular scoliosis. *Spine Surg Relat Res*. 2018;2(4):278–82.
18. Johari J, Sharifudin MA, Ab Rahman A, et al. Relationship between pulmonary function and degree of spinal deformity, location of apical vertebrae and age among adolescent idiopathic scoliosis patients. *Singapore Med J*. 2016;57(1):33–8.
19. Kang GR, Suh SW, Lee IO. Preoperative predictors of postoperative pulmonary complications in neuromuscular scoliosis. *J Orthop Sci*. 2011;16(2):139–47.
20. Huh S, Eun LY, Kim NK, et al. Cardiopulmonary function and scoliosis severity in idiopathic scoliosis children. *Korean J Pediatr*. 2015;58(6):218–23.
21. Dhuper S, Ehlers KH, Fatica NS, et al. Incidence and risk factors for mitral valve prolapse in severe adolescent idiopathic scoliosis. *Pediatr Cardiol*. 1997;18(6):425–8.
22. Bhutia MP, Pandia MP, Rai A. Anaesthetic management of a case of Duchenne muscle dystrophy with Moyamoya disease. *Indian J Anaesth*. 2014;58(2):219–21.
23. Gibson PRJ. Anaesthesia for correction of scoliosis in children. *Anaesth Intensive Care*. 2004;32(4):548–59.
24. Ma LL, Yu XR, Zhu B, et al. Difficult airway for patients undergoing spine surgeries. *Chin Med J (Engl)*. 2016 20;129(6):749–50.
25. Reames DL, Smith JS, Fu KM, et al. Scoliosis research society morbidity and mortality committee. Complications in the surgical treatment of 19,360 cases of pediatric scoliosis: A review of the scoliosis research society morbidity and mortality database. *Spine*. 2011;36(18):1484–91.
26. De la Garza Ramos R, Goodwin CR, Abu-Bonsrah N, et al. Patient and operative factors associated with complications following adolescent idiopathic scoliosis surgery: An analysis of 36,335 patients from the Nationwide Inpatient Sample. *J Neurosurg Pediatr*. 2016;25(6):730–6.
27. *Cochrane Database Syst Rev*. 2014;2:CD006058./*Cochrane Database Syst Rev*. 2015;10:CD010356.
28. Yin S, Tao H, Du H, et al. Postoperative pulmonary complications following posterior spinal

instrumentation and fusion for congenital scoliosis. *PLOS ONE*. 2018;13(11):e0207657.

29. Wu L, Zhang XN, Wang YS, et al. Risk factors for pulmonary complications after posterior spinal instrumentation and fusion in the treatment of congenital scoliosis: A case-control study. *BMC Musculoskelet Disord*. 2019;20(1):331.

30. Marsh S, Ross N, Pittard A. Neuromuscular disorders and anaesthesia. Part 1: General anaesthetic management. doi:10.1093/bjaceaccp/mkr020.

31. Yuan N, Fraire JA, Margetis MM, et al. The effect of scoliosis surgery on lung function in the immediate postoperative period. *SPINE*. 30(9):2182–5.

32. Al Rafai Z, Mulvey D. Principles of total intravenous anaesthesia: Practical aspects of using total intravenous anaesthesia. *BJA Educ*. 2016;16(8):276–80. doi: 10.1093/bjaed/mkv074

33. Edgcombe H, Carter K, Yarrow S. Anaesthesia in prone position. *Br J Anaesth*. 2008;100(2):165–83.

34. McSwain JR, Yared M, Doty JW. Perioperative hypothermia: Causes, consequences and treatment. *World J Anesthesiol*. 2015;4(3):58–65.

35. Dick AG, Pinder JP, Lyle SA, et al. Reducing allogenic blood transfusion in pediatric scoliosis surgery: Reporting 15 years of multidisciplinary, evidence-based quality improvement project. *Glob Spine J*. 2019;9(8):843–9.

36. Hassan H, Halasnki M, Wincek J, et al. Blood management in pediatric spinal deformity surgery: Review of a 2 year experience. *Transfusion*. 2011;51(10):2133–44.

37. Peters A, Verma K, Diefenbach C, et al. Preoperative autologous blood donation does not affect pre-incision hematocrit in AIS patients. A retrospective cohort of a prospective randomized trial. *Spine J*. 2013;13(9):S110–1.

38. Kelly MP, Zebala LP, Kim HJ, et al. Effectiveness of preoperative autologous blood donation for protection against allogeneic blood exposure in adult spinal deformity surgeries: A propensity-matched cohort analysis. *J Neurosurg Spine*. 2016;24(1):124–30.

39. Hasan MS, Choe NC, Chan CY, et al. Effect of intraoperative autologous transfusion techniques on perioperative hemoglobin level in idiopathic scoliosis patients undergoing posterior spinal fusion: A prospective randomized trial. *J Orthop Surg*. 2017;25(2):2309499017718951.

40. Batista MF, Costa CO, Vialle EN, et al. Acute normovolemic hemodilution in spinal deformity surgery. *Rev Bras Ortop*. 2019;54(5):516–23.

41. Epstein NE. Bloodless spinal surgery: A review of the normovolemic hemodilution technique. *Surg Neurol*. 2008;70(6):614–8.

42. Johnson DJ, Johnson CC, Goobie SM, et al. High-dose versus low-dose tranexamic acid to reduce transfusion requirements in pediatric scoliosis surgery. *J Pediatr Orthop*. 2017;37(8):e552–7.

43. Grant JA, Howard J, Luntley J, et al. Perioperative blood transfusion requirements in pediatric scoliosis surgery: Efficacy of tranexamic acid. *J Pediatr Orthop*. 2009;29(3):300–4.

44. Neilipovitz DT, Murto K, Hall L, et al. A randomized trial of tranexamic acid to reduce blood transfusion for scoliosis surgery. *Anesth Analg*. 2001;93(1):82–7.

45. Sethna NF, Zurakowski D, Brustowicz RM, et al. Tranexamic acid reduces intraoperative blood loss in pediatric patients undergoing scoliosis surgery. *Anesthesiology*. 2005;102(4):727–32.

46. Dutton RP. Controlled hypotension for spinal surgery. *Eur Spine J*. 2004;13(Suppl. 1):S66–71.

47. Sadeh YS, Smith BW, Joseph JR, et al. The impact of blood pressure management after spinal cord injury: A systematic review of literature. *Neurosurg Focus*. 2017;43(5):E20.

48. Li G, Lin L, Xiao J, et al. Intraoperative physiological ranges associated with improved outcomes after major spine surgery: An observational study. *BMJ Open*. 2019;9(5):e025337. doi: 10.1136/bmjopen-2018-025337

49. Alexandre Campos Moraes A, Stolf NAG. Anatomy of spinal blood supply. *J Vasc Bras*. 2015;14(3):248–52.

50. Hoehmann CL, Hitscherich K, Cuoco JA. The artery of Adamkiewicz: Vascular anatomy, clinical significance and surgical considerations. *J Cardiovasc Res*. 2016;5:6.

51. Bracken MB. Steroids for acute spinal cord injury. *Cochrane Database Syst Rev*. 2012;1:Art no: CD001046.

52. Wheatley BM, Nappo KE, Christensen DL, et al. Effect of NSAIDs on bone healing rates. *J Am Acad Orthop Surg*. 2018;1. doi: 10.5435/jaaos-d-17-00727

53. Boezaart AP, Eksteen JA, Spuy GV, et al. Intrathecal morphine. Double-blind evaluation of optimal dosage for analgesia after major lumbar spinal surgery. *Spine*. 1999;24(11):1131–7.

54. Pendi A, Acosta FL, Tuchman A, et al. Intrathecal morphine in spine surgery: A meta-analysis of randomized controlled trials. *Spine*. 2017;42(12):E740–7.

55. Pendi A, Lee YP, Farhan SAB, et al. Complications associated with intrathecal

morphine in spine surgery: A retrospective study. *J Spine Surg.* 2018;4(2):287–94.

56. Kinnear WJ, Johnston ID. Does Harrington instrumentation improve pulmonary function in adolescents with idiopathic scoliosis? A meta-analysis. *Spine.* 1993;18(11):1556–9.

57. Kumano K, Tsuyama N. Pulmonary function before and after surgical correction of scoliosis. *J Bone Joint Surg Am.* 1982;64(2):242–8.

58. Lenke LG, Bridwell KH, Baldus C, et al. Analysis of pulmonary function and axis rotation in adolescent and young adult idiopathic scoliosis patients treated with Cotrel-Dubousset instrumentation. *J Spinal Dis.* 1992;5(4):16–25.

59. Lindh M, Bjure J. Lung volumes in scoliosis before and after correction by the Harrington instrumentation method. *Acta Orthop Scand.* 1975;46(6):934–48.

60. Pehrsson K, Danielsson A, Nachemson A. Pulmonary function in adolescent idiopathic scoliosis: A 25 year follow up after surgery or start of brace treatment. *Thorax.* 2001;56(5):388–93.

61. Vedantam R, Lenke LG, Bridwell KH, et al. A prospective evaluation of pulmonary function in patients with adolescent idiopathic scoliosis relative to the surgical approach used for spinal arthrodesis. *Spine.* 2000;25(1):82–90.

62. Lenke LG, Bridwell KH, Blanke K, et al. Analysis of pulmonary function and chest cage dimension changes after thoracoplasty in idiopathic scoliosis. *Spine.* 1995;20(12):1343–50.

63. Shneerson JM, Edgar MA. Cardiac and respiratory function before and after spinal arthrodesis in adolescent idiopathic scoliosis. *Thorax.* 1979;34(5):658–61.

64. Lamarre A, Hall JE, Weng TR, et al. Pulmonary function in scoliosis one year after surgical correction [Abstract]. *Proceedings of the Scoliosis Research Society. J Bone Joint Surg Am.* 1971;53:195.

65. Kim YJ, Lenke LG, Bridwell KH, et al. Pulmonary function in adolescent idiopathic scoliosis relative to the surgical procedure. *JBJS.* 2005;87(7):1534–41.

8a Biomechanics of Surgical Intervention Associated with Early-Onset Scoliosis

Aakash Agarwal

CONTENTS

INTRODUCTION

There exists an understanding of how a scoliotic curve progresses with time, but the main biological catalysts that initiate, progress, or halt the curve are uncertain. Therefore, the biomechanics of surgical intervention relies solely on our mechanistic understanding of the progression of a growing curve. To understand the biomechanics of surgical intervention, it helps to bear in mind the complex three-dimensional (3D) nature of spinal curvature and possible mechanisms of its initiation and progression [1]. Scoliosis appears to develop in two stages: curve initiation and subsequent progression [2].

INITIATION

According to the Hueter–Volkmann principle, the strain rate of axial growth in long bones, including vertebral bodies at the period of skeletal immaturity, is retarded by mechanical compression on growth plates. The opposite is true when tension is applied, i.e. accelerated strain rate of axial growth. Because of the physiologic curvature in the normal thoracic spine, compressive forces are delivered on the ventrally located part of the vertebral column, whereas distractive forces are delivered on the dorsally located part. The process that leads to abnormal spinal curvature is thought to be initiated by the rotation of the vertebral bodies in the axial plane, which causes discrepant axial loading between the ventrally and dorsally located portions of the involved vertebrae. Over time, this discrepancy manifests as a change in the directionality of spinal curvatures, i.e. the ventrally located part of the vertebral column becomes the convex side and the dorsally located part becomes the concave side leading to the onset of scoliosis [3–5]. It still remains unclear what leads to such instability. A 70% confluence rate among identical twins for the presence of scoliosis makes a direct genetic relationship difficult to establish. Therefore, there must be factors that work together or in place of each other resulting in different outcomes [6, 7]. From a biomechanical standpoint, an upright spinal column with curvatures is exposed to shear forces in multiple planes, which may contribute to the rotational instability from which scoliosis originates [8, 9]. Nevertheless, a number of factors also suggest the major role of spinal growth mechanisms in the occurrence of scoliosis. Besides the velocity and age of growth, there could also exist a fault in the symmetry of growth in the neurocentral Schmorl cartilage [6, 10]. As scoliosis is related to the onset of puberty, scoliosis might be the visible aspect of a metabolic or endocrinal disease accounting for a specific morphotype. Observation of sporadic cases of scoliosis development during growth hormone treatment has led to consideration of the possible role of the growth hormone in the process. That said, no anomaly in growth hormone blood concentration has been reported in scoliosis patients. Low bone mineral density in young female scoliosis patients suggests that estrogen disorders may engender osteopenia, which would account for a particularly high susceptibility to deformation of the bone matrix. Despite all these theories, one of the main difficulties encountered in this area of research consists in determining whether all these observed anomalies are the causes or concurrences of scoliosis. For example, any modification of the volume, activity, and nature of the spinal muscles observed in the convexity of the scoliosis is subject to the same question as to whether the symptoms should be considered as causes or a parallel observation.

PROGRESSION

After a critical degree of curvature has developed, a vicious mechanical cycle drives the progression of scoliosis, which accelerates during periods of rapid spinal growth. Therefore, the effects of both time and 3D structural distortions must be considered during the management of scoliosis. Biomechanical curve progression parallels spinal growth. Hence, irrespective of type, scoliosis mainly progresses only during growth and ceases when skeletal maturity is reached, provided that the final curvature is not severe. The rates of spine-related symptoms and

mortality among patients who have a curve with a Cobb angle of less than 50° are similar to those among patients without scoliosis; by contrast, patients who have a curve with a Cobb angle of more than 50° have higher rates of back pain and mortality associated with cardiopulmonary complications [11]. The progression of idiopathic scoliosis after skeletal maturity depends on the severity of curvature. If the Cobb angle is less than 30° after the cessation of skeletal growth, the scoliotic curve tends not to progress, regardless of the pattern of curvature. Curves with a Cobb angle of 30°–50° at skeletal maturity progress 10°–15° during a normal lifetime, whereas curves with a Cobb angle of 50°–75° at skeletal maturity progress at a rate of 1° per year. The frequency of curve progression differs according to the cause and type of scoliosis. Congenital scoliosis progresses in 75% of cases. Among patients with idiopathic scoliosis, progression is most common in the juvenile group (70%–95% of patients) [12]. Adolescent idiopathic scoliosis also progresses less often than juvenile idiopathic scoliosis and congenital scoliosis. Only 5% of adolescent patients with idiopathic scoliosis experience curve progression beyond a Cobb angle of 30°. The factors that have the greatest effect on the probability of progression of adolescent idiopathic scoliosis are spinal growth velocity and magnitude of the curve at initial presentation [13]. Because growth velocity is the main factor that affects curve progression, accurate estimation of the growth phases is important for managing scoliosis [14].

CORRECTION STRATEGIES

For curves in the range of 20°-40°, bracing can be an effective means of controlling some forms of early-onset scoliosis (EOS), such as idiopathic scoliosis and some syndromic forms of the condition; however, bracing is not appropriate for neuromuscular or congenital scoliosis. Most braces, a plaster or foam copy of the patient's body fitted by straps to the patient, could help prevent scoliosis from rapidly worsening in a patient [15]. At best, it could avoid surgery and, at worst, it could delay surgery; however, compliance to wearing the brace on a permanent basis is necessary to achieve satisfactory results. Bracing works via application of multidirectional pressure (rotational and lateral) on the spine-rib-pelvic complex using multiple pads aimed at halting or slowing the progression of deformity. In contrast, body casts are not removable. It is done in series of up to five or more in infantile idiopathic scoliosis cases to increase the amount of correction, and at an interval of 8 weeks to 24 weeks, depending upon the changes observed in the curve [16, 17]. Casting could correct or delay surgery in appropriate patients and is usually more effective than bracing. Currently many researchers and entrepreneurs are focussed on the concept of dynamic bracing. If this research translates from bench to bedside, it could change the landscape of the conservative treatment modalities. Such bracing would rely on an electronic feedback loop and use pressure sensors to monitor and change the corrective forces, thus actively limiting the progression of scoliosis. However, the reality today is that most progressing curves eventually undergo surgical intervention. The objectives of surgical correction strategies include 1) growth sustenance and 2) limiting the extent of deformity.

STANDALONE SURGICAL PHILOSOPHIES

Distraction-based growth rods have been the mainstay of surgical intervention in EOS for more than a decade [18]. The concept uses distraction to create additional soft-tissue space in-between the vertebrae for the bone to later grow into. Its universal application was thrusted through the use of traditional growth rods which required repeated invasive surgeries every 6–12 months for the sustenance of growth via distraction. There are many problems with traditional growth rods, but the most obvious problem is that it requires repeated surgeries. The trauma of repeated surgery is a nightmare for both the patients and the surgeons, from increased complications with each subsequent surgery to infections and unplanned surgeries [19]. This limitation in the surgical technique led to the invention of MAGEC (MAGnetic Expansion Control, Nuvasive) rods [20]. The main benefit of the MAGEC rod is that it allows for a noninvasive mode of distraction in the growth rods. This benefit is theoretically realised by a drastic reduction in the number of consecutive

surgeries. Despite this transition in technology, the majority of surgeries performed in countries with limited resources relies on the use of traditional growth rods. This is in part due to the very high initial cost associated with the use of MAGEC rods in such countries [21]. The section below delves further into the modes of failure associated with these two devices and how to reduce such adverse events.

Guided-growth techniques are the second most common surgical intervention [22, 23]. This relies on axial stabilisation of the spine with natural allowance for growth. The most well-known technique, SHILLA, falls under this category. The SHILLA technique could be performed both using rods and SHILLA screws (Medtronic), however, in the absence of SHILLA screws, this technique can be performed using a sliding rod-dominos construct.

And the third most common technique in scoliosis intervention is compression-based vertebral modulation. This technique employs the Hueter–Volkmann principle through mechanical compression on the convex sides of the growth plates, thus allowing a higher relative growth rate at the concave side to reduce wedging. This has traditionally been thought to be applied via anterior-body tethering (a flexible cord that is under tension to compress the convex side) or staples [24–26]. Although earlier intervention is necessary to achieve success in such cases. This is because the technique only halts the potential leftover growth on the convex end of the curve, thereby relying on the passive correction mode via normal growth on the contralateral sides, i.e. the concave side to achieve long-term correction.

BIOMECHANICS OF FAILURE MODES

Rod Fracture and Screw Loosening with Distraction-Based System

Rod fracture is a common complication among all the long and rigid constructs used in the management of scoliosis and has been highlighted in several studies [27, 28]. It is known that the risk of rod fracture increases with single rods, stainless steel rods and smaller diameter rods [29]. The same study also found that rod fracture was more prevalent among patients with preoperative ability of ambulation. However, rod fracture has also been reported in nonambulatory patients. The mean time reported for rod fracture was 25 ± 21 months and the mean time after distraction (for distraction-based systems) was 5.8 ± 3 months. Hence fracture could occur at any time [29]. Furthermore, a retrieval analysis study performed by the U.S. Food and Drug Administration (FDA) on failed growth rods revealed that these rods fracture only at specific sites on the rods. They concluded that the posterior surface of the rod is the fracture initiation point, with mid-construct, adjacent to distal connector, and adjacent to tandem connector as the common fracture sites [30]. The fatigue strength of most medical grade metals, e.g. 510 MPa at 10 million cycle of medical grade titanium alloy (Ti6Al4V) is high enough to withstand a juvenile patient's upper body weight and muscle forces; however, the innate fatigue strength reduces drastically if there are notches on the rods [31]. Therefore, these fractures could easily be accelerated by surgical (contouring, notching, etc.) or patient (traumatic and sudden exposure to uncommon physical undertakings, accidents, etc.) specific variables that are unrelated to the construct's geometry and may not typically occur under normal circumstances [32]. Nevertheless, lowering the stresses on the rods will help in reducing the occurrence of failure, especially in distraction-based systems. Distraction-based systems have an added disadvantage of residual distraction stresses when considering the fatigue life of its construct in human body. Using representative biomechanical models (**Figure 8a.1**), optimised for lowest distraction forces and sustained growth, it was found that forces greater than 100N on the concave side and 75 N on the convex side resulted in unnecessary growth at the expense of increased complication, i.e. higher stresses on the rod [33–35]. Long-standing clinical literature suggests that distraction forces stimulate apophyseal growth of the axial skeleton compared to normal growth rate [36, 37]. Based on the Hueter–Volkmann principle, this could occur only by applying a higher distraction force than physiologically necessary. This mechanism was simulated in the biomechanical models using representative scoliotic spines corroborating the trends similar to what was observed in previous clinical studies [20, 37, 38].

With traditional dual growth rods, changing the frequency of distraction is not an option, but, with the use of MAGEC, it is feasible. Multiple representative biomechanical models have been simulated to look at the frequency of distraction of growth rods and its effect on the stresses generated on growth rods over a period of 2 years. The stresses on the rod for the duration of 24 months decreased with an increase in frequency of rod distraction. The shorter distraction period may not be required in all patients, but it may prove tremendously helpful for patients with stiffer spines or patients who need higher magnitude of distraction to improve lung function (by stimulation of growth). Biomechanical data have shown that frequent distractions would require smaller distraction forces and thus will induce

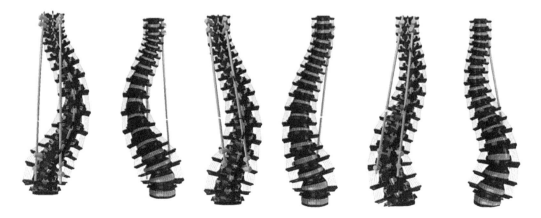

FIGURE 8A.1   Few of the representative biomechanical models that previously simulated the distraction forces and frequency associated with distraction-based surgical intervention [34].

lower stresses in the rods [31, 33–35]. It is crucial to apply these risk-mitigation strategies in clinical practise. A significant amount of information has been obtained from previous biomechanical studies on lowering the incidence of growth rod fracture. As with all surgical procedures, patient selection is an important factor that affects the efficacy of any risk-mitigation technique. A distraction frequency that is ideal for one patient may not be suitable for another. Therefore, previous study has used a graphical representation, based on variances in spinal stiffnesses among different patients instead of a single number representing an ideal distraction frequency [39]. It is conferred that the distraction frequency and distraction forces are integrated, i.e. for every distraction frequency there is an optimal distraction force. Therefore, reducing the distraction interval with the aim of reducing the propensity of rod fracture also requires a reduction in the distraction force. This concept has been previously misunderstood, and clinicians solely relied on changes in distraction frequency without changing the amount of distraction force (**Figure 8a.2**) [40]. Therefore, it is of paramount importance that clinicians understand the mechanical reasons behind such concepts. Theoretically, the distraction force of approximately zero magnitude would ideally mean a growth rod technology in which the growth rod is able to sense the change in compressive stresses and undergoes automated lengthening as a negative feedback

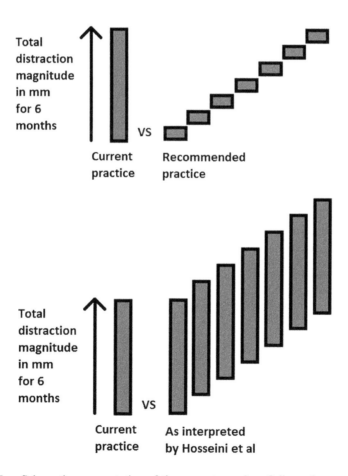

FIGURE 8A.2 *Top:* Schematic representation of the current practise of distraction vs the recommended practise from Agarwal et al., through their findings [31, 33–35, 39]. In this example, the current practise shows one distraction in 6 months, while the recommended practise shows seven smaller distractions in 6 months, hence the term smaller distraction intervals. *Bottom:* Schematic representation of the current practise vs. Hosseini et al. interpretation of our work. and the comparison made in their published article [40].

mechanism. In absence of such a technology, we need to apply as small an increment of distraction as possible to sustain height at equivalently smaller intervals of time. For example, 1.5 mm–2.0 mm every month, instead of 4.5 mm–6.0 mm every 3 months.

Screw loosening is one of the other common complications that is often clinically observed [41, 42]. The concept of reducing stresses on the rod via smaller increments of distraction at smaller intervals of time has been tested in both using biomechanical models and *in vitro* settings. The pull-out forces increased significantly with lower distraction forces at frequent intervals. The pull-out results of *in vitro* studies have also corroborated the significance of the reduction of high loads at screw-bone interface by using smaller distraction forces at smaller intervals as a method to lower the incidence of screw loosening [34].

AUTOFUSION AND LAW OF DIMINISHING RETURNS WITH DISTRACTION-BASED SYSTEM

Previous clinical studies have characterised the distraction forces and lengths observed during distraction episodes in EOS patients implanted with growth rods [43, 44]. The studies showed a law of diminishing return, i.e. the distraction forces increased, whereas the distraction amount decreased with consecutive distraction episodes (**Figure 8a.3**). Cumulatively, the distraction force increased by an amount of 268%, with 120% increase in the early stages (distraction episodes 1–6) and 68% increase in the later stages (distraction episodes 6–11), whereas the cumulative decrease in the length over 11 distraction episodes was 47%, with 34% and 20% in the early and later stages, respectively. Furthermore, in the late stages of distractions (6–11), the trend did not result in significant differences between each consecutive episode for both the distraction force and the length [44]. The reason for this could be multifold. It could either be because of a decrease in the sample size, hence an increase in variance, a plateau in the growth velocity, a sustained distraction-trauma causing the stiffness of the spine to plateau, or a combination of thereof. The phenomenon of increased spinal stiffness could be a result of several factors: reduction in laxity of the soft tissues due to damages incurred at every

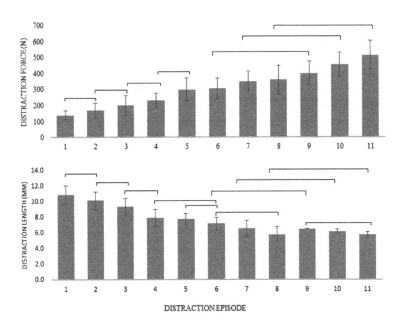

FIGURE 8A.3 *Top:* Distraction forces at each distraction episode. The error bar represents two SDs, the 95% confidence interval. *Bottom:* Distraction length at each distraction episode. The error bar represents two SDs, the 95% confidence interval. The brackets represent a p value of <0.05, i.e. significant difference existed between consecutive episodes [44].

distraction, development of fusion mass due to exposure, or a reduction in motion [45, 46]. The qualitative element of this has been highlighted previously by demonstrating mitigation of auto-fusion due to 'smaller' but frequent distraction [47]. Therefore, to date, the most accepted reasoning for this phenomenon is the trauma caused to the soft tissues due to excessive distraction forces, which, in turn, leads to reduced flexibility via fibrogenesis or osteogenic response. This adds to the benefits of using smaller distractions at smaller intervals, as recommended in the previous section for reducing rod fracture and screw loosening. However, the term 'smaller distraction' is just a qualitative nomenclature in a clinical setting for lower distraction forces in the absence of a clinically available force measuring devices. As patient's curve stiffness, weight, etc. vary, so will the forces (and stresses) generated in them with the same distraction length (applied through MAGEC rods). This implies that for a very stiff curve, autofusion, rod fracture, etc. may still occur despite frequent supposedly 'smaller' distractions (generating high forces and stresses because of the high stiffness of the curve). In this regard (to assess the stiffness of a scoliotic curve), it is important to use gravity-based techniques in which the patient lies sideways with a fulcrum at the apex instead of taking x-rays while the patient stands and bends to the side to assess curve-flexibility (and thus determining the frequency of distraction). The standing side-bend technique does not provide the correct flexibility of the curve because of nonspecific bending moments, which varies from patient to patient. Furthermore, it would be a major technological advancement if MAGEC or some other technology can measure the distraction forces during the distraction episodes.

Failure to Lengthen MAGEC Rods

The main benefit of MAGEC rod's main benefit is that it allows for the noninvasive distraction of the growth rods. However, the failure of this attribute, i.e. the noninvasive distraction mechanism, reduces the overall efficacy of the device with newer studies even questioning if there is a real quality-of-life difference with use of MAGEC rods [48]. It was recently shown that the most frequent clinical problem associated

with the MAGEC rod is the failure of noninvasive distraction mechanism, which leads to invasive revision surgeries required to replace the device [49]. These results also highlight the exponential increase in such failure rates (**Figure 8a.4**). Furthermore, the 'Manufacturer and User Facility Device Experience' (MAUDE) record on the top five failure modes associated with standard instrumentation usage in spinal fusion proves that such failures are substantially underreported [49]. Studies continue to suggest a growing number of distraction mechanism failures associated with MAGEC rods [50]. Better technical and clinical controls need to be set in place to avoid such adverse events, which leads to unplanned open surgeries. A higher distraction magnitude results in the generation of higher distraction forces, and this, in combination with off-axis loading (exemplified by 'growth marks'), result in wear and breakage of the MAGEC rod's components. Therefore, one hypothesised method to reduce the propensity of such failures would be to apply minimum distraction at higher frequency, as described in previous sections. This would also reduce tissue trauma and its effects, such as autofusion [31, 34, 40, 43, 44, 47].

Wear and Metallosis in MAGEC and Guided-Growth Techniques

Most cases of metallosis have been observed during necessary procedures for other clinical reasons. The voluntary nature of such reporting also presents a challenge against excluding infrequently reported complications, such as necrosis, which although is present in all cases (off-axis loading and wear), has only been reported 10 times in total [49]. A previous study concluded that 91% of the MAGEC rods showed measurable wear of the extending bar toward the magnet end [50]. This is similar to the result of other studies where MAGEC presented with metallosis, pseudo-capsule surrounding the actuator, and abrasive circumferential markings around the rod [51]. They also showed a significant amount of metal debris when the actuators were carefully cut open. Analytical studies demonstrated metal fragments of predominantly titanium with a mean particle size of 3.36 microns. Similarly, during revisional

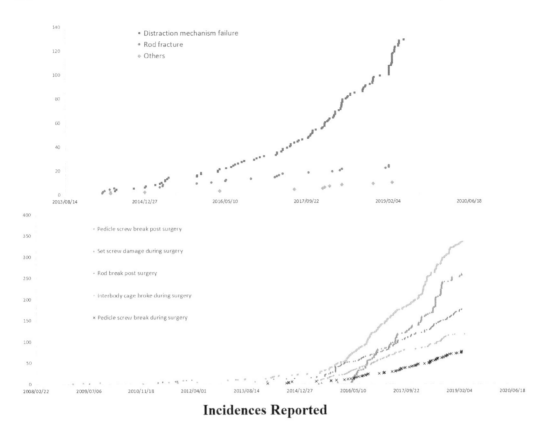

Incidences Reported

FIGURE 8A.4 *Top:* Adverse event reporting from MAUDE database for MAGEC rod usage up till June 2019. *Bottom:* Adverse event reporting from MAUDE database for top five failure modes associated with standard instrumentation usage in spinal fusion up till June 2019 [49].

surgery with guided-growth systems, signs of implant wear and metallosis were observed at the location of the unconstrained interfaces [52]. In sum, the histological evaluation confirmed chronic inflammation with encapsulated foreign body granules. Although not much research has been done on reducing metallosis, few technical controls, such as ceramic coating at wear-generating surfaces, has been suggested [49].

CRANKSHAFTING, ADDING-ON, AND DISTAL MIGRATION WITH GUIDED-GROWTH TECHNIQUES

A factor that contributes to curve progression is called crankshaft phenomenon. This can develop in skeletally immature children after spinal fusion as a result of continued spinal growth with increased axial rotation of the fixed spine. The clinical evidence of crankshaft phenomenon is often subtle, whereas the

radiographic findings are considered more apparent [53, 54]. However more recent studies with longer follow-up time presents another curve evolution theory after SHILLA implantation. Results suggest that the apex of the fused primary curve shifts in approximately 62% of patients, with nearly all of these (92%) involving a distal migration. Overall, these findings represent adding on or distal migration of the apex after a guided-growth technique rather than a crankshaft phenomenon about the apex [55].

HYBRID SURGICAL PHILOSOPHY

The failure of most of these standalone techniques has shown that the concept of 'one size fits all' is not applicable for the surgical management of EOS. Therefore, newer concepts employing two or more of the above philosophies, i.e. various combinations of distraction-based, guided-growth, and compression-based

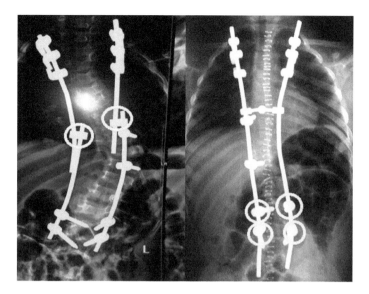

FIGURE 8A.5 Radiograph of two patients exemplifying the two types of, but analogous, modified SHILLA procedure. Left: the modified SHILLA approach using dominos (4.5 mm rod in 5.5 mm domino hole) for sliding with growth. Right: the modified SHILLA approach using pedicle screw-rod clearance for sliding with growth. Yellow circles identify the sliding units of this SHILLA construct for sustenance of overall longitudinal growth of the spine until puberty.

approaches might be more suitable and, biomechanically speaking, a more optimal surgical intervention. One such combination currently used for surgery includes active apex correction (APC), **Figure 8a.5** [56, 57]. It is a hybrid of guided-growth and compression-based management of deformity. The technique simply consists of replacing the apical fusion (of traditional SHILLA) with unilateral compression (via pedicle screws or any other means) on the convex side. This compression is meant to halt the growth on the convex side and thus allow the ratio of concave-to-convex height to increase overtime, thus reducing the vertebral wedging at the apex of the curve. Biomechanically it allows for an active compression-based intervention at the apex of the curve, alongside passively restrained guided-growth height allowance of the entire scoliotic curvature. The result of clinical studies on this technique provides evidence of reverse vertebral modulation at the apex of the curve in patients with scoliosis and kyphoscoliosis when modifying the traditional SHILLA technique with APC [56]. Furthermore, when comparing the correction parameters and height gain between APC and long-established traditional growth rod systems, the two techniques

did not show any clinically significant distinction at their current follow-up period [57]. Nevertheless, the latter presented an obvious disadvantage because it required multiple surgeries to regularly distract the spine. Another example of such a combination is a hybrid of guided-growth and distraction-based system, called the spring distraction system [58]. It is similar to passively restrained guided-growth technique, however, it replaces the apical fusion with an energised mechanical spring to add an active component driving the growth in a singular direction (along the height). This energised spring provides a low distraction force, which further continues to reduce with spinal growth (**Figure 8a.6**). Both of these techniques rely on a single surgery, and the short-term results are encouraging. Long-term follow-up will be necessary to establish these as biomechanically superior techniques.

CONCLUSION

Progression of an EOS curve is inevitable in cases in which the device undergoes breakage due to fatigue or trauma. Alternatively, curves have also progressed (for example in

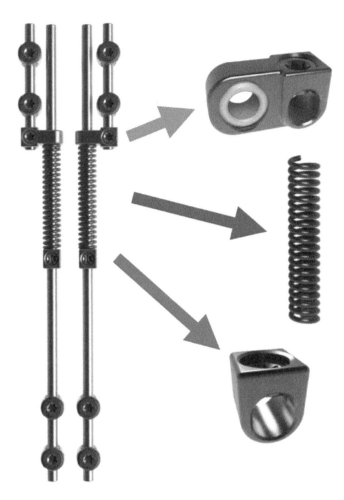

FIGURE 8A.6 Spring distraction system (SDS): A hybrid of guided-growth and distraction-based technique [58].

guided-growth systems) without device failure. Unlike treatment of nonspecific low back pain, the surgical intervention of EOS involves long-term understanding of the surgical principles, biomechanics surrounding the failure modes, and growth. At present most surgical interventions rely on a one of the three methods of correction, such as distraction-based, guided-growth, and compression-based. This results in a lot of limitations because each of these philosophies suffers from a distinct biomechanical disadvantage, including but not limited to excessive distraction-force led fracture and autofusion, repeated open surgeries, failure of noninvasive distraction mechanism, progression of deformity due to apex migration, metallosis and tissue encapsulation, and inefficacy with need for early intervention. Nevertheless,

such limitations can be tackled using a combination of two or more of these techniques, and future work should focus on understanding and implementing hybrid surgical philosophies for unprecedented biomechanical advantage.

REFERENCES

1. Kotwicki T. Evaluation of scoliosis today: Examination, X-rays and beyond. *Disability and Rehabilitation*. 2008;30(10):742–751.
2. Hoh DJ, Elder JB, Wang MY. Principles of growth modulation in the treatment of scoliotic deformities. *Neurosurgery*. 2008;63(suppl_3):A211–A221.
3. Stokes I. Mechanical effects on skeletal growth. *Journal of Musculoskeletal and Neuronal Interactions*. 2002;2(3):277–280.

4. Stokes IA, Burwell RG, Dangerfield PH. Biomechanical spinal growth modulation and progressive adolescent scoliosis–a test of the 'vicious cycle' pathogenetic hypothesis: Summary of an electronic focus group debate of the IBSE. *Scoliosis*. 2006;1(1):16.

5. Stokes IA, Spence H, Aronsson DD, et al. Mechanical modulation of vertebral body growth: Implications for scoliosis progression. *Spine*. 1996;21(10):1162–1167.

6. Ahn UM, Ahn NU, Nallamshetty L, et al. The etiology of adolescent idiopathic scoliosis. *American Journal of Orthopedics (Belle Mead, NJ)*. 2002;31(7):387–395.

7. Lowe TG, Edgar M, Margulies JY, et al. Etiology of idiopathic scoliosis: Current trends in research. *Bone and Joint Surgery*. 2000;82(8):1157.

8. Acosta FL, Buckley JM, Xu Z, et al. Biomechanical comparison of three fixation techniques for unstable thoracolumbar burst fractures. *Journal of Neurosurgery: Spine*. 2008;8(4):341–346.

9. Parent S, Newton P, Wenger D. Adolescent idiopathic scoliosis: Etiology, anatomy, natural history, and bracing. *Instructional Course Lectures*. 2005;54:529–536.

10. Yamada K, Yamamoto H, Nakagawa Y, et al. Etiology of idiopathic scoliosis. *Clinical Orthopaedics and Related Research*. 1984;184(184):50–57.

11. Weinstein SL, Zavala D, Ponseti I. Idiopathic scoliosis: Long-term follow-up and prognosis in untreated patients. *Journal of Bone and Joint Surgery*. 1981;63(5):702–712.

12. Kim H, Kim HS, Moon ES, et al. Scoliosis imaging: What radiologists should know. *RadioGraphics*. 2010;30(7):1823–1842.

13. Ylikoski M. Growth and progression of adolescent idiopathic scoliosis in girls. *Journal of Pediatric Orthopaedics – Part B*. 2005;14(5):320–324.

14. Van Goethem J, Van Campenhout A, Van den Hauwe L, et al. Scoliosis. *Neuroimaging Clinics of North America*. 2007;17(1):105–115.

15. Fletcher ND, Bruce RW. Early onset scoliosis: Current concepts and controversies. *Current Reviews in Musculoskeletal Medicine*. 2012;5(2):102–110.

16. D'Astous JL, Sanders JO. Casting and traction treatment methods for scoliosis. *Orthopedic Clinics of North America*. 2007;38(4):477–484.

17. Fletcher ND, McClung A, Rathjen KE, et al. Serial casting as a delay tactic in the treatment of moderate-to-severe early-onset scoliosis. *Journal of Pediatric Orthopaedics*. 2012;32(7):664–671.

18. Thompson GH, Akbarnia BA, Campbell Jr RM. Growing rod techniques in early-onset scoliosis. *Journal of Pediatric Orthopaedics*. 2007;27(3):354–361.

19. Akbarnia BA, Breakwell LM, Marks DS, et al. Dual growing rod technique followed for three to eleven years until final fusion: The effect of frequency of lengthening. *Spine*. 2008;33(9):984–990.

20. Akbarnia BA, Cheung K, Noordeen H, et al. Next generation of growth-sparing techniques: Preliminary clinical results of a magnetically controlled growing rod in 14 patients with early-onset scoliosis. *Spine*. 2013;38(8):665–670.

21. Agarwal A TO THE EDITOR: Letter to Editor for: 'Harshavardhana NS, Noordeen MH, Dormans JP. Cost analysis of magnet-driven growing rods for early-onset scoliosis at 5 years. Spine 44 (1): 60–67'. *Spine*. 2019;44(18):E1108–E1108.

22. McCarthy RE, McCullough FL. Shilla growth guidance for early-onset scoliosis: Results after a minimum of five years of follow-up. *Journal of Bone and Joint Surgery*. 2015;97(19):1578–1584.

23. Bumpass DB, McCullough L, McCarthy RE. Shilla growth guidance—Evolution of a new procedure: Rate of complications in the first two years following implantation in the first 80 patients. *The Spine Journal*. 2017;17(10):S106–S107.

24. Braun JT, Akyuz E, Ogilvie JW, et al. The efficacy and integrity of shape memory alloy staples and bone anchors with ligament tethers in the fusionless treatment of experimental scoliosis. *Bone and Joint Surgery*. 2005;87(9):2038–2051.

25. Lavelle WF, Samdani AF, Cahill PJ, et al. Clinical outcomes of nitinol staples for preventing curve progression in idiopathic scoliosis. *Journal of Pediatric Orthopaedics*. 2011;31:S107–S113.

26. Samdani AF, Ames RJ, Kimball JS, et al. Anterior vertebral body tethering for idiopathic scoliosis: Two-year results. *Spine*. 2014;39(20):1688–1693.

27. Gillingham BL, Fan RA, Akbarnia BA. Early onset idiopathic scoliosis. *JAAOS. Journal of the American Academy of Orthopaedic Surgeons*. 2006;14(2):101–112.

28. Gomez JA, Lee JK, Kim PD, et al. "Growth friendly" spine surgery: Management options for the young child with scoliosis. *Journal of the American Academy of Orthopaedic Surgeons*. 2011;19(12):722–727.

29. Yang JS, Sponseller PD, Thompson GH, et al. Growing rod fractures: Risk

factors and opportunities for prevention. *Spine*. 2011;36(20):1639–1644.

30. Hill G, Nagaraja S, Akbarnia BA, et al. Retrieval and clinical analysis of distraction-based dual growing rod constructs for early-onset scoliosis. *The Spine Journal*. 2017;17(10):1506–1518.

31. Agarwal A, Agarwal AK, Jayaswal A, et al. Smaller interval distractions may reduce chances of growth rod breakage without impeding desired spinal growth: A finite element study. *Spine Deformity*. 2014;2(6):430–436.

32. Agarwal A. *Mitigating Biomechanical Complications of Growth Rods in Juvenile Idiopathic Scoliosis*. University of Toledo; 2015.

33. Agarwal A, Agarwal AK, Jayaswal A, et al. Effect of distraction force on growth and biomechanics of the spine: A finite element study on normal juvenile spine with dual growth rod instrumentation. *Spine Deformity*. 2014;2(4):260–269.

34. Agarwal A, Agarwal AK, Jayaswal A, et al. Outcomes of optimal distraction forces and frequencies in growth rod surgery for different types of scoliotic curves: An in silico and in vitro study. *Spine Deformity*. 2017;5(1):18–26.

35. Agarwal A, Zakeri A, Agarwal AK, et al. Distraction magnitude and frequency affects the outcome in juvenile idiopathic patients with growth rods: Finite element study using a representative scoliotic spine model. *The Spine Journal*. 2015;15(8):1848–1855.

36. Olgun ZD, Ahmadiadli H, Alanay A, et al. Vertebral body growth during growing rod instrumentation: Growth preservation or stimulation? *Journal of Pediatric Orthopaedics*. 2012;32(2):184–189.

37. Demirkiran G, Yilgor C, Ayvaz M, et al. Effects of the fusionless instrumentation on the disks and facet joints of the unfused segments: A pig model. *Journal of Pediatric Orthopaedics*. 2014;34(2):185–193.

38. Rong T, Shen J, Kwan K, et al. Vertebral growth around distal instrumented vertebra in patients with early-onset scoliosis who underwent traditional dual growing rod treatment. *Spine*. 2019;44(12):855–865.

39. Agarwal A, Jayaswal A, Goel VK, et al. Patient-specific distraction regimen to avoid growth-rod failure. *Spine*. 2018;43(4):E221–E226.

40. Agarwal A, Jayaswal AK, Goel VK, et al. Letter to the Editor concerning "Rod fracture and lengthening intervals in traditional growing rods: is there a relationship?" by P. Hosseini et al. Eur Spine J (2016). *European Spine Journal*. 2017;26(6):1696–1697.

41. Li Q-y, Zhang J-g, Qiu G-x, et al. Primary effect of dual growing rod technique for the treatment of severe scoliosis in young children. *Chinese Medical Journal*. 2010;123(2):151–155.

42. Yu Z, Qiu G-x, Wang Y-p, et al. Comparison of initial efficacy between single and dual growing rods in treatment of early onset scoliosis. *Chinese Medical Journal*. 2012;125(16):2862–2866.

43. Noordeen HM, Shah SA, Elsebaie HB, et al. In vivo distraction force and length measurements of growing rods: Which factors influence the ability to lengthen? *Spine*. 2011;36(26):2299–2303.

44. Agarwal A, Goswami A, Vijayaraghavan GP, et al. Quantitative characteristics of consecutive lengthening episodes in early-onset scoliosis (EOS) patients With dual growth rods. *Spine*. 2019;44(6):397–403.

45. Cahill PJ, Marvil S, Cuddihy L, et al. Autofusion in the immature spine treated with growing rods. *Spine*. 2010;35(22):E1199–E1203.

46. Rohlmann A, Zander T, Burra N, et al. Flexible non-fusion scoliosis correction systems reduce intervertebral rotation less than rigid implants and allow growth of the spine: A finite element analysis of different features of orthobiom™. *European Spine Journal*. 2008;17(2):217–223.

47. Cheung JPY, Bow C, Samartzis D, et al. Frequent small distractions with a magnetically controlled growing rod for early-onset scoliosis and avoidance of the law of diminishing returns. *Journal of Orthopaedic Surgery*. 2016;24(3):332–337.

48. Bauer JM, Yorgova P, Neiss G, et al. Early onset scoliosis: Is there an improvement in quality of life with conversion from traditional growing rods to magnetically controlled growing rods? *Journal of Pediatric Orthopaedics*. 2019;39(4):e284–e288.

49. Agarwal A, Kelkar A, Agarwal AG, et al. Device-related complications associated with MAGEC rod usage for distraction-based correction of scoliosis. *Spine Surgery and Related Research*. 2019.

50. Joyce TJ, Smith SL, Rushton PR, et al. Analysis of explanted magnetically controlled growing rods from seven UK spinal centers. *Spine*. 2018;43(1):E16–E22.

51. Teoh K, Von Ruhland C, Evans SL, et al. Metallosis following implantation of magnetically controlled growing rods in the treatment of scoliosis: A case series. *The Bone and Joint Journal*. 2016;98(12):1662–1667.

52. Yang JH, Ham CH, Hwang YG, et al. Metallosis: A complication in the guided growing rod system used in treatment of scoliosis. *Indian Journal of Orthopaedics*. 2017;51(6):714.

53. Dubousset J, Herring J, Shufflebarger H. The crankshaft phenomenon. *Journal of Pediatric Orthopedics*. 1989;9(5):541–550.

54. Murphy RF, Mooney III JF. The crankshaft phenomenon. *Journal of the American Academy of Orthopaedic Surgeons*. 2017;25(9):e185–e193.

55. Wilkinson JT, Songy CE, Bumpass DB, et al. Curve modulation and apex migration using shilla growth guidance rods for early-onset scoliosis at 5-year follow-up. *Journal of Pediatric Orthopaedics*. 2019;39(8):400–405.

56. Agarwal A, Aker L, Ahmad AA. Active apex correction with guided growth technique for controlling spinal deformity in growing children: A modified SHILLA technique. *Global Spine Journal*. 2019:2192568219859836.

57. Agarwal A, Aker L, Ahmad AA. Active apex correction (modified SHILLA technique) versus distraction-based growth rod fixation: What do the correction parameters say? *Spine Surgery and Related Research*. 2019.

58. Lemans J, Kodigudla M, Kelkar A, et al. Spring distraction system for early onset scoliosis provides continuous distraction without a potential increase in rod fractures, compared to traditional growing rods. *Spine Deformity*. 2018;6(6):819–820.

8b Principles of Surgical Management

Michael Grevitt

CONTENTS

INTRODUCTION

Patients with early-onset scoliosis (EOS) form a small but heterogeneous group. This makes study of the natural history and outcomes of treatments difficult given the paucity of large patient cohorts. With the latter problem, there is no consensus based on evidence-based research on what is the optimal treatment in any given clinical scenario. Matters are further complicated by the absence of outcome assessment tools or agreed-upon criteria to measure success. Thus, although growth preservation is an often-stated aim of all treatment modalities, there is a poor understanding of the fundamental relationships between spinal longitudinal growth, chest wall morphometry, and pulmonary function.

CURRENT SURGICAL STRATEGIES

Given all the uncertainties outlined above, the management of children with EOS is often empirical and guided by a surgeon's clinical experience and heuristic reasoning.

This bespoke approach is exemplified by the study of Yang et al. [1]. The authors conducted a case-based survey of members of the Growing Spine Study Group to examine attitudes and thresholds for certain treatment strategies. These results were then related to actual practice based on a database of 265 EOS patients treated by growing rods over 4.7 +/– 2.1 years. The survey indicated a preference for growing rod surgery over nonoperative, rib-based distraction (vertical expandable prosthetic titanium rib – VEPTR), growth guidance (Shilla), and primary arthrodesis techniques. The majority indication for growing rod insertion was a curve of over 60° and a patient younger than 8–10 years of age. In practice, the mean Cobb angle at time of rod insertion was 73° and mean age was 6 years. Other factors favouring rod insertion were curve rigidity, brace intolerance, and syndromic scoliosis.

Given the often poor bone quality in EOS patients, gracile rib structure, and tenuous method of attachment to rib and pelvis, there is an expected rate of complications in the surgery of EOS. The magnitude of the risk and factors that might predispose to the same has been made clearer in several published reports.

Sankar et al. [2] reviewed the charts of 36 EOS children treated by standard dual growing rods, hybrid growing rods (rib-spine attachments), and the VEPTR device. There were 72 unplanned surgeries in 26 patients (72%

complication rate or 2.77 per patient). The main causes were rod breakage (18), migrated anchors (31), and treatment of deep wound sepsis (18). The standard dual rod construct had a complication rate of 2.30, hybrid construct 0.86, and VEPTR 2.37 per patient. In this study, there was no relationship in rate of complications and preoperative Cobb angle, kyphosis, age, and body mass index.

Bess et al [3] published data from the Growing Spine Study Group database. The study included 140 patients with a mean age and follow-up similar to the previously mentioned report; 81 (58%) had a minimum of one complication. Their data suggested that a single growing rod construct had a higher complication rate than dual rods (27% versus 10%), and that subcutaneous rod insertion had more wound problems, implant prominence, and unplanned surgeries. Older age at time of rod insertion seemed to have a lower risk (reduced by 13% for each additional year of age) but increased by 24% for each additional surgical procedure performed.

EOS SURGICAL TREATMENT IN LOW- AND MIDDLE-INCOME COUNTRIES

Matters are further complicated in low- and middle-income countries (LMIC) where problems of funding expensive implants, logistics of follow-up visits, and expeditious management of complications all require an alternative strategy.

The latter requires a synthesis of principles that include the essential goals of surgery and an acknowledgment of the restricted circumstances of LMIC patients. These are:

1. Growth-preservation of the immature spine to maximise T1–T12 length.
2. Control of the spinal deformity (and the adverse effects of the Heuter-Volkmann principle in progressive vertebral wedging).
3. Use of less-expensive and potentially locally derived implants.
4. Less dependence on regular follow-up clinic visits.
5. Avoidance of a high complication rate.

By following the above principles, it is hoped these children will have satisfactory outcomes, acceptance of the care-pathway by the family, and treatment that is sensitive to the socioeconomic circumstances and constraints of climate and geography.

The following sections will focus on growth modulation (convex epiphysiodesis, anterior vertebral staples) and growth guidance (Luque Trolley and SHILLA) techniques and determine how well they respect the above principles:

CONVEX EPIPHYSIODESIS

Epiphysiodesis has been extensively used in the management of limb-length discrepancies and angular deformities of long bones. Convex hemiepiphysiodesis remains one of the most used methods for scoliosis. This is a relatively easy procedure with a short learning curve [4, 5]. These procedures address the curve by reducing growth on the convex side and continuing growth on the concave side, provided there is enough growth potential. Progression is prevented (with potential regression of the deformity) by slowing down the growth of the curve convexity by the destruction of the growth plate. Presently the most common indication is in children with multisegment congenital deformities in which fusion is undesirable (for fear of aggravating potential thoracic insufficiency syndrome through trunk shortening), particularly when the anomalies are hemivertebrae. However, it may be applied in idiopathic EOS in combination with growth-guiding instrumentation.

The results are better in younger children with greater growth potential and enough time for correction. Several authors modified the original technique with better results [6]. However, unpredictability of the correction and curve progression, slowly evolving outcomes, are the requirement of occasional anterior surgery are drawbacks [6].

Several authors documented a growth tether effect in the majority of curves, but the demonstrable correction of curve is less frequent [7,8]. In a study by Marks et al. [9], 53 patients with congenital scoliosis were analysed. Results showed reduction in the rate of change of Cobb angles in patients with unsegmented bars. In complex anomalies, there was a decrease in the rate of progression of the curve, but the final deformity was more than that just prior to surgery. However, in the hemivertebrae group, 97% of patients showed reduction in the final Cobb angle. The author concluded that convex epiphysiodesis has an important role in the surgical management of congenital scoliosis, particularly for hemivertebra [9]. Demirkiran et al. [10] proposed a modified technique of convex epiphysiodesis with instrumented fusion. He studied 13 patients who underwent this procedure in which there was acute correction of the curve by end plate destruction and fusion by pedicle screws and gradual correction later by concave growth. The average curve magnitude was $49°\pm10.9°$ (range, $34°–68°$) preoperatively, $38.3°\pm9.7°$ (range, $28°–58°$) early postoperatively, and $33.5°\pm12.4°$ ($16°–52°$) at last follow-up [10].

These results suggest that procedures to arrest convex growth can be used with great effect in children with growth potential, particularly in complex multisegment curves. The results in lumbar curves are more advantageous than thoracic counterparts. Various local modifications can be applied in these patients, but long-term follow-up is extremely important to prevent failures.

ANTERIOR VERTEBRAL STAPLES

The inspiration for stapling the spine for scoliosis grew out of the success obtained in lower extremity deformity conditions in children. It is minimally invasive, avoids the need for fusion, and is potentially reversible with the correction starting immediately upon insertion [11]. Vertebral body stapling attempts to reverse the wedging caused by Hueter–Volkmann law.

Vertebral body stapling is an option for the growing child with progressive scoliosis as an alternative to bracing. Indications include a scoliosis deformity that would be considered for brace treatment or may have failed or refused bracing with at least 1 year of growth remaining. Poor results are seen with curves over $45°$ and with kyphosis greater than $40°$.

Initial reports of the use of staples in the spine were in canine models by Nachlas and Borden [12]. They first created and then tried to correct the deformity in animals using staples. Some of the staples failed because they spanned three vertebrae, and there were concerns regarding the staple design. The enthusiasm for this novel treatment waned after the application of their stapling technique in three children with progressive scoliosis yielded poor results. Later, Smith et al. [13] presented disappointing results in patients with congenital scoliosis. Its use in severe curves with significant rotational components and in children with little remaining growth limited the amount of potential correction.

Initial staples used for spinal deformities were similar to those used in long bones and made of stainless steel. Being rigid, they were prone to dislodge due to motion in the spine. To overcome this, special staples made up of Nitinol (Nickel Titanium Naval Ordnance Laboratory) were designed. Nitinol is a biocompatible metal alloy of 50% titanium and 50% nickel. The uniqueness of this staple is that it is made out of a shape memory alloy in which the prongs are straight when cooled but assume a C-clamp shape in the bone for secure fixation when the staple returns to body temperature. The temperature at which the staples will undergo the shape transformation can be controlled by the manufacturing process [13]. Nitinol has a low corrosion rate, has been used extensively in orthodontic implants and cardiovascular stents, and found to be safe. It does not lead to significant elevations in the nickel levels in the tissues or blood, and its properties are not altered with any sterilization methods used in the operating room [14,15]. The US Food and Drug Administration has given 510(k) approval for Nitinol shape memory staples for fixation of a bone screw in the anterior spine as well as for hand and foot osteotomies. The staples are not approved for use across the disc space and are used off-label [16].

Betz et al. [17] demonstrated the feasibility, safety, and utility of vertebral body stapling for the treatment of AIS in a group of 21 patients (Figure 8b.1). Only minor complications were noted, with no cases of staple dislodgement. In 2005, the same group [18] reported on 39 patients and their increased experience with the procedure. Stabilization of the curve was seen in 87% of those patients older than 8 years at the time of stapling who had a curve of $50°$ or less with at least 1 year of follow-up. No curve less than $30°$ at the time of stapling progressed more than $10°$ at follow-up.

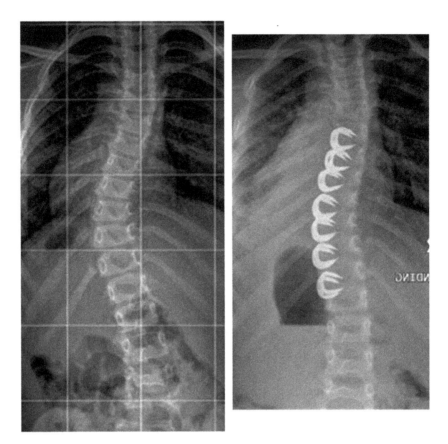

FIGURE 8B.1   X-rays demonstrating anterior vertebral staples.

Indications for stapling include:

a. Age less than 13 years for girls and less than 15 for boys.
b. Risser 0 or 1.
c. At least 1 year of growth remaining by wrist x-ray, or Sanders digital stage less than or equal to 4.
d. Thoracic curves 25–35°, and lumbar coronal curves less than or equal to 45°, with minimal rotation and flexible to less than or equal to 20°.
e. Thoracic kyphosis less than or equal to 40° (due to the theoretic potential of the staples to induce kyphosis).

Contraindications to stapling are preoperative curves greater than 50°, kyphosis greater than 40°, any medical contraindication to general anaesthesia, reduced pulmonary function, or a known hypersensitivity to nickel [19–21].

The technique of convex side staple insertion is either via thoracoscopic or open insertion in the thoracic spine and the use of minimal access tubes for thoracolumbar or lumbar curves. Using these minimally invasive techniques, scoliotic vertebrae from T3 to L4 can be stapled while limiting the total scar length. Staples are allowed to cool for at least 45 minutes. Once adequately cooled, the staples are placed onto their inserters, where they remain in iced cardioplegia solution prior to insertion. The transfer of staples from ice-water bath to vertebral bodies should be as quick as possible to prevent staple warming. Staples are placed anterior to the rib heads, and if the patient has severe hypokyphosis or thoracic lordosis, the staples can be placed more anterior on the vertebrae to help produce kyphosis with the patient's growth. In the lumbar spine, the staples should be placed as far posteriorly on the vertebral body as possible, at least in the posterior half of the body, to maintain a normal lordosis [19]. All vertebral bodies included in the Cobb angle of the curve are instrumented. Two single staples (two prongs) or one double staple (four prongs) is placed at each level except when an additional two-prong staple is inserted anterior to these to induce further kyphosis.

Although the technique does not require a large inventory or complex instrumentation, the alloy and manufacture of Nitinol staples are expensive and, therefore, probably not relevant to LMIC. However, staples may be used as an adjunct to brace therapy. Whilst the curve is still flexible, the brace produces some curve correction and reduces the stresses on the implanted staples giving the latter time to exert its growth modulating effect.

SHILLA TECHNIQUE

This technique was devised by McCarthy and named after the hotel where he first conceived the concept. Fundamental to the technique is correction of the apical deformity and rotation with instrumentation. There is a limited arthrodesis over the apical segments and nonsecured 'sliding' pedicle screws above and below the fused segments. The remainder of the spine may, therefore, passively elongate over the rods that function as a growth-guidance construct.

Andras [19] compared the results of the SHILLA with dual-spine growing rods (GR). The study compared 36 matched pairs, and the GR group had a greater improvement in Cobb angle and T1–S1 length but had more surgeries. However, those in the SHILLA group were more likely unplanned or emergent.

That same year (2015), McCarthy [20] published the results of the first 40 patients treated by his technique. The average age was 6 years and 11 months, with an average follow-up interval of 7 years. The mean curve size presurgery was 69°, and at the latest follow-up it was 38.4°; however, the complication rate was 73%.

The same study group [21] compared the results of GR with SHILLA technique at definitive fusion/removal of implants or final lengthening, after average intervals of 6–7 years. Age at first surgery was similar at 7.7 and 7.9 years, respectively. The SHILLA group had a better initial Cobb correction, but both groups were similar in terms of the initial increase in the

T1–T12 length and subsequent increase growth-related increases. In contrast to the earlier studies, complication rates were similar, but GR had a three-fold greater number of surgeries.

McCarthy published his longer term results in 2019 [22] and found that, although there was no crankshaft phenomenon, there was distal add-on beneath the fused apex in over two-thirds of cases. The mean growth was 45 mm (i.e. not dissimilar to normal growth).

The latest evidence [23], however, contradicts the latter finding. In their group of 20 patients, a growth rate of 4.2mm/year was achieved; this being a third of normal growth. Once again, the complication was high (75%), with the majority being implant related.

In summary, the SHILLA technique has the advantage of limited implant density using pedicle fixation and sliding screws that are neither complex nor necessarily expensive to produce. The passive nature of the construct and avoidance of need for frequent returns to the clinic are obvious attractions in LMIC health systems. However, the data on the outcomes are conflicting with nondeveloper reports suggesting less growth and initial correction than distraction rods. Moreover, the high complication rate would also be challenging to overcome or deal with in more disadvantaged settings.

LUQUE TROLLEY

Luque was the first to develop multisegmental instrumentation in the post-Harrington rod era. The need arose from having to treat a cohort of patients with postpoliomyeltic deformities. Given the local circumstances, the usual prolonged postsurgical confinement in bed and need for a plaster jacket were unacceptable. Advantages included rapid postoperative mobilisation discharge from hospital and relative cheapness of the implants. His initial report [24] showed an average of 72% correction.

Winter's [25] experience of 100 patients of sublaminar wiring for scoliosis fusion emphasised the need for care in passing the wires. There were no cases of broken wires or rods but 'disturbing loss of correction' in idiopathic scoliosis. Pseudarthrosis was common in fusions to the sacrum except where Luque-Galveston fixation was used.

The first description of this technique in EOS was in 1992 [26]. There were only nine cases, with an average age of 9 at the time of surgery. All patients had at least one revision procedure, which was technically difficult due to extensive fibrosis. Average gain in height was 5.8 cm, but little occurred in the instrumented segments. There was no effective control of the spinal deformity.

Webb et al [27] performed a retrospective analysis of the 5-year follow-up data from patients instrumented with Luque Trolley with or without convex epiphysiodesis for management of progressive infantile and juvenile idiopathic scoliosis. For Luque Trolley alone, Cobb angle worsened for all patients. For progressive infantile scoliosis managed with Luque Trolley and convex epiphysiodesis, Cobb angle worsened in seven, remained unchanged in four, and improved in two patients. Mean age at operation was 3.1 years and instrumented spinal growth was 32% of expected growth. Average preoperation Cobb angle was 65°; at the 5-year follow-up, it was 32°. For juvenile idiopathic scoliosis managed with Luque Trolley and convex epiphysiodesis, Cobb angle worsened in three patients and improved in one. This study concluded that the Luque Trolley alone was insufficient to prevent curve progression; a convex epiphysiodesis was required to prevent the crankshaft phenomenon.

In a more recent report of the technique, Rosenfeld et al. [28] used 13 children with low-tone EOS. The mean age at surgery was 7.4 years. On average, 15 segments (13–16) were instrumented; none of the children went on to a spontaneous fusion, and the average growth rate per year from T1–T12 and T1–S1 was 0.9 cm/y and 1.5 cm/y, respectively. The mean total growth from T1–T12 and T1–S1 was 22.3 cm and 37.5 cm, respectively. A total of three additional surgeries were needed in two children to address complications.

In summary, the use of the Luque Trolley in EOS has been used for more than 20 years. The need for an adjuvant convex epiphysiodesis remains unclear because of insufficient data. The growth rates using the procedure range from near normality to approximately one-third. There are also conflicting data regarding the spontaneous fusion and complication rate.

The technique is technically demanding (which may account for the varied results in the literature) and, therefore, some tips and tricks are necessary:

The Luque Trolley procedure is technically demanding not just in the care and dexterity required to safely pass the wires in small children, but also in the careful extraperiosteal exposure of the spine. Only sufficient spine should be exposed to create the small laminotomies for wire passage.

The laminae in small and syndromal children may be soft and should not be unduly stressed by forceful tightening of the wires (e.g. as part of a cantilever reduction manoeuvre) to secure to the rods.

Where a large curve exists, a significant reduction of the deformity may be achieved by the adjuvant use of halo-femoral traction during the operation.

The use of pedicle screws as a caudal foundation provides for a better fixation, and less distal junctional kyphosis and caudal migration of the lower rods as described in the original Luque technique (see case example, Figures 8b.1–8b.5).

Proximal fixation is also challenging using pedicle screws in the upper thoracic spine in EOS patients. Use of wires alone to secure the proximal rod (cf. unit rod procedure) is acceptable in very small infants. For the larger child, hooks or hook-screw devices may be useful.

To maximise the construct rigidity, there should be maximal overlap of the proximal and distal rods, as well as allowing the greatest length to accommodate growth (Figures 8b.3-8b.7).

In an effort to reduce the necessary dissection to pass the sublaminar wires, a pedicle-screw based adaptation of the Luque Trolley system has been developed (DePuy Synthes, Raynham, US). Pairs of proximal and distal rods secured cephalad and caudad with conventional pedicle screws or hooks are interlinked with gliding vehicles (GV) that have polyetheretherketone (PEEK) cable ties (Figure 8b.8).

The advantage is that less exposure of the spine is required to insert the GVs and, therefore, reduces the risk of spontaneous fusion. However, there are fewer intermediary anchor points and, therefore, the instrumentation is likely less suited for stiff curves or associated

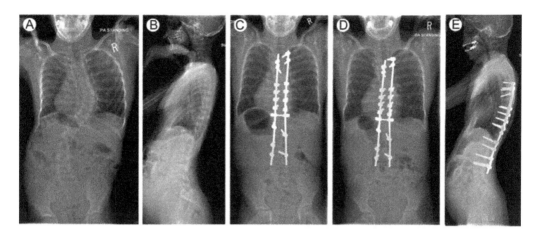

FIGURE 8B.2 X-rays demonstrating SHILLA technique (A–E).

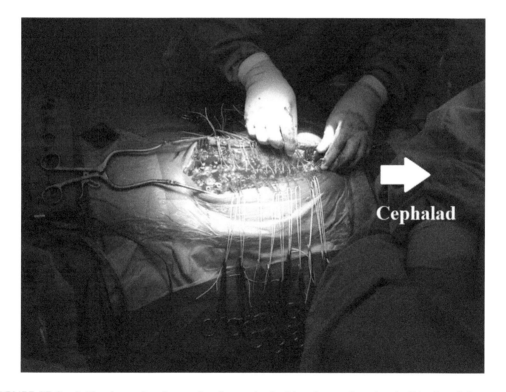

FIGURE 8B.3 Sublaminar wires inserted and organised with polypropylene bands. Distal pedicle screws are inserted.

hyperkyphosis (see case example, Figures 8b.9, 8b.10 and 8b.11).

Ouellet [29] described the initial results of the above system at a mean follow-up of 4 years. The primary curve was corrected from 60° to 21° and was maintained at 21°. An average of 10 vertebrae was spanned, allowing the spine to grow a mean of 3 cm over 4 years, representing a mean of 77% of the expected growth. Two of the five cases outgrew the construct requiring lengthening of rods. One patient had gradual recurrence of deformity without substantial axial growth that required revision surgery after 4 years.

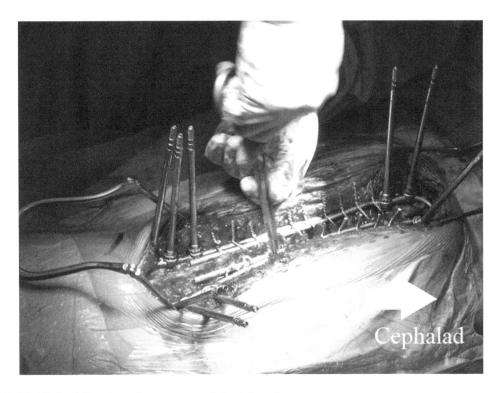

FIGURE 8B.4   Sublaminar wires are sequentially tightened.

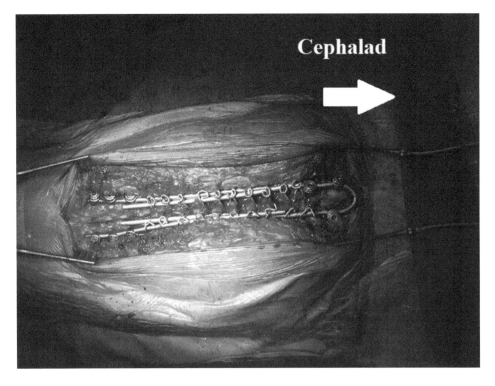

FIGURE 8B.5   Final construct – upper thoracic hook-screws inserted. Note majority overlap of rods.

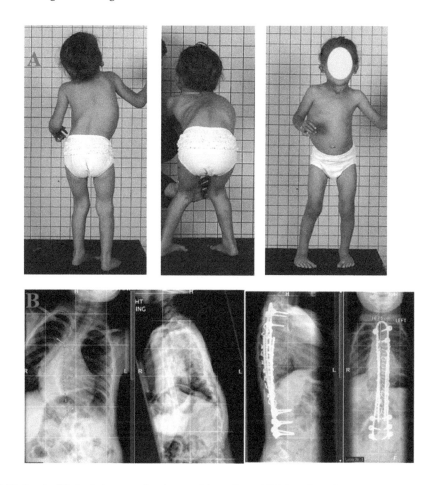

FIGURE 8B.6 A. Clinical photographs; 4-year-old syndromal EOS patient. B. Pre- and immediate postoperative x-rays.

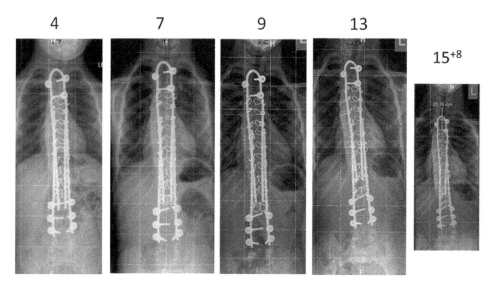

FIGURE 8B.7 12-year follow-up – no revision procedures or additional surgeries required. Postpubertal final follow-up x-ray aged 15+8 years.

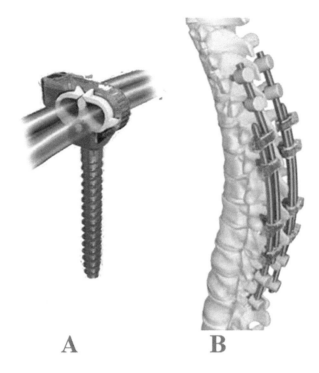

FIGURE 8B.8 Updated trolley system (DePuy Synthes). A. Pedicle screw with PEEK cable tie securing rods. B. Construct with proximal and distal pedicle screws and intermediate gliding vehicles.

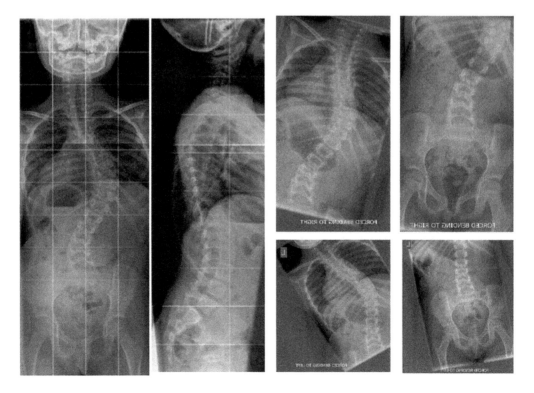

FIGURE 8B.9 7-year-old syndromal EOS patient. Preoperative and bending x-rays.

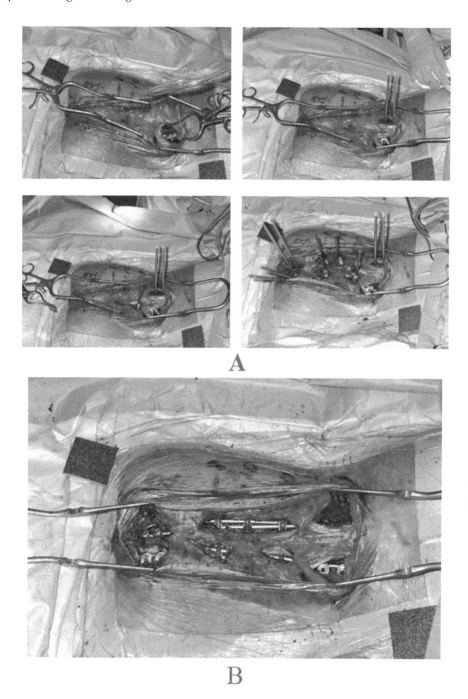

FIGURE 8B.10   A. Insertion of proximal and distal pedicle screws. B. Intermediate GVs with protruding cable ties.

THE CHALLENGE OF EOS SURGERY IN LMICS

Conventional distraction-based growing rod systems are inappropriate given the repeated visits and need for frequent lengthening required. Apart from the reported considerable complication rate, there is also the affordability. The latter refers not just to the cost of implants but the socioeconomic cost of this treatment

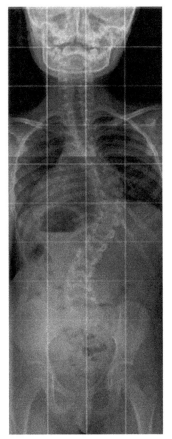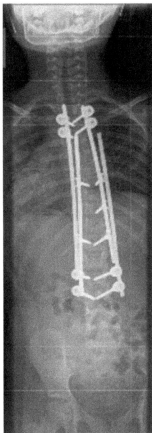

FIGURE 8B.11 Pre- and postoperative x-rays.

regimen. Repeated distraction procedures are also resource intensive.

The growth guidance or modulating procedures are thus theoretically more attractive. An idealised care pathway is a single surgical intervention, negligible complications, and easier conversion to a definitive fusion.

The data for all the above techniques demonstrate that the above ideal is not met in the majority. The complication rates are not inconsiderable and may not be easy to manage both from a logistical perspective (i.e. timely revision) as well as being technically challenging.

The fact that there are such diverse procedures for surgical management of EOS implies that there is no single 'catch-all' choice. Each case requires a bespoke approach that addresses the surgical challenge and the socioeconomic circumstances of the family.

From a technical perspective, epiphysiodesis, at an early stage, is a safe option and may

be combined with cast or brace therapy. Where the latter is practically difficult because of geographical and organizational constraints, then some form of internal brace is required. In these instances, and where implants are restricted, judicious use of apical screws to control the apex, with limited use of sublaminar wires at the caudal and cephalad limits of the construct, may control the curve with some growth-guidance capability. Alternatively, if screw availability is challenging then an all-wire construct may be employed (Figure 8b.12).

Whilst some of the implants might be more affordable or have local equivalents, there are fundamental challenges to the system of postoperative care and surveillance required to deliver the best outcomes.

The challenges are considerable. A study published in January 2018 [30], followed 11,422 postoperative patients in 25 African nations. The report found that 1 in 5 patients developed

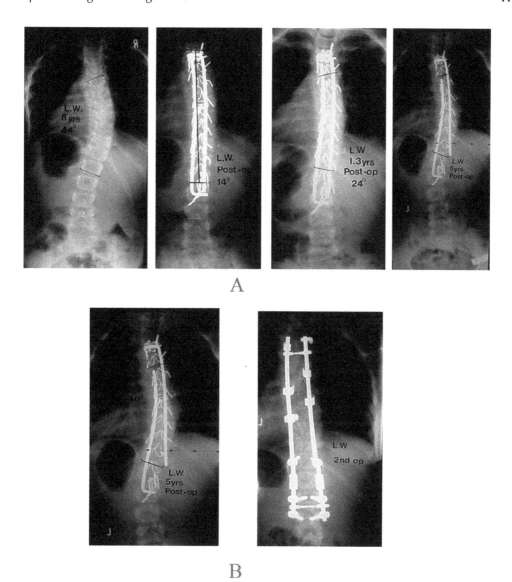

FIGURE 8B.12   A. All-wire Luque trolley construct in juvenile idiopathic EOS. B. Definitive fusion 6 years later aged 14 years.

postoperative complications and had a 5.6% chance of dying. The lead researchers of the study pointed to the inadequate and under-staffed postoperative care offered in most hospitals as the cause of this phenomena.

Many patients also live a significant distance from hospitals, which means that they struggle to follow up on postoperative visits and cannot reach help in time if there are complications.

If EOS surgery is to be safely delivered, there needs to be a framework of local care and clinical surveillance from nonmedical or allied health professionals. Telemedicine and the use of video call to consult with specialists in the spinal hub hospitals are the minimum requisites.

CONCLUSION

Surgical management of EOS in LMICs poses considerable challenges. The procedure chosen is less important than the system of care (and the feasibility of timely follow up). The technique is dependent on the latter and the available implants. Epiphysiodesis and bracing is the least implant dependent procedure but requires longer fusion length to adequately control the deformity. Anterior stapling and vertebral body tethering are attractive options; however, there are resource issues related to the thoracotomy approach and unpredictable nature of the growth guidance principle. Posterior approaches may use sublaminar wires either as a SHILLA or Luque Trolley strategy.

REFERENCES

1. Yang JS, McElroy MJ, Akbarnia BA, et al. Growing rods for spinal deformity: Characterizing consensus and variation in current use. *Journal of Pediatric Orthopedics.* 2010;30(3):264–70.
2. Sankar WN, Acevedo DC, Skaggs DL. Comparison of complications among growing spinal implants. *Spine (Phila Pa 1976).* 2010;35(23):2091–6.
3. Bess S, Akbarnia BA, Thompson GH, et al. Complications of growing-rod treatment for early-onset scoliosis: Analysis of one hundred and forty patients. *Journal of Bone and Joint Surgery.* 2010;92(15):2533–43.
4. Roaf R. The treatment of progressive scoliosis by unilateral growth-arrest. *The Journal of Bone and Joint Surgery, British Volume.* 1963;45(4):637–51. PubMed PMID: 14074311.
5. Thompson AG, Marks DS, Sayampanathan SR, et al. Long-term results of combined anterior and posterior convex epiphysiodesis for congenital scoliosis due to hemivertebrae. *Spine.* 1995;20(12):1380–5. PubMed PMID: 7676336.
6. Alanay A, Dede O, Yazici M. Convex instrumented hemiepiphysiodesis with concave distraction: A preliminary report. *Clinical Orthopaedics and Related Research.* 2012;470(4):1144–50. PubMed PMID: 21484474. Pubmed Central PMCID: 3293962.
7. Kieffer J, Dubousset J. Combined anterior and posterior convex epiphysiodesis for progressive congenital scoliosis in children aged <or = 5 years. *European Spine Journal.* 1994;3(2):120–5. PubMed PMID: 7874550.
8. Andrew T, Piggott H. Growth arrest for progressive scoliosis. Combined anterior and posterior fusion of the convexity. *The Journal of Bone and Joint Surgery, British Volume.* 1985;67(2):193–7. PubMed PMID: 3980524.
9. Marks DS, Sayampanathan SR, Thompson AG, et al. Long-term results of convex epiphysiodesis for congenital scoliosis. *European Spine Journal.* 1995;4(5):296–301. PubMed PMID: 8581531.
10. Demirkiran G, Yilmaz G, Kaymaz B, et al. Safety and efficacy of instrumented convex growth arrest in treatment of congenital scoliosis. *Journal of Pediatric Orthopedics.* 2014;34(3):275–81. PubMed PMID: 24045587.
11. Blount WP. A mature look at epiphyseal stapling. *Clinical Orthopaedics and Related Research.* 1971;77:158–63. PubMed PMID: 5140445.
12. Nachlas IW, Borden JN. The cure of experimental scoliosis by directed growth control. *The Journal of Bone and Joint Surgery. American Volume.* 1951;33A(1):24–34. PubMed PMID: 14803474.
13. Smith AD, Von Lackum WH, Wylie R. An operation for stapling vertebral bodies in congenital scoliosis. *The Journal of Bone and Joint Surgery. American Volume.* 1954;36(A:2):342–8. PubMed PMID: 13152142.
14. Sanders JO, Sanders AE, More R, et al. A preliminary investigation of shape memory alloys in the surgical correction of scoliosis. *Spine.* 1993;18(12):1640–6. PubMed PMID: 8235844.
15. Randal R, Betz JA, Samdani Amer F. Non-fusion anterior stapling. In: AKbarnia B. Aea, editor. *The Growing Spine.* 1st ed. Heidelberg: Springer; 2011:560–78.
16. Betz RR. Non-fusion anterior stapling. In: AKbarnia B. Aea, editor. *The Growing Spine.* 1st ed. Heidelberg: Springer; 2011:569–78.
17. Betz RR, Kim J, D'Andrea LP, et al. An innovative technique of vertebral body stapling for the treatment of patients with adolescent idiopathic scoliosis: A feasibility, safety, and utility study. *Spine.* 2003;28(20):S255–65. PubMed PMID: 14560201.
18. Betz RR, D'Andrea LP, Mulcahey MJ, et al. Vertebral body stapling procedure for the treatment of scoliosis in the growing child. *Clinical Orthopaedics and Related Research.* 2005;434(434):55–60. PubMed PMID: 15864032.
19. Andras LM, Joiner ER, McCarthy RE, et al. Growing rods versus Shilla growth guidance: Better cobb angle correction and T1-S1 length increase but more surgeries. *Spine Deformity.* 2015;3(3):246–52.
20. McCarthy RE, McCullough FL. Shilla growth guidance for early-onset scoliosis: Results after a minimum of five years of follow-up. *Journal of Bone and Joint Surgery.* 2015;97(19):1578–84.
21. Luhmann SJ, Smith JC, McClung A, et al. Radiographic outcomes of Shilla growth guidance system and traditional growing rods through definitive treatment. *Spine Deformity.* 2017;5(4):277–82.
22. Wilkinson JT, Songy CE, Bumpass DB, et al. Curve modulation and apex migration

using Shilla growth guidance rods for early-onset scoliosis at 5-year follow-up. *Journal of Pediatric Orthopedics.* 2019;39(8):400–5.

23. Nazareth A, Skaggs DL, Illingworth KD, et al. Growth guidance constructs with apical fusion and sliding pedicle screws (SHILLA) results in approximately 1/3rd of normal T1-S1 growth. *Spine Deformity.* 2020;Feb 24:1–5.

24. Luque ER. Segmental spinal instrumentation for correction of scoliosis. *Clinical Orthopaedics and Related Research.* 1982;163(163):192–8.

25. Winter RB, Anderson MB. Spinal arthrodesis for spinal deformity using posterior instrumentation and sublaminar wiring. A preliminary report of 100 consecutive cases. *International Orthopaedics.* 1985;9(4):239–45.

26. Mardjetko SM, Hammerberg KW, Lubicky JP, et al. The Luque trolley revisited. Review of nine cases requiring revision. *Spine (Phila Pa 1976).* 1992;17(5):582–9.

27. Pratt RK, Webb JK, Burwell RG, et al. Luque trolley and convex epiphysiodesis in the management of infantile and juvenile idiopathic scoliosis. *Spine (Phila Pa 1976).* 1999;24(15):1538–47.

28. Rosenfeld S, Schlechter J, Smith B. Achievement of guided growth in children with low-tone neuromuscular early-onset scoliosis using a segmental sublaminar instrumentation technique. *Spine Deformity.* 2018;6(5):607–13.

29. Ouellet J. Surgical technique: Modern Luqué trolley, a self-growing rod technique. *Clinical Orthopaedics and Related Research.* 2011;469(5):1356–67.

30. Biccard BM, Madiba TE, Kluyts HL, et al. African surgical outcomes study (ASOS) investigators. Perioperative patient outcomes in the African surgical outcomes study: A 7-day prospective observational cohort study. *Lancet.* 2018;391(10130):1589–98.

8c Preoperative Diagnosis and Management

Mohamed Fawzy Khattab

CONTENTS

INTRODUCTION

Early-onset scoliosis (EOS) is not a diagnosis; it defines the structural coronal and/or sagittal spinal deformity that started before the age of 10 years. It has different aetiologies, including congenital, neuromuscular, syndromic, or idiopathic. The diagnosis determines the natural history and helps in decision-making. Diagnosis relies on a multidisciplinary approach with a team consisting of a spine deformity surgeon, paediatric orthopaedic surgeon, neurologist, paediatrician, pulmonologist, nutrition specialist, genetic specialist, radiologist, physiotherapist, and neurosurgeon.

EOS remains a challenging scenario because natural history varies according to the aetiology, there is no globally agreed-upon method for treatment, and outcomes rely on the patient's comorbidities, diagnosis, and management protocols. In limited-resource countries, the situation has special considerations, including limited perinatal examinations of pregnant mothers in rural areas, limited infant-screening methods, late presentations of the deformity, limited diagnostic tools, a limited number of deformity surgeons, a limited number of well-equipped hospitals, the economic and psychological burden on poor families, and a lack of multidisciplinary team approach.

In Egypt, there is a difference in the available resources, availability of healthcare professionals, and the degree of healthcare offered to the EOS cases based on geographical location. In order for a child with EOS to receive effective treatment, a multidisciplinary approach to reach the diagnosis is necessary. The author works with a multidisciplinary team, led by a senior professor of paediatric neurology, at a university in Egypt that is considered to be referral centre. The team utilised the Khattab EOS Checklist (Table 8c.1), which was developed to help fulfil the patient diagnosis requirements, and the WhatsApp messaging application to notify team members about newly discovered cases. The team started some live and online seminars to increase community awareness and to help patients and families psychologically. This

TABLE 8C.1
Khattab EOS Checklist

Personal Data	Symptoms	Alarming Symptoms	Previous Paediatric Consultation	
Family History	Known Syndromes	Siblings		
General Examination	Growth and Development	Face/Skin/Possible Syndromatic	Cardiac and Respiratory Systems	Gastrointestinal and Renal
Musculoskletal	Spine	Lower limb/LLD/Hip/Pelvis	Upper Limb	Spine/Balance
Neurological State	Sensory	Motor/Walker/Nonwalker	Abdominal Reflexes	Reflexes
Laboratory	Routine	Specific		
Radiology	Plain X-Ray	MRI	CT	DEXA/Pelvic Abdominal Ultrasound/
Remarks				
Team/Multidisciplinary Approach	Spine Deformity Surgeon/Paediatric Orthopaedic Surgeon	Paediatric Cardiologist, Pulmonologist, Paediatrician, Neurologist, Genetic Paediatrician	Neurosurgeon, Nutrition Specialist, Physiotherapy Specialist	Radiologist, Anaesthesiologist, Psychologist
Team Decision				

group of healthcare professionals is working to launch a special paediatric deformity care unit.

HISTORY-TAKING

The preoperative assessment starts with proper history-taking with analysis of the parents' complaint, followed by proper examination of the musculoskeletal system, neurological state, pulmonary state, and syndromic assessment. The team then must gain parental approval to conduct the proper investigations. Diagnosis can be achieved through proper history-taking, which requires parents of EOS patients to answer some questions regarding the natal, family, and spine deformity history.

For the natal history, the parents are asked about difficulties during pregnancy, ultrasound examination, type of labour, postnatal neonatal care unit admission, and length of physiological jaundice. The parents are asked to give a detailed history about the patient's Apgar score if possible.

The multidisciplinary team also gathers information regarding the patient's history of:

- Motor milestones development.
- Any significant postnatal events that may have affected the child's growth.
- Activity.
- Exertional dyspnoea.
- Exercise intolerance.
- Failure to gain weight.
- Gastroesophageal reflux.
- Night cough.
- Vomiting or gagging.
- Refusing food.
- Drug history.
- Allergic reactions.
- Urine and stool incontinence.
- Mental state.
- Psychosocial problems.
- School problems encountered.

Pain (onset, course, duration, what increased, and what decreased) as a symptom should be analysed. It is also important to identify similar cases in the family, as some syndromes or neuromuscular disorders may be present in other family members. Spinal deformity analysis is important, as the onset, course and duration of the deformity, previous hospital admission, treatment, and medical comorbidities may help to diagnosis of some syndromes.

The main problem the team encountered in history-taking is that the software and systems needed to connect healthcare providers is not available. Physicians rely on their own computers or patient files to document the related data, which is time-consuming and often does not provide a complete picture, especially if the parents are not cooperative or literate.

PHYSICAL EXAMINATION

A physical examination of patients with EOS deformity is mandatory. This usually requires cooperation between the team of physicians and the patient's family. The physical examination should look for characteristic features of vertebral anomalies, anorectal malformations, congenital cardiac defects, tracheoesophageal anomalies, renal anomalies, and limb defects, as people with three or more of these anomalies are typically diagnosed with VACTREL association.

Once the patient presents, a complete general physical examination is conducted and followed by a local spinal and neurological examination. If the examination reveals abnormal physical signs or increases suspicion of syndromic or congenital pathology, then the EOS team should be consulted. The EOS team members include a paediatric orthopaedic surgeon, spine deformity surgeon, paediatrician, pulmonologist, cardiologist, neurologist, neurosurgeon, nutrition specialist, genetic specialist, physiotherapist, anaesthesiologist, and radiologist.

1. **General Examination (Face, Skin, Chest, Cardiac, Renal, Gastrointestinal)**

The general examination starts by having the patient undress. The patient's face and mouth are examined to see if there are abnormal facial manifestations or a high-arched palate that indicates syndromic manifestation of EOS. Abnormal walking should trigger proper

neurological and other investigations for the child. Physically, the patient's nutritional state, gastrointestinal system, respiratory system, cardiovascular system, endocrinal, neurological, and musculoskeletal system should be evaluated. Some symptoms should encourage the paediatric spine surgeon to address these systems via examination, investigation, and other specialty consultation. This mandates EOS teamwork approach.

Symptoms that warrant respiratory system assessment:

1. Increased respiratory rate.
2. Exertional dyspnoea.
3. Exercise intolerance.
4. Failure to gain weight.
5. Retraction and diaphragmatic breathing.
6. Recurrent chest infection.

Symptoms that warrant consultation from nutrition and paediatrician specialists:

- History of gastroesophageal reflux.
- Vomiting or gagging.
- Night cough.
- Refusing food.
- Anthropometric measures:
  - Weight for age <5th percentile.
  - Body mass index <10th percentile.

If the child is under weight and malnourished, the patient may need a gastrostomy or nasogastric tube for feeding. This is important to help ensure adequate soft tissue coverage for the implants, encourage wound healing, and prevent postoperative complication as infection.

CARDIOLOGICAL ASSESSMENT

A cardiological consultation should be requested in EOS patients and an echocardiogram considered a routine preoperative investigation in the preoperative evaluation [1], especially for patients with

1. Connective tissue disorders, such as Marfan syndrome characterised by ocular, cardiac, and skeletal abnormalities.

2. Neuromuscular scoliosis and myopathy patients [2].
3. Cases with severe curves.
4. Echocardiography confirming that 13.6%–24.4% of patients with idiopathic scoliosis may have valvular anomalies [3].
5. Congenital cases, as 7%–26% have congenital heart disease [4].

Urogenital

Up to 25% of cases with congenital scoliosis have renal problems, such as renal hypoplasia, single kidney, megaureter, horseshoe kidney, pelvic kidney, hypospadias, urethral anomalies, cloacal anomaly, exstrophy of the bladder, and undescended testis [2]. Urinary tract infections, especially in neuromuscular cases, increase the risk of surgical site infection; therefore, consulting with a urologist is a must to assess a child's ability to withstand major correction surgery and can help optimise the child's renal function [5].

Trophic Changes in the Skin

Skin pigmentations, axillary or inguinal freckling, skin scaring, ulcers, skin defects, abnormal skin stigmata, café au lait patches, and soft cystic swellings may indicate neurofibromatosis or meningocele. Neurocutaneous signs of intraspinal pathologies (spinal dysraphism) can appear from history or examination; it is common with congenital cases that these include hairy patches and dimples overlying the spine and may denote the presence of bladder symptoms (Figure 8c.1) [6, 7, 8].

Neurological Examination

EOS cases can be presented with asymptomatic neural axis abnormality (NAA). These NAA may include Arnold-Chiari malformation, syringomyelia, and tethered cord syndrome. Undiagnosed NAA carries the risk of postoperative neurological deficit due to instrumented correction of the deformity [9, 10]. Detailed neurological examination, including information on history of headaches, backaches, and the presence of neurologic signs and symptoms, should be documented.

The sensory, motor, and reflexes neurological examination should be done, noting abdominal

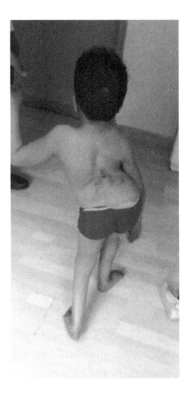

FIGURE 8C.1 Male child 7 years old presented with congenital EOS, coronal imbalance, and skin stigmata; for neural arch defect and flat feet deformity, he flexed knee to compensate.

reflexes and the absence of or unequal bilateral reflexes, such as ankle or knee jerk, as motor or sensory deficits may highlight the presence of intrathecal pathology. Abnormal walking should trigger proper neurological and other investigations for the patient. If there are neurological signs and proved intrathecal anomalies, a neurosurgeon should be consulted for possible early neurosurgical intervention (Figure 8c.2). The preoperative and postoperative neurological state of the EOS child should be documented.

Musculoskeletal Examination

The coronal and sagittal profile of the back should be assessed. In cases with dystrophic neurofibromatosis, sharp, angular, rapidly progressive kyphoscoliosis can be suspected. Limb length discrepancy, equinus, and pelvic obliquity should be properly assessed. A thorough musculoskeletal examination should be conducted, including examination of the hips and feet, to see if there is any hip dysplasia or

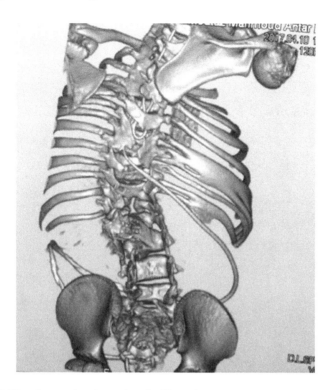

FIGURE 8C.2 CT 3D reformat for the patient in Figure8c.1 after shunt application by neurosurgeon to help the child with Arnold-Chiari malformation, multiple fused ribs, congenital vertebral malformation, and unsegmented bar.

foot deformity. Having the patient perform the Adam's forward bending test and the use of cubes for short limbs will help to assess the patient clinically. Hand and ligamentous laxity need to be assessed to exclude syndromatic cases, and legs and forearms should be examined for dystrophic skeletal changes as anticipated in neurofibromatosis. If the facility does not have a scoliometer, assessment of rib hump may be assessed by appearance, meaning that rotation is more than 30°. Chest expansion is evaluated by measuring chest wall circumference with a tap below the nipple.

It is important to assess the weight, height, spine balance, and rib hump, as these parameters are documented every visit to assess spine growth, deformity progression, and nutritional state. If the patient cannot stand, sitting height can be measured. In limited-resource countries, data archives are rare, so every doctor must document his or her own cases. If possible, patients may be asked to take and save clinical photos using their smart phones to compare them at each visit. The clinical photos include posteroanterior

(PA), anteroposterior (AP), lateral (right- and left-sided) views, and views of the lumbar and thoracic prominences present during an Adam's forward bending test. (Figure 8c.3)

Developmental hip dysplasia has been diagnosed more frequently in patients with early onset idiopathic scoliosis than in normal children. Other skeletal abnormalities with idiopathic EOS include isthmic spondylolisthesis, hereditary exostosis, and slipped capital femoral epiphysis (SCFE) [11]. Sprengel's deformity, upper and lower limb hypoplasia, wasting of one leg, club feet, and other pedal deformities can be associated with congenital EOS [4].

PREOPERATIVE LABORATORY TESTS TO COMPLETE

Laboratory investigations are tailored according to the provisional diagnosis, and the EOS team is involved in the interpretation of these investigations. Complete blood count, alanine transaminase (ALT), serum creatinine, prothrombin time (PT), partial thromboplastin time

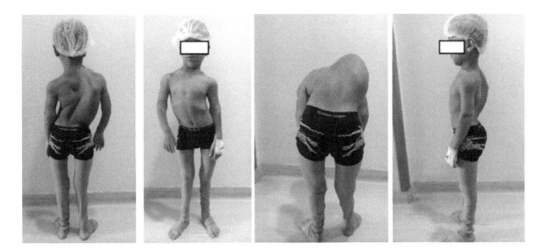

FIGURE 8C.3   Clinical photos PA, AP, Adam's forward bending test, Lateral views of male patient with achondroplasia.

(PTT), international normalised ratio (INR), hepatitis markers, HIV (especially if frequent blood transfusions or previous surgery was done), and morning midstream urine analysis are the author's routine preoperative investigations. Investigations according to certain syndromes could be requested. For the paediatric spine deformity surgeon, taking the preoperative HbA1C for diabetic patients is important. Correction of anaemia and identification of the patient's ABO system should be done preoperatively for possible preparation of blood units.

RADIOLOGICAL INVESTIGATIONS

PLAIN RADIOGRAPHS

Images of the patient standing posteroanterior and lateral should be taken, and both need to span the lower cervical vertebrae to the femoral heads. Preoperative supine right- and left-bending films are mandatory. Fulcrum-bending films are helpful to measure curve flexibility. Traction film can be used to assess curve flexibility. Lead shields is not available, so it is important to limit children's exposure to this ionised radiation from x-rays (**Figure 8c.4**).

MAGNETIC RESONANCE IMAGING

While magnetic resonance imaging (MRI) is not a routine investigation in general, it needs to be done in EOS children because more than 30% have associated spinal dysraphism, such as diastematomyelia, tethered cord syndrome, syringomyelia, and other intrathecal anomalies. Tethered cord is the most common MRI-detected intraspinal anomaly in congenital EOS, syringomyelia is the second, then thickened fatty filum terminal, low-seated conus medullaris, diastematomyelia, intradural lipoma, extradural space occupying lesions, Arnold-Chiari malformation, arachnoid cystic lesions, and Dandy–Walker malformation [4, 12]. Large spinal canal caused by intraspinal tumours or dural ectasia is common, causing vertebral scalloping due to erosion of the ligamentous and bony structures. Meningoceles, pseudo-meningoceles, and dumbbell lesions are related to neurofibroma [14]. Screening by doing whole spine MRI in EOS cases is recommended at the time of presentation, especially with a Cobb angle of more than 20°, even if the findings of the neurological examination are normal [13].

Usually, the child needs sedation or anaesthesia to do such investigations, which may increase economic burden and psychological stress to the family, but it is advisable for congenital curvature. In Egypt, MRI is available and cheaper than developed countries, but the MRI machines may be older. For best results, engage a musculoskeletal radiologist on the team.

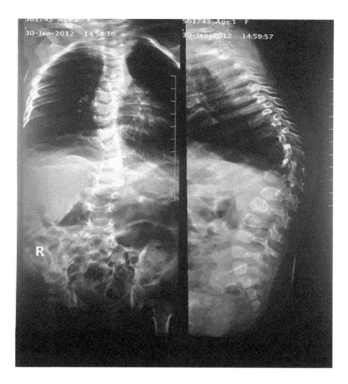

FIGURE 8C.4 Plain x-ray long film of female patient with congenital EOS.

COMPUTERISED TOMOGRAPHY (CT)

Computerised tomography (CT) scans are usually used as a preoperative radiological investigation to assess the bony anatomy. It is indicated in congenital scoliosis to assess vertebral failure of formation or segmentation and pedicle shape. Dural ectasia can be diagnosed in Marfan syndrome through CT by showing anterior meningoceles, wide interpediculate distance, vertebral scalloping, and increased sagittal diameter [3, 15]. Dural ectasia was reported in 63% of Marfan syndrome patients [8].

In scoliosis associated with neurofibromatosis, CT scans are the most sensitive radiological investigative tool to diagnose intraspinal rib dislocation [8]. CT scans can be used to assess pathology at the cervicodorsal junction or at the dorsal spine. If MRI is contraindicated, such as for patients with cochlear implants, the use of intrathecal dye prior to the CT scan may help in diagnosis of intrathecal anomalies. Bone mineral density (BMD) may be requested for patients with osteogenesis imperfect and Marfan syndrome [5]. Pelvic abdominal ultrasound can be used to assess gastrointestinal and renal abnormalities with the help of a radiologist who has experience in that.

CONCLUSION

Taking a full, detailed patient history, family involvement, clinical examination, EOS team consultations, and the results of radiological investigations form the foundation of decision-making for the surgical or nonsurgical treatment plan. Spinal sagittal and coronal alignment should be documented clinically, which should include taking and saving photographs and radiographs of each visit, and should be mandatory for the treatment plan.

Countries with limited resources can manage the preoperative evaluation in a good way according to the available resources. An EOS team and experienced mentors for the spine deformity surgeon should be available. The use of social media and artificial intelligence will help to change medical service. The Khattab EOS checklist can help spine deformity surgeons follow good diagnostic protocol. Developed countries should cooperate and donate new medical technology and medical instrumentation to less developed countries, helping to create a standard of care all over the world.

REFERENCES

1. Basu PS, Elsebaie H, Noordeen MH. Congenital spinal deformity: A comprehensive assessment at presentation. *Spine*. 2002;27(20):2255–9.

2. Ahn NU, Sponseller PD, Ahn UM, et al. Dural ectasia is associated with back pain in Marfan syndrome. *Spine*. 2000;25(12):1562–8.

3. Colomina MJ, Puig L, Godet C, et al. Prevalence of asymptomatic cardiac valve anomalies in idiopathic scoliosis. *Pediatric Cardiology*. 2002;23(4):426–9.

4. Ogilvie JW, Braun J, Argyle V, et al. The search for idiopathic scoliosis genes. *Spine*. 2006;31(6):679–81.

5. Do T, Fras C, Burke S, et al. Clinical value of routine preoperative magnetic resonance imaging in adolescent idiopathic scoliosis: A prospective study of three hundred and twenty-seven patients. *Bone & Joint Surgery*. 2001;83(4):577.

6. Ahn NU, Sponseller PD, Ahn UM, et al. Dural ectasia in the Marfan syndrome: MR and CT findings and criteria. *Genetics in Medicine*. 2000;2(3):173–9.

7. Porter RW. The position of the cerebellar tonsils and the conus in patients with scoliosis. *Journal of Bone & Joint Surgery. (British Volume)*. 2000;82:286.

8. Suh SW, Sarwark JF, Vora A, Huang BK. Evaluating congenital spine deformities for intraspinal anomalies with magnetic resonance imaging. *Journal of Pediatric Orthopaedics*. 2001;21(4):525–31.

9. Gillingham BL, Fan RA, Akbarnia BA. Early onset idiopathic scoliosis. *Journal of the American Academy of Orthopaedic Surgeons*. 2006;14(2):101–12.

10. Inoue M, Minami S, Nakata Y, et al. Preoperative MRI analysis of patients with idiopathic scoliosis: A prospective study. *Spine*. 2005;30(1):108–14.

11. Buttermann GR, Mullin WJ. Pain and disability correlated with disc degeneration via magnetic resonance imaging in scoliosis patients. *European Spine Journal*. 2008;17(2):240–9.

12. Van Karnebeek Naeff MSJ, Mulder BJM, Mulder BJ, et al. Natural history of cardiovascular manifestations in Marfan syndrome. *Archives of Disease in Childhood*. 2001;84(2):129–37.

13. Dobbs MB, Lenke LG, Szymanski DA, et al. Prevalence of neural axis abnormalities in patients with infantile idiopathic scoliosis. *Bone & Joint Surgery*. 2002;84(12):2230–4.

14. Crawford AH, Herrera-Soto J. Scoliosis associated with neurofibromatosis. *Orthopedic Clinics of North America*. 2007;38(4):553–62.

15. Prahinski JR, Polly Jr DW, McHale KA, et al. Occult intraspinal anomalies in congenital scoliosis. *Journal of Pediatric Orthopaedics*. 2000;20(1):59.

8d Principles of Intraoperative Management of Early-Onset Scoliosis

Ashok N. Johari, Rashid Anjum, and Vrushali Ponde

CONTENTS

INTRODUCTION: CAN EARLY-ONSET SCOLIOSIS (EOS) BE MANAGED IN RESOURCE-LIMITED SETTINGS?

The management of early-onset scoliosis (EOS) has seen tremendous advancement in the past decade. EOS is frequently associated with obstructive pulmonary disease and dyspnoea, among others, and these are considered more troublesome than the deformity itself [1, 2]. Thoracic cage abnormalities pose the greatest risk for developing restrictive pulmonary disease [3]. The lung parenchyma and bronchial tree are fully developed by 8 years of age, and by 10-years, thoracic volume is half that of an adult [4, 5]. To allow continued growth of the spine and thorax while controlling progression of deformity, growth-friendly surgical options emerged, such as traditional growing rods, VEPTR (vertical expandable prosthetic titanium rib), and, recently, the magnetically controlled growing rods (MCGR). The goal of treatment in EOS is not only deformity correction, but also allowing continued growth [5, 6]. The recent shift from fusion to fusionless surgery has promised the same, but it is not without complications. Hence, the most important consideration is to have an absolute indication for the surgery prior to evaluation of other parameters. The management of EOS is quite possible in resource-limited conditions, provided the proper preoperative evaluation, intraoperative and post operative management is meticulously undertaken. There should be a proper operative setup (Figure 8d.1) with all the required equipment and personnel for the safe and effective treatment of EOS patients.

PREOPERATIVE CONSIDERATIONS THAT WILL HAVE A BEARING ON INTRAOPERATIVE MANAGEMENT

The preoperative evaluation for patients with EOS comprises of a series of assessments. This is to ensure that the patient is an appropriate candidate for the selected treatment method. A preoperative visit to assess the risk, such as a difficult airway and identification of preexisting pulmonary disease; optimise through physiotherapy and bronchodilator; provide a detailed explanation of the intraoperative wake-up test (very unlikely that neuromuscular monitoring will be implemented in limited-resources setting); and connect with the family is indispensable. History of effort tolerance in terms of the child's playing ability or stamina and the breath-holding time (BHT) should give an apt clinical judgment of the cardiopulmonary reserve. Collection of the complete blood count, cross matching, coagulation profile, and urea electrolytes is mandatory.

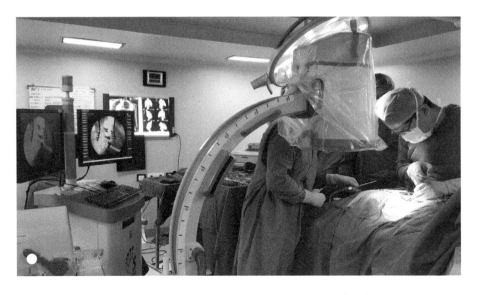

FIGURE 8D.1   A well-equipped operation theatre allows peaceful spine deformity surgery.

RESPIRATORY SYSTEM

The pulmonary system may be the main indication for intervention; therefore, its preoperative status is likely to be impaired in many patients, requiring a chest physician and an anaesthesiologist consultation preoperatively [7]. The most important measure of respiratory system function is a pulmonary function test (PFT) and should be obtained whenever possible; however, it is not possible to perform PFTs in children younger than 5 years of age. A PFT helps to provide objective criteria for active treatment and is well documented as the best prognostic test for postoperative respiratory morbidity. In circumstances in which a PFT cannot be performed, magnetic resonance imaging (MRI) or fluoroscopy to evaluate diaphragm or chest wall movement are important predictors of possible postoperative respiratory status [8]. Adequate measures should be taken to prevent reflux aspiration. A tracheostomy should be considered for patients with anomalies of the cervical spine that limit neck motion, which may make intubation difficult, or have an increased risk of spinal cord compression if occult instability is present.

CURVE TYPE AND CORD STATUS

Preoperative evaluation of the curve type, length, flexibility, and instrument construct is pivotal. Anteroposterior (AP) and lateral x-ray scanogram of the whole spine are needed to describe the curve pattern and sagittal and coronal balance. Bending films are also taken to elicit the flexibility of curve and finalisation of anchor points. The status of the spinal cord is ascertained with an MRI to rule out occult spinal dysraphism (OSD) with intraspinal anomalies such as diastematomyelia and tethering of the cord. If a neurosurgical intervention is required, it is undertaken prior to any planned deformity correction or along with it.

ASSOCIATED CONDITIONS

The patients should be evaluated for any associated anomalies to avoid any last-minute surprises, especially in cases of EOS that include the congenital types as well. Associated cardiac, renal, and other anomalies in congenital scoliosis can be seen in up to a third of cases. Neuraxial abnormalities, including occult spinal dysraphism, is seen in as many as 50% of the cases of congenital scoliosis, whereas its incidence in infantile idiopathic scoliosis is less than 20% [9–10].

NUTRITIONAL STATUS

The next crucial factor in planning is to assess the nutritional status of the patient, as it affects the postoperative recovery and wound healing. Nutritional status is assessed using parameters such as the absolute lymphocyte count, total proteins, haemoglobin, and overall caloric intake. All routine investigations, including coagulation profile, that are required for general anaesthesia must be obtained.

BONE QUALITY

Osteopenia is another important factor that has a bearing on intraoperative events and should be assessed by dual-energy x-ray absorptiometry (DEXA) scan. Osteopenia can be reversed by giving bisphosphonates, or it can point to some underlying metabolic conditions and evaluation thereof. Preoperative administration of bisphosphonates or inclusion of additional vertebrae in the anchor region is recommended in cases of osteopenia.

INTRAOPERATIVE MANAGEMENT

Positioning

The patient are placed in the prone position (Figure 8d.2) on the Jackson table or with padding under the chest and pelvis. The abdomen should be kept free to minimise venous pressure and bleeding from the surgical sites. The use of the reverse-Trendelenburg position at a mild angle aids venous drainage. This also prevents oedema of face, tongue, and eyes due to prolonged prone position. Adequate padding of pressure points such as eyes, face, forehead, elbow, wrists, knees, and ankles with cotton pads or any material available as per the work environment should be used. Each aspect shall have its repercussions in due course. The arms are abducted, and elbows flexed, and a blanket

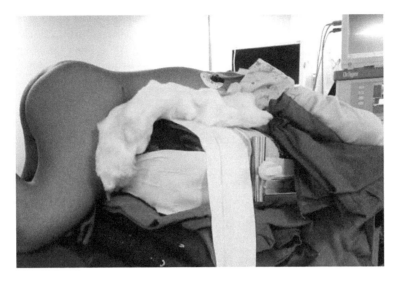

FIGURE 8D.2   Positioning of the patient on bolsters with adequate padding.

or available padding is placed under the thigh and lower leg to keep the knee and ankles off the table. Visual impairment (ischaemic optic neuropathy) as a consequence of increased intraocular pressure is a major concern. Meticulous placement of the face along with the endotracheal tube (ET) in the head rest is crucial.

ANAESTHESIA CONSIDERATIONS

Anaesthesia for EOS in a limited-resource setting is steered by a clear understanding of what is mandatory and otherwise. Thoughtful planning to achieve a hypovascular field while minimising any major complications intraoperatively that result in early extubation is required. This decides 'the must haves' and the so called 'may consider' drugs, equipment and strategies. Interestingly, the medication and anaesthesia equipment that are often deemed mandatory for EOS seem to fit well in a limited-resource environment.

Intravenous access by two large bore IV lines, one on each hand, are enough to run fluids, blood, blood products, and even certain infusions through the drip sets if required (obviates the need for syringe pumps). The central venous access cannulation may be used with discretion. We believe that the radial artery cannulation must be done. The cost consuming transducers and continuous intraoperative invasive arterial monitoring as such can be initiated if required. A cannulated radial artery can be

a ready access for sample collections in case of any eventuality. Strict adherence to fasting guidelines goes a long way in having a well-hydrated and satisfied patient. Tranquilisers, such as oral or intravenous midazolam, antisialogogues, bronchodilators, H2 blocking agents, or proton pump inhibitors may be administered as per their availability. Intraoperatively, cost-effective induction agents, such as thiopentone, propofol, opioids, ketamine, muscle relaxant (whichever is available), could be selected. The cost benefits of expensive inhalational agents, such as sevoflurane and desflurane, should be considered. More economical alternatives, such as isoflurane for maintenance and halothane for induction, are viable and more practisable alternatives. At a minimum, it is mandatory to monitor electrocardiogram (ECG), oxygen saturation (SPO$_2$), end tidal carbon dioxide (ETCO$_2$), and noninvasive blood pressure (NIBP), and by no means should this monitoring be compromised on. An ETCO$_2$ graph can provide a wealth of information about the perfusion status and blood volume [11–12].

ANTIBIOTIC PROPHYLAXIS

The prophylactic antibiotic dose, such as injectable cefuroxime, is given half an hour prior to the incision in the operation room or preoperative ward. The choice of antibiotic depends upon the local hospital policy. The dose is calculated as per the body weight of the child. The antibiotic is repeated if the surgery takes more than 4 hours or there is excessive blood loss.

HYPOTHERMIA PREVENTION

Temperature can be maintained by warming the fluids in a warm water basin or with a simple in-line warmer if available; however, warming blankets are ideal. Electrical heaters, although not very expensive, should be avoided because they may lead to burns, as they do not have a temperature control. The temperature in the operating theatre should be kept comfortable. Hypothermia can deter early extubation and increase cost.

BLOOD-LOSS MANAGEMENT

Scoliosis surgery requires extensive dissection of tissue and, therefore, can cause excessive blood loss. Many centres around the world use autologous blood donations prior to surgery, which removes the risk of transmitted disease as well as any transfusion reaction associated with homologous transfusion [13]. However, the guidelines for the use of autologous blood transfusion are not clear at present. Homologous blood, which is cross matched and arranged prior to the surgery, is generally used.

CELL SAVER SYSTEM

Many centres around the world use a cell saver system to salvage the patient's red cells during surgery with the rationale that it decreases the need for transfusion during scoliosis surgery. The cell saver system is estimated to salvage 40%–50% of red blood cells during spine surgery, the salvage is less in spinal surgery compared to extremity surgery, owing to a lack of blood pooling in the spine and use of a narrow diameter suction tip that results in larger damage of red blood cells. There is conflicting literature on the benefit of using a cell saver system with many surgeons emphasising that it does not reduce the need for transfusions [14, 15]. It can be considered when a heavy blood loss is anticipated. The added cost of the cell saver system, setup, and associated personnel add further to the expenses and, moreover, are not readily available in resource-limited conditions.

HYPOTENSIVE ANAESTHESIA

The blood loss during a scoliosis surgery can be reduced by using a hypotensive anaesthesia technique, which means keeping the mean arterial pressure (MAP) at 65mm Hg. An arterial line is a must if using hypotensive anaesthesia. Hypotensive anaesthesia should not be considered in patients with heart disease or spinal cord compression because of increased risk of ischaemic injury of the spinal cord. Normovolemic haemodilution can also be used to reduce the need for homologous blood transfusion by an experienced anaesthetist. Coagulation cascade can be manipulated by tranexamic acid bolus followed by infusion if available. Simple strategies to minimise intraoperative blood loss other than positioning are dense analgesia with ketamine, opioids, intravenous Mgso4, and lignocaine [12]. A conservative approach toward transfusion is recommended. A drop in Hb to 7 g/dl is well tolerated in otherwise healthy children. A smooth intraoperative course without major fluid shifts and blood loss should result in early recovery.

DRUGS

The most common drug used to reduce blood loss is tranexamic acid, an omega amino carboxylic analogue of lysine and epsilon-aminocaproic acid (EACA), both of which act as antifibrinolytics. Intravenous desmopressin acetate, a synthetic analogue of vasopressin, has been shown to be effective in reducing the blood loss in scoliosis surgery.

NEUROPHYSIOLOGIC MONITORING

Intraoperative spinal cord monitoring is a must in scoliosis surgery (Figure 8d.3). Muscle relaxants are avoided if intraoperative neuromonitoring (NM) is used and anaesthesia is finely balanced with intravenous agents, such as propofol with ketamine infusions, morphine, or fentanyl combined with propofol. A clear communication amongst the surgeons, the NM monitoring team, and the anaesthesiologist is crucial to achieve the best results. Cord monitoring can be accomplished using the Stagnara wake-up test, in which the anaesthesia is lightened or

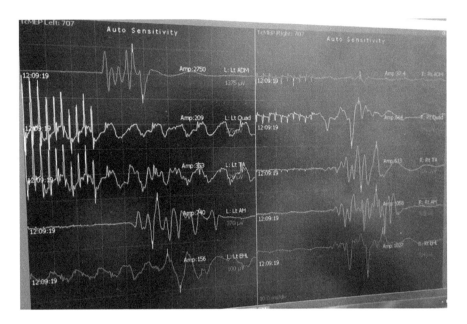

FIGURE 8D.3   Neuromonitoring with SSEP and MEPs has become a standard of care.

reversed to elicit a motor response. It can detect only the active movement of distal extremity to assess motor response and cannot check the sensory system. The test is usually done only once after correction of deformity and cannot be easily repeated, there is possibility of anaesthetic complications as well [16]. In addition to the inherent disadvantages of the wake-up test, the use of a wake-up test in children is not suitable. Neurophysiologic monitoring using somatosensory evoked potentials (SSEP) and motor evoked potentials (MEP) is considered as a standard of care in scoliosis surgery. Preoperative neuromonitoring for a baseline is recorded for intraoperative comparison. Transcranial stimulation of the motor cortex produces an electrical impulse that is carried through the corticospinal tract, terminating in the peripheral muscle where it is recorded. The combination of SSEP and MEP has significantly reduced the frequency of unrecognised spinal cord injury. The available anaesthesia agents used can be fine-tuned to obtain the desired response. The bispectral index (BIS Index) monitor, available as a part of neuromonitoring, can be a good guide to manage this with precision.

Neuromonitoring using SSEP and MEP is very effective in assessing the spinal cord function, but it is not fool proof, and false positive and negative results have been reported in literature. The availability of neuromonitoring in most of the centres in resource-limited conditions is a point of concern, as it has become a standard of care.

FLUID MANAGEMENT

A well-hydrated patient to begin with and intraoperative fluid management guided by real-time clinical monitoring is advisable, including measurement of hourly urine output. Balanced salt solutions, such as Ringer's lactate, is the choice of IV fluid. Ideally, dextrose should be given if hypoglycaemia is documented. It is usual for children to receive 100ml/kg fluid after a prolonged scoliosis surgery.

NEUROLOGICAL INJURY

Neurological injury is the most feared complication for surgeons and patients alike. The most common cause of an intraoperative neurological deficit or injury is rod distraction causing an ischaemic injury of cord, or direct compression by a hook/wire or very low MAP in select patients. It is essential to recognise the high-risk cases, such as congenital kyphosis, skeletal dysplasia, and congenital scoliosis, with the possibility of OSD. Immediate intervention for a deficit is undoing any distraction or correction manoeuvre and adjustment or removal of hook or wire to prevent a permanent neurological injury. The patient's blood pressure and oxygenation should be optimised by the anaesthesiologist, and a wake-up test should be performed in case neuromonitoring is not available. In the past, many surgeons used to administer methylprednisolone, however, there is limited evidence on its role.

TRADITIONAL GROWING RODS

Growth rods are implants used in a technique on the posterior spine in EOS patients that allows continued longitudinal growth of the spine in addition to halting the progression of deformity. It is usually employed when the curve is greater than 60° in a child of less than 10 years of age [17]. A repeat surgery for lengthening is required every 6 months, and the family should be counselled regarding the needed follow-up visits. The complete technique with tricks and pitfalls of single and dual traditional growth rods (TGR) will be discussed elsewhere in the book.

TECHNIQUE AND INTRAOPERATIVE CARE

After positioning the patient, a midline incision is made over the levels that need to be instrumented as per preoperative planning. The proximal and distal foundation sites are exposed and confirmed on radiography for levels. Ideally, one level above and below the planned anchors should be exposed. However, it is crucial to limit the subperiosteal dissection to the foundation vertebrae levels only to avoid any inadvertent fusion. Subcutaneous tissue and fascia are dissected for placement of rod as close to the spine as possible. The distal foundation is prepared first, preferably with pedicle screws, the proximal foundation is prepared next with pedicle screws or laminar hooks (sublaminar/over the top). The size of the rod is selected depending upon the patient aesthetics, generally a 5.5 mm rod (single rod) is used in most children. The length of the rod is measured with a suture and additional length of 5 cm–7cm is added for planned initial distraction and for future

lengthening. The rod is properly contoured and placed, the rods are rotated appropriately to achieve normal sagittal balance, the proximal construct is tightened, and the rod is distracted distally. This step should be done with neurophysiologic monitoring wherever possible or should be followed by a wake-up test. The technique for dual rods mostly remains the same: low profile 4.5 mm rods are cut into four pieces. The rods can be connected by side-to-side connector with an overlap of 5 cm–6 cm for future lengthening or using tandem connectors (Figure 8d.4). The proximal foundation or anchor is made with hooks in a claw fashion, including at least two vertebrae or with pedicle screws. Complete sagittal correction should not be achieved in a single go to avoid anchor breakage. The rods can be tunnelled subfascially if only two incisions are made over proximal and distal foundation sites or under direct vision in case of complete exposure. After locking of rods in the anchors, the tandem connectors or the side-to-side connectors are placed, usually in the thoracolumbar region to maintain the balance, as they are rigid and do not deform easily. The deformity correction and lengthening are performed at this point, taking care of all the necessary precautions. The wound is closed back in layers.

EVIDENCE AND COMPLICATIONS

The largest series of dual growing rods was published by Bess et al. [18]. In their patients, the mean curve severity improved from 82° before surgery to 38° after the first surgery and 36° by final follow-up. A mean of 6.6 lengthenings were required for a T1–S1 increase of 1.2 cm/y, and lung space ratio increased from 0.87 to 1 [18]. Complications are frequent and are related to the prolonged treatment required. A comprehensive analysis of complications reported that 58% of patients had at least one complication, and the complication rate increased by 24% for each additional procedure performed [19]. The complication rate decreased by 13% for each year of increased patient age at treatment initiation. Fewer instrumentation complications were reported in dual rods as opposed to single rods, and more wound complications, prominent implants, and unplanned procedures were

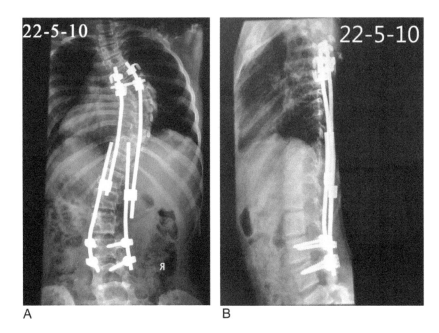

FIGURE 8D.4   A. Postoperative x-rays AP and Lat views of a traditional growth rod insertion. B. The rods are in four parts with overlap and a proximal and distal foundation with side-to-side connectors.

reported in patients with subcutaneous rods than in those with submuscular rods. Wound complications were more frequent when lengthenings were performed at more frequent intervals, whereas implant-related complications occurred more often when lengthenings were performed at longer intervals [17]. Flynn et al. [6] reported that less than half of the patients achieve additional correction and more than 80% had some areas of autofusion, spine stiffness, or a completely fused spine [6]. Sankar et al. [20] reported a 'law of diminishing returns' for repeated lengthening of growing rods, noting progressively less T1–S1 length gain in their 38 patients with subsequent procedures. Their study also mentioned that fusion of the upper thorax, as is performed for the upper growing rod anchors, adversely affected pulmonary function. Hybrid systems utilising standard hooks avoid this fusion by using ribs for anchorage [20]. Skaggs et al. [21] showed that, on average, bilateral hybrid growing rods produced 1.2 cm/y of T1–S1 growth comparable to that found with dual growing rods and superior to that of VEPTR. Suken et al. [22] showed that growth rods had a positive effect on the sagittal vertical axis, which returned the spine to a more neutral alignment through the course of treatment.

Magnetic Growing Rods

The very first magnetic growing rod (MGR) was the Phenix device developed by Jean Dubousset and Arnaud [23] in 2004. Currently MAGEC (Ellipse Technologies, United States) is the only approved device available in United States. The MAGEC includes an implantable rod, a manual distractor, MAGEC magnet locator, and external remote control. The rod consists of an expanded actuator portion housing the magnet, which is 70 mm or 90 mm in length and an additional 5 mm length on either end is nonmalleable.

TECHNIQUE AND INTRAOPERATIVE CARE

The positioning, exposure, and techniques of preparation of proximal and distal foundation points remains the same as it is for TGR (Figure 8d.5).

ROD PLACEMENT AND CONTOURING

The maximum distraction possible with 90 mm and 70 mm actuator is 48 mm and 28 mm

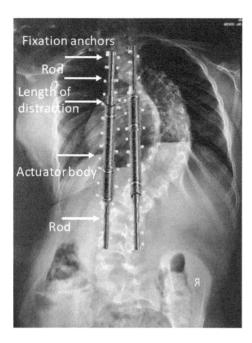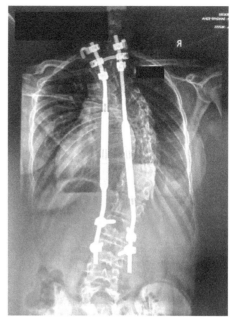

FIGURE 8D.5 Planning and execution for a dual magnetic growth rod.

respectively. A rod template is used to measure the length of the rod, and additional length should be taken keeping in mind the intraoperative distraction and deformity correction. Many surgeons first apply the convex rod temporarily to have a better idea of length. The actuator and 5 mm on either end of rod is nonmalleable and care should be taken to avoid any bending in this area. In small children the short actuator (70 mm) should be used so as to have more rod length available for bending. Bending the rod in small children with congenital scoliosis at junctional regions can be particularly problematic.

ROD TESTING AND ORIENTATION

After contouring but prior to placement of the rods, it is suggested that the rods should be tested for distraction by the MAGEC manual distractor, in which four full counterclockwise rotations are done to confirm proper functioning, followed by three clockwise turns to avoid jamming. In dual rods, both rods can be standard if the surgeon intends to lengthen both the rods simultaneously and in the same direction otherwise a standard and an offset rod can be selected. In any case, both actuators should be at the same level for optimum functioning.

ROD TUNNELLING

Generally, a long clamp is used to make a passage for subfascial tunnelling of the rod, but many surgeons use a chest tube for the same purpose. The concave rod is placed first, especially in single curves, followed by the second rod and they are attached to the proximal anchor maintaining the sagittal balance. The rods are then attached to the lower foundation loosely, and the concave rod is distracted first, followed by the convex rod. The correction, positioning, and sagittal balance is assessed radiographically and confirmed. The wound is closed in layers after thorough washing. The immediate postoperative care and rehabilitation is the same as it is for other techniques and is discussed elsewhere.

EVIDENCE AND COMPLICATIONS

Dannawi et al. [24] reported 34 children (mean age of 8 years) with EOS and a mean Cobb angle of 69° who underwent correction with either single or dual MGR. At a mean follow-up of 15 months, both groups had a statistically significant improvement in mean preoperative, immediate postoperative, and final Cobb angles and a significant increase in the mean T1–S1 distance. No patient developed a postoperative fusion. The complications included superficial infection and rod breakage in two (one in each group), loss of distraction in two (single rod; rectified subsequently), and hook pull-out in one patient with a dual rod. One patient had hardware prominence and required trimming of the rod. Overall, complications were fewer than those that occurred with TGR [21, 22]. Keskinen et al. [25] compared the efficacy of using dual MGR in the primary surgery or during a conversion surgery from a previously placed TGR and found that scoliosis can be equally controlled after conversion from TGR to dual MGR, but the growth from baseline was less in the conversion group. Teoh et al. [26], with the longest follow-up study to date, reported a 43% correction of scoliosis in primary surgeries, whereas it was only 2% in the conversion surgeries, but the curves were maintained at last follow-up. These authors reported that six of eight patients required revision surgeries, four of which were for rod problems and one for proximal junctional kyphosis [26].

There has been an increase of treatment options for young children with scoliosis; however, no single algorithm for treating EOS has been proposed. Small heterogeneous patient populations and regulatory challenges in prospectively studying off-label use of devices have made rigorous clinical research challenging; therefore, comparative effectiveness of various treatment strategies is not well elucidated. Potential adverse outcomes of growth rods or VEPTR for EOS include failure to prevent progression of thoracic insufficiency syndrome, a short or stiff spine, deformed thorax, increased burden of care, and possible negative psychological effects from repeated surgical interventions. Neither technique reliably corrects all deformities over the entire spine during growth. Infections are common to both treatment types. Rod breakage and spontaneous premature spinal fusion beneath rods are troublesome complications in growth rods, and drift of rib attachments and chest wall scarring are possible complications with the use of the VEPTR. The indications for growth rods and VEPTR overlap, but thoracogenic scoliosis and severe upper thoracic kyphosis are best treated by VEPTR and TGR, respectively [15].

REVERSAL AND EXTUBATION

A fast-track recovery with on-table extubation and the minimisation or reduction of time spent in intensive care aids in decreasing the healthcare cost. Good postoperative pain management (POPM) and postoperative nausea vomiting (PONV) management is worthwhile to foster a faster recovery. A multimodal pain management with local anaesthesia (LA) infiltration, NSAIDS, paracetamol, and oral opioids is the way to go. Furthermore, mobilisation, physiotherapy, and pain management complement each other. Availability of resources is as per the circumstances; however, training of the anaesthesiologist to work in limited-resource countries is not. Grooming through real-time hands-on work goes a long way in ensuring patients' safety and pain management.

IMMEDIATE POSTOPERATIVE CARE

The patient should be kept in an intensive care unit for the initial 24–36 hours after surgery with vital monitoring. Postoperative blood profile should be ordered after 24 hours to assessing for the need for transfusion. Postoperative respiratory support in patients with neuromuscular disease, such as spinal muscular atrophy, cerebral palsy, and chest wall or diaphragm dysfunction, must be anticipated. Respiratory system problems are the most common complications seen in the immediate postoperative period. Ventilator support and intermittent positive pressure ventilation may be required. Fluid balance should be monitored carefully and any overload should be avoided, especially in neuromuscular scoliosis patients who have an increased antidiuretic hormone (ADH) secretion leading to oliguria. The need for a brace/cast is decided on a case-by-case basis, depending upon the treatment given, implant used, and quality of bone.

POSTOPERATIVE PAIN MANAGEMENT

Generally, a multimodal approach is preferred, which consists of local anaesthetic infiltration, an indwelling epidural catheter, bilateral erector spinae single shot, catheters with continuous infusion of local anaesthetic, patient-controlled analgesia (PCA) pumps with opioids (if available), injectable paracetamol, and NSAIDS. Furthermore, mobilisation, physiotherapy, and pain management complement each other.

POSTOPERATIVE NAUSEA AND VOMITING

Dexamethasone along with ondansetron is generally enough to address the issue. Pantoprazole avoids the gastric irritation, which may set in from taking NSAIDS. Opioids can increase the incidence explaining the importance of a multimodal approach.

CONCLUSION

In conclusion, the management of EOS can be challenging but quite possible in resource-limited conditions. The importance of an absolute indication for surgery, meticulous preoperative planning, perioperative care of the patient, and an experienced team cannot be discounted. A team approach should be adopted for the care of such children, the positioning of patient and monitoring should be assessed by both the surgeon and anaesthetist to avoid any preventable complications. The need for a well-equipped operating room is ideal, but a setup with the minimum requirements including an experienced anaesthesiologist and surgeon is essential for the optimum care of children with spinal deformity undergoing treatment in developing countries with limited resources and trained manpower.

REFERENCES

1. Nnadi C. *Early Onset Scoliosis.* Stuttgart, Germany: Thieme; 2015.
2. Dimeglio A, Canavese F. The growing spine: How spinal deformities influence normal spine and thoracic cage growth. *Eur Spine J.* 2012;21(1):64–70.
3. Zeltner TB, Burri PH. The postnatal development and growth of the human lung. II. Morphology. *Respir Physiol.* 1987;67(3):269–282.
4. Karol LA, Johnston C, Mladenov K, et al. Pulmonary function following early thoracic fusion in non-neuromuscular scoliosis. *J Bone Joint Surg Am.* 2008;90(6):1272–1281.
5. Johari AN, Maheshwari SK, Nemade A, et al. Management of early onset scoliosis. *Curr Orthop Pract.* 2017;28(1):31–37.
6. Flynn JM, Tomlinson LA, Pawelek J, et al. Growing-rod graduates: Lessons learned from ninety-nine patients who completed lengthening. *J Bone Joint Surg Am.* 2013;95(19):1745–1750.
7. Johnston CE. Preoperative medical and surgical planning for early onset scoliosis. *Spine.* 2010;35(25):2239–2244.
8. Campbell RM Jr. Spine deformities in rare congenital syndromes: Clinical issues. *Spine.* 2009;34(17):1815–1827.
9. Chan G, Dormans JP. Update on congenital spine deformities. Preoperative evaluation. *Spine.* 2009;34(17):1766–1774.
10. Pahys JM, Samdani AF, Betz RR. Intraspinal anomalies in infantile idiopathic scoliosis: Prevalence and role of MRI. Paper presented at: *The 44th Annual Meeting of Scoliosis Research Society*; September 23–26, 2009; San Antonio, TX. Paper number 37.
11. Kulkarni AH, Ambareesha M. Scoliosis and anaesthetic considerations. *Indian J Anaesth.* 2007;51:486–495.
12. Jabbour H, Naccache N, Jawish R, et al. Ketamine and magnesium association reduces morphine consumption after scoliosis surgery: Prospective randomised double-blind study. *Acta Anaesthesiol Scand.* 2014;58(5):572–579.
13. Anand N, Idio JF, Remer S, et al. The effects of perioperative blood salvage and autologous blood donation on transfusion requirements in scoliosis surgery. *J Spinal Disord.* 1998;11(6):532–534.
14. Reitman CA, Watters III WC, Sassard WR. The cell saver in adult lumbar fusion surgery: A cost-benefit outcomes study. *Spine.* 2004;29(14):1580–1583.
15. Weiss JM, Skaggs D, Tanner J, et al. Cell saver: Is it beneficial in scoliosis surgery? *J Child Orthop.* 2007;1(4):221–227. doi:10.1007/s11832-007-0032-6.
16. Chen B, Chen Y, Yang J, et al. Comparison of the wake-up test and combined TES-MEP and CSEP monitoring in spinal surgery. *J Spinal Disord Tech.* 2015;28(9):335–340. doi:10.1097/BSD.0b013e3182aa736d.
17. Johari AN, Nemade AS. Growing spine deformities: Are magnetic rods the final answer? *World J Orthop.* 2017;8(4):295–300. Published 2017 Apr 18. doi: 10.5312/wjo.v8.i4.295.
18. Bess S, Akbarnia BA, Thompson GH, et al. Complications of growing-rod treatment for early-onset scoliosis: Analysis of one hundred and forty patients. *J Bone Joint Surg Am.* 2010;92(15):2533–2543.
19. Akbarnia BA, Asher MA, Bagheri R, et al. *Complications of Dual Growing Rod Technique in Early Onset Scoliosis: Can We*

Identify Risk Factors. Miami, FL: 41st Annual Meeting of the Scoliosis Research Society; 2006.

20. Sankar WN, Acevedo DC, Skaggs DL. *Comparison of Complications among Growing Spinal Implants*. Las Vegas, NV: Annual Meeting of the Pediatric Orthopaedic Society of North America; 2009.

21. Skaggs DL, Myung KS, Yazici M, et al. *Hybrid Growth Rods Using Spinal Implants on Ribs*. Toronto, Canada: The 4th International Congress on Early Onset Scoliosis and Growing Spine; 2010.

22. Shah SA, Karatas AF, Dhawale AA, et al. The effect of serial growing rod lengthening on the sagittal profile and pelvic parameters in early-onset scoliosis. *Spine*. 2014;39(22):E1311–E1317.

23. Arnaud S, Lotfi M, Jacques G, et al. A technical report on the Phenix m-rod, an expandable rod linkable to the spine, ribs or the pelvis and controllable at home by hand through the skin with a palm size permanent magnet. *J Child Orthop*. 2009;3(2):145–168.

24. Dannawi Z, Altaf F, Harshavardhana NS, et al. Early results of a remotely-operated magnetic growth rod in early-onset scoliosis. *Bone Joint J*. 2013;95-B(1):75–80.

25. Keskinen H, Helenius I, Nnadi C, et al. Preliminary comparison of primary and conversion surgery with magnetically controlled growing rods in children with early onset scoliosis. *Eur Spine J*. 2016;25(10):3294–3300.

26. Teoh KH, Winson DMG, James AH, et al. Magnetic controlled growing rods for early-onset scoliosis: A 4 year follow up. *Spine J*. 2016; 16(4 Suppl):S34--S39.

8e Postoperative Management for EOS Children

Kaustubh Ahuja, Bhavuk Garg

CONTENTS

INTRODUCTION

Surgical management of early-onset scoliosis (EOS) includes growth-friendly nonspine fusion surgeries. As stated by Skaggs et al. [1], growth-friendly spine implant systems fall into three categories. First, and the most widely used implant systems, are the distraction-based growing implants, including traditional growth rods, vertically expandable prosthetic titanium rib prosthesis (VEPTR), and magnetic-controlled growth rods (MCGR). Next are the compression-based growth modulation systems, including stapling and tethering techniques. The third category is the growth guidance systems, including the SHILLA procedure and Luque Trolleys. Postoperative management and rehabilitation of the patients after these complex surgical procedures is of extreme importance, not only from a medical perspective, but also from a mental and social standpoint. Postoperative management of these patients begins as early as the patient is turned supine after surgery, till complete rehabilitation and restoration of near preoperative functional status. The postoperative period can be divided into three phases on the basis of time since primary intervention and management priorities.

- Immediate postoperative period: from Postoperative Day 0 (POD 0) until discharge from hospital.
- Early postoperative period: from discharge to 3 months.
- Late postoperative period: from 3 months to 1 year.

Apart from certain postoperative considerations specific to some procedures, general postoperative management principles remain more or less the same for all the surgical techniques.

IMMEDIATE POSTOPERATIVE PERIOD

The immediate postoperative period is the most crucial period after a scoliosis surgery. Optimum management during this period is paramount to improve function outcome by facilitating early rehabilitation while reducing postoperative morbidity and complications. Although, the majority of patients who undergo surgery for EOS are extubated immediately, some patients with associated congenital abnormalities or syndromic affections may need intensive care support. The major emphasis in the immediate postoperative period lies in maintaining haemodynamic stability, pain management, preventing avoidable perioperative complications, and early mobilisation and rehabilitation. 'Accelerated discharge' (AD) protocols have replaced the traditional discharge pathways in most of the major centres aimed at early mobilisation, transition to oral analgesics and oral feeding, and early discharge from the hospital. AD pathway implementation has shown significant reduction in the economic burden on the family with no significant increase in complication rate [2, 3]. AD protocols must be formulated in accordance with the available hospital resources and accessibility for follow-up (Table 8e.1).

EOS comprises of a variety of different diagnoses ranging from idiopathic to congenital to syndromic patients with significant systemic affections making this population susceptible to perioperative complications. Recognising these patients and being proactive can significantly reduce postoperative morbidity.

Haemodynamic Recovery

Patients undergoing spine surgery for scoliosis are at a high risk for haemodynamic compromise due to perioperative blood loss, hypothermia, and deleterious effects of prone positioning. Moreover, because of preexisting restrictive pulmonary disease, associated cardiac abnormalities, and young age, even a small amount blood loss may lead to severe haemodynamic compromise. A number of authors have reported the presence of left ventricular hypertrophy in patients with EOS, leading to hypotension and arrythmias on prone positioning [4]. In the postoperative period, samples for complete blood count, renal function test, and electrolytes should be taken for all patients. Arterial blood gas analysis should be kept reserved for patients needing intensive care (ICU) or high dependency unit (HDU) support.

The threshold level of postoperative haemoglobin for blood transfusion varies according to the hospital guidelines [5, 6]. Rouette et al. [6] compared blood transfusion in patients with postoperative haemoglobin level 9.5 gm versus 7 gm and reported comparable results in terms

of 28-day mortality and organ system dysfunction. In fact, longer hospital stays were recorded in patients with transfusion at higher thresholds. The authors recommend a packed red blood cell (RBC) transfusion when postoperative haemoglobin is less than 8 gm or packed cell volume is less than 24. Maintaining adequate mean arterial blood pressure during the postoperative period by administration of crystalloids and adequate blood products is important to avoid complications such as prerenal failure. On the other hand, overhydration may lead to complications such as pulmonary oedema and electrolyte abnormalities. Therefore, in the immediate postoperative period, kidney function should be monitored closely with urine output and daily fluid requirement should be calculated accordingly.

Pain Management

Inadequate pain management can lead to significant haemodynamic disturbance and poor postoperative recovery. A suitable balance between adequate pain management and minimal adverse effects of various pharmacological agents is essential for optimal clinical outcome. Therefore, most authors suggest the use of multiple analgesic agents concurrently. Multimodal pain management includes the use of intravenous (IV) acetaminophen, NSAIDs, narcotics in the form of patient-controlled anaesthetic pumps (PCA), or intrathecal morphine, intravenous benzodiazepines, and continuous epidural analgesia [7–10]. Recently, the use of erector spinae block has significantly reduced the analgesic requirement on the first postoperative day (POD 1). AD protocols advocate the usage of morphine via PCA and intravenous benzodiazepines on POD 0 with or without gabapentin and ketorolac [11]. All intravenous analgesics are discontinued on POD 1 once the patient starts accepting oral feeds while intravenous narcotics are kept reserved for cases in which pain is inadequately managed with oral acetaminophen and tramadol (Table 8e.1).

In a retrospective study comparing PCA with intrathecal morphine injection and continuous epidural infusion, Milbrandt et al. [8] concluded that PCA with intrathecal injection provides the best pain management with minimal adverse effects. The author's choice of regimen for pain management includes PCA and

TABLE 8E.1
Accelerated Discharge Protocol

POD 0

- Check for any injury (including eye) due to positioning as soon as patient is turned supine.
- Check for neurological status as soon as patient is extubated.
- Maintenance fluid and supplemental oxygen to continue overnight to maintain Spo2 above 95 and mean arterial pressure above 70.
- Head end elevation to 30° in postoperative room.
- Send blood samples for complete blood count, renal function tests. and serum electrolytes.
- Incentive spirometry every 2 hours when awake.
- Intravenous morphine via PCA pump and 1000 mg intravenous acetaminophen every 8 hours.
- Oral gabapentin 75 mg starting from the night of the surgery.
- Intravenous cefixime 200 mg twice a day until POD 2
- DVT prophylaxis with DVT pumps.
- PT assisted sitting in a PVC custom-fit brace if tolerated.
- Clear fluids 6 hours after surgery followed by juices and coconut water.
- If well digested, semisolid food including mashed potatoes, bananas, or lentil soup for dinner.
- Transfusion considered if postoperative haemoglobin is less than 8 gm %

POD 1

- Start normal breakfast if no nausea.
- Discontinue intravenous fluids once accepting well orally.
- Discontinue PCA. Switch to intravenous tramadol with acetaminophen.
- Fentanyl/Morphine to be kept reserved for breakthrough doses.
- Urinary catheters to be removed.
- PT assisted standing/walking with brace.
- Bed to chair transfer three times a day, preferably after every meal.
- Commence using toilets for urination and defecation.
- Postoperative radiographs after ambulation.

POD 2

- Discontinue all intravenous medications.
- Start oral acetaminophen and tramadol.
- Intravenous morphine/fentanyl kept for breakthrough doses.
- Wound dressing and evaluation.
- Remove drain.
- Unassisted walking and standing with the help of parents and PT.
- Assisted stair climbing.
- Start laxatives if incontinence.

POD 3

- Parent education, training, and counselling.
- Evaluation of the patient for fitness of discharge.

intravenous acetaminophen on POD 0, intravenous acetaminophen and tramadol on POD 1, and switching to oral pain medications on POD 2 (Table 8e.1).

Minimising Complications

Patients undergoing surgery for EOS are at an increased risk of pulmonary, urinary, and haematological complications. Longer duration of surgery, preexisting hepatorenal compromise, higher American Society of Anaesthesiologists (ASA) grade, and patients with cognitive impairment are at a higher risk for postoperative complications and longer hospital stays [12, 13]. Wenger et al. [14] recommended measures to reduce these complications during hospital stay. Head end elevation to 30° starting from the night of surgery for better lung expansion, frequent use of incentive spirometry, and steam inhalation can significantly reduce the pulmonary complications. Removal of urinary catheters, wound site drains and central lines, and having a low threshold for aspirating wound site haematomas or collections while maintaining strict asepsis have proven beneficial in reducing iatrogenic urinary tract and surgical site infections (SSI). For early identification of SSIs six hourly temperature readings should be charted with early wound inspection and dressing on POD 2 is important. Persistence of pyrexia more than 39° beyond POD 2 warrant search for an infective focus or SSIs. The need for formulation a protocol for postoperative days cannot be overemphasised for proper implementation of the above-mentioned recommendations (Table 8e.1).

Switching to Oral Diet

Early switching to oral diet is beneficial for promoting gut motility, providing essential nutrients, and allowing the surgeon to prescribe oral pain medications. AD pathways generally recommend clear fluids and juices on the day of surgery itself and switching to a normal oral diet on the following day. Ileus is a common complication following spine surgery. Colonic motility takes the longest to return and can be improved by oral laxatives [15]. Aggressive and well-planned oral feeds is an essential factor in reestablishing gut motility. Early switching to oral medications also helps in removal of the intravenous lines and PCA, which improves the general outlook of the patient and promotes early mobilisation. Additionally, oral medications have longer half-life and fewer adverse effects compared to intravenous analgesics [11]. Clear fluids are recommended as early as 6 hours following surgery. If this is tolerated well, gradual stepping up to juices and semisolid food, including mashed banana and lentil soup on the night of surgery and a complete balanced meal on the following morning is the recommended practice.

Early Mobilisation

Early mobilisation is the key to optimal surgical outcome [16, 17]. Postoperative pain management, reduction of perioperative complications, and early oral feeding are important prerequisites for early mobilisation and rehabilitation, and their benefits are mutually reinforcing. Early mobilisation, in turn, reduces pulmonary complications, improves gut motility, promotes self-dependence and confidence, and improves the general outlook of the patient, thus leading to a faster transition to 'normalcy'.

A multidisciplinary approach is followed at most centres combining the surgeons, physicians, physical medicine and rehabilitation (PMR) specialists, and physical therapists for a planned rehabilitation protocol. Patients can be assisted to sit at the bedside in a polyvinyl chloride (PVC) brace on the POD 1 for as long as the patient tolerates. Once comfortable, patients are made to stand with support and assisted with bed to chair transfers. In-bed mobilisation and passive and active joint mobilisation is continued for the entire duration the patient is in bed. Walking in a brace with support begins on the POD 2 followed by stair training and unsupported walking on POD 3 (Table 8e.1).

Early Postoperative Period

This period begins from the discharge of the patient from the hospital to 3 months following surgery. In a normal surgery without any complications, AD protocols recommend discharge on the third or fourth postoperative day irrespective of bowel motility. In a resource-limited setting, the hospital stay may have to be increased in cases with poor accessibility to health services. The early postoperative period aims to regain the spinal mobility while still protecting the instrumentation. Optimal functional outcome depends on adequate rehabilitation in the early postoperative period.

Patients are commonly discharged on oral analgesic medications including acetaminophen, tramadol, pregabalin, and, in some cases with inadequate analgesia, ketorolac patches. Discharging patients on 1000mg of acetaminophen every 8 hours and 50mg of tramadol every 12 hours is recommended. Patients are usually called for their first follow-up around the 14th day for suture removal. After the first 2 weeks, the majority of the patients are prescribed analgesics only if required.

The major emphasis in the early postoperative period is early and full-time return to school and daily activities while providing maximum protection to spine. Most patients return to school part time at the end of 6 weeks and full time at the end of 10 weeks [15]. After discharge, rehabilitation advice is usually sought on an out-patient basis. The following activities are recommended in the early postoperative period supported by an orthosis (**Figures 8e.1, 8e.2,** and **8e.3**).

• Standing up from bed – For transfer, hips and knees are bent to 90° and body is made to rotate such that the legs dangle at the edge of the bed. With the help of arms and hands, the patient then lifts his or her body into sitting and then standing position.

• Leaning forward – In order to pick up an object, the patient is taught first to bend the knees down for lesser strain on the back.

• Sitting – Sitting on a high, firmly cushioned chair with waist support is preferred. The duration of sitting should be gradually increased as tolerated by the patient with brief intervals of walking in between.

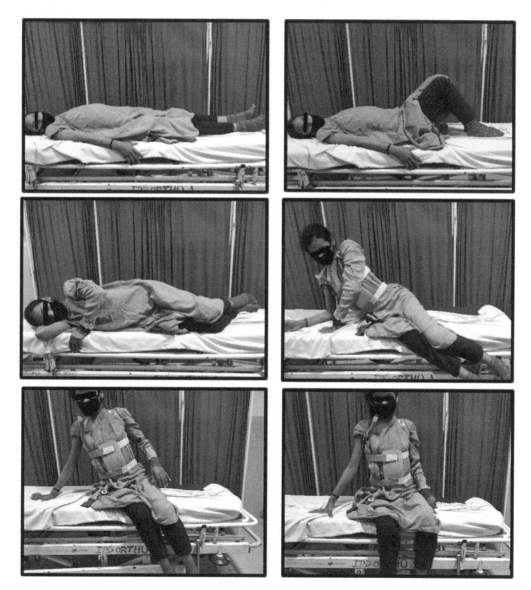

FIGURE 8E.1   Sitting up from lying down position.

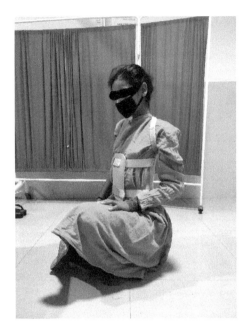

FIGURE 8E.2 Picking up an object from the ground.

- Standing from sitting – While standing from sitting position, the patient is taught to slide to the edge of the chair followed by transferring the weight on his or her legs gradually without leaning forward too much. Patients may need assistance with this for the first 2 weeks.
- Going to bathroom and toilet – Patients need assistance while going to the bathroom and the toilet in the first few weeks. Use of supporting railings while sitting on the toilet seat or while in a shower significantly unload the spine and help bear the stress.
- Climbing stairs – In the first 2 weeks, the patients are assisted while climbing stairs followed by independent stair climbing one step at a time in the next 2 weeks.

Follow-up visits occur on a monthly basis after the initial visit. Most surgeons recommend orthosis until 6 months after surgery, as most intended fusion levels at the top and bottom end of instrumentation fuse by 6 months.

LATE POSTOPERATIVE PERIOD

The late postoperative period is an extension of the early postoperative period. By the end of the early postoperative period, the patient is expected to do most of the activities of daily life unassisted. The late postoperative period serves to build on the attained activity level in the first 3 months and aims at regaining strength, flexibility,

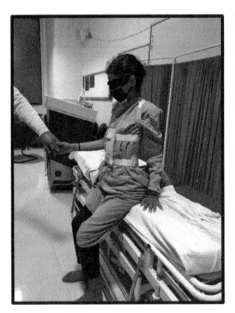
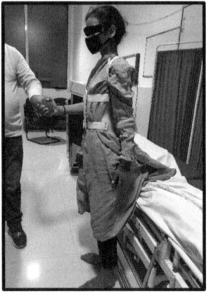

FIGURE 8E.3 Standing up from sitting position.

and self-confidence. Also, patients managed with growing rods or VEPTR may have to undergo their first distraction during this period.

Special Considerations

Growth-friendly implants, including traditional growing rods, magnetically controlled growing rods, and VEPTR need repeated lengthening to accommodate for increases in the length of the spine. The current trend is to perform lengthening every 4 months in very small children, every 6 months in patients from 4 to 10 years of age and every 9 months if the instrumented spine segment is short [18]. Distraction procedures for traditional growth rods are conducted using general anaesthesia by distracting between rod holder and domino when using side-to-side connectors or between rods when using a tandem connector. Apart from frequent exposure to radiation and general anaesthesia, other complications include metallosis, autofusion, and neurological complications. Magnetically controlled growth rods offer a significant advantage by avoiding repeated exposure to general anaesthesia, as it is an out-patient procedure. Additionally, the frequency of distraction is not dictated by limitation of resources, occupational therapy (OT) slots, or general anaesthesia exposure. However, distraction frequency of greater than 2 months is associated with higher reoperation rate. Also, complications seen with traditional growth rods can be present with magnetic growth rods too.

VEPTR is indicated in cases with thoracic insufficiency syndrome due to spinal and thoracic deformities. Active phase of VEPTR include serial expansion surgeries until skeletal maturity is reached.

CONCLUSION

Young age, limited bone stock, pulmonary considerations, and associated congenital and syndromic affections make postoperative management an extremely crucial part of the surgical management of patients with EOS. Each institute should have well-formed guidelines for perioperative management of these patients in accordance with the available resources within the institute. Early mobilisation and rehabilitation is important for AD protocols. In countries with limited resources, AD protocols may limit expenses in the postoperative period while reducing the risk of hospital-acquired infections at the same time.

REFERENCES

1. Skaggs DL, Akbarnia BA, Flynn JM, et al. A classification of growth friendly spine implants. *J Pediatr Orthop.* 2014;34(3):260–74.
2. Fletcher ND, Andras LM, Lazarus DE, et al. Use of a novel pathway for early discharge was associated with a 48% shorter length of stay after posterior spinal fusion for adolescent idiopathic scoliosis. *J Pediatr Orthop.* 2017;37(2):92–7.
3. Sanders AE, Andras LM, Sousa T, et al. Accelerated discharge protocol for posterior spinal fusion patients with adolescent idiopathic scoliosis decreases hospital postoperative charges 22. *Spine.* 2017;42(2):92–7.
4. Soliman DE, Maslow AD, Bokesch PM, et al. Transoesophageal echocardiography during scoliosis repair: Comparison with CVP monitoring. *Can J Anaesth J Can Anesth.* 1998;45(10):925–32.
5. Fletcher ND, Marks MC, Asghar JK, et al. Development of consensus based best practice guidelines for perioperative management of blood loss in patients undergoing posterior spinal fusion for adolescent idiopathic scoliosis. *Spine Deform.* 2018;6(4):424–9.
6. Rouette J, Trottier H, Ducruet T, et al. Red blood cell transfusion threshold in postsurgical pediatric intensive care patients: A randomized clinical trial. *Ann Surg.* 2010;251(3):421–7.
7. Klatt JWB, Mickelson J, Hung M, et al. A randomized prospective evaluation of 3 techniques of postoperative pain management after posterior spinal instrumentation and fusion. *Spine (Phila Pa 1976).* 2013;38(19):1626–31.
8. Milbrandt TA, Singhal M, Minter C, et al. A comparison of three methods of pain control for posterior spinal fusions in adolescent idiopathic scoliosis. *Spine.* 2009;34(14):1499–503.
9. Blanco JS, Perlman SL, Cha HS, et al. Multimodal pain management after spinal surgery for adolescent idiopathic scoliosis. *Orthopedics.* 2013;36(2 Suppl):33–5.
10. Seki H, Ideno S, Ishihara T, et al. Postoperative pain management in patients undergoing posterior spinal fusion for adolescent idiopathic scoliosis: A narrative review. *Scoliosis Spinal Disord.* 2018;13(1):1–14.
11. Borden TC, Bellaire LL, Fletcher ND. Improving perioperative care for adolescent idiopathic scoliosis patients: The impact of a

multidisciplinary care approach. *J Multidiscip Healthc.* 2016;9:435–45.

12. Pugely AJ, Martin CT, Gao Y, et al. The incidence and risk factors for short-term morbidity and mortality in pediatric deformity spinal surgery: An analysis of the NSQIP pediatric database. *Spine.* 2014;39(15):1225–34.

13. Basques BA, Bohl DD, Golinvaux NS, et al. Patient factors are associated with poor short-term outcomes after posterior fusion for adolescent idiopathic scoliosis. *Clin Orthop.* 2015;473(1):286–94.

14. Wenger DR, Mubarak SJ, Leach J. Managing complications of posterior spinal instrumentation and fusion. *Clin Orthop.* 1992;284:24–33.

15. Nachlas MM, Younis MT, Roda CP, et al. Gastrointestinal motility studies as a guide to postoperative management. *Ann Surg.* 1972;175(4):510–22.

16. Sanders JO, Haynes R, Lighter D, et al. Variation in care among spinal deformity surgeons: Results of a survey of the shriners hospitals for children. *Spine.* 2007;32(13):1444–9.

17. Leider LL, Moe JH, Winter RB. Early ambulation after the surgical treatment of idiopathic scoliosis. *J Bone Joint Surg Am.* 1973;55(5):1003–15.

18. Akbarnia BA, Emans JB. Complications of growth-sparing surgery in early onset scoliosis. *Spine.* 2010;35(25):2193–204.

8f Principles of Management of Long-Term Complications in EOS

Meric Enercan, and Azmi Hamzaoglu

CONTENTS

INTRODUCTION

Early-onset scoliosis (EOS) in very young children is an extremely difficult problem that requires thorough knowledge of normal spine development as well as the aetiology, natural history, clinical evaluation, and available treatment options. Unlike adolescent spinal deformity, untreated progressive deformity can cause significant health problems for young children and later in their adult life [1, 2].

EOS is often associated with other comorbid conditions, and this increases the complexity in managing the spinal deformity. The management of EOS requires consideration of inter-related growth of spine and thorax and their impact on the lung development. The spine grows most rapidly in the first 5 years, with an average T1–S1 segment length increase of 10 cm during this time (>2 cm/year) followed by a deceleration to 0.5 cm/year between 6 to 10 years of age and increases again during adolescent growth spurt (2 cm/year). The number of alveoli and lung volume also increase most rapidly in the first several years, and the total alveoli number completes development by 8 years of age [3, 4]. The progressive early-onset spinal deformity occurs during this critical time of lung development and may result in pulmonary dysfunction and cardiopulmonary compromise. Early recognition and proper treatment is essential for the management of EOS deformity [5,6].

The main goals of the treatment of EOS are to obtain and maintain curve correction while simultaneously preserving the spinal, trunk, and lung growth. Treatment options include conservative treatment and surgical interventions. Surgical treatment should be considered for patients with progressive deformity when cast or brace treatment have failed or is contraindicated [1, 2, 7].

Surgical treatment options include early definitive surgery or temporary surgery. Early definitive fusion before the age of 10 endangers thoracic growth and pulmonary functions and may not prevent the progression of deformity, development of crankshaft phenomenon, and/or thoracic insufficiency syndrome [5, 6, 8].

Many nonfusion options have been proposed, and various types of spinal implants have been used to control deformity while allowing spinal and thoracic growth in immature spines. Although growth potential is preserved in growth-friendly surgeries, complications are a common and inevitable part of the surgical treatment [9, 10, 11]. Complications increase the financial burden of the healthcare system and this can be even more challenging in resource-limited settings. Dealing with the challenges of EOS treatment requires a long-term commitment by the surgeon, the family, and the healthcare system.

Skaggs et al. [12] had classified these systems into three categories based on the forces of correction: distraction-based systems, compression-based systems, and guided-growth systems.

DISTRACTION-BASED SYSTEMS

Distraction-based implants are the most common devices used in EOS. Moe et al. [13] first described the distraction-based growing rod system in 1984. Four types of implants have been used: the traditional growing rod (TGR), vertical expandable prosthetic titanium rib (VEPTR) device, hybrid systems, and magnetically controlled growing rod (MCGR). With the development of dual rods, strong upper and lower anchors, and expandable connectors, TGR became a powerful tool and gold standard in the treatment of EOS. Several studies have shown growing rods to be effective for achieving spinal length increase on the immature spine [14, 15]. Regardless of the implant used for distraction-based treatment of the growing spine, all strategies have their own disadvantages and are associated with high complication rate [7].

The main disadvantage of distraction-based implants is the lack of apical and intermediate anchors along the main curve. These systems try to correct the spinal deformity by applying distractive forces across the apical segments of the deformity between proximal and distal anchors. As anterior spinal growth continues in the immature spine, rotational deformity at the apical and intermediate segments will continue to progress. Because there are no apical and intermediate anchors along the main curve, correction and control of the main deformity will be limited during treatment [16]. Xu et al. [17] evaluated the effects of TGR on apical vertebra rotation (AVR) using computerised tomography (CT) scans. They reported significant AVR can be achieved after inital surgery; however, TGR could not prevent progression of AVR during long-term follow-up [17].

Another limitation of the distraction-based systems is the need for multiple surgeries for repeated lengthening procedures. The rods are periodically lengthened as the child grows to maintain spine curve correction every 6 to 8 months [14, 15]. The length gained from serial lengthening has also been shown to follow a law of diminishing returns, with decreased spinal length gained after each lengthening [18]. The prolonged immobilisation between lengthening intervals creates a static fixation and may result in autofusion after repeated lengthenings [19]. The utility of lengthening may decrease significantly after the sixth or seventh lengthening procedure, limiting the potential spinal growth to 4–5 years after initial surgery. Multiple surgeries for repeated lengthening procedures require repeated exposure to general anaesthesia. In addition to the physical effects on the spine, repetitive surgeries leads to increased anxiety and significant psychological effects on the patient. Patients with repeated surgery demonstrate abnormal psychosocial scores with a positive correlation between behavioural problems and the number of repetitive surgeries [20].

TGRs are associated with a high complication rate. Implant failure, rod breakage, junctional kyphosis, spontaneous fusion, wound problems, and infection are the most common complications of TGRs [21]. The overall complication rate of TGRs can occur in 58%–86% with a 20% procedural complication rate. Forty percent of these complications required treatment with an unplanned procedure [22]. Another study demonstrated that each lengthening surgery increases the risk of deep infection 3.3 times in EOS [23]. Upasani et al. [24] tried to identify the preoperative factors that contribute to complications in 110 EOS patients treated with TGR. They reported that 79% of the patients had complications resulting in 84 unplanned surgeries. The most common complications were implant-related (49%), surgical site infection (23%), medical (19%), alignment (6%), and neurologic (3%). Earlier age at implantation, greater thoracic kyphosis (>40°), and larger major curves (>85°) increased the probability of complications following TGR [24].

Management of the long term complications is challenging. Optimal treatment strategy should minimise the complications that lead to unplanned surgical interventions and minimise the psychological effects on the patient and decrease the total cost of treatment and financial burden on the healthcare system.

MAGNETICALLY CONTROLLED GROWING RODS

Magnetically controlled growing rods (MCGR) were designed as an alternative to TGR to eliminate the need for repeated surgical lengthenings and minimise the total number of exposures to anaesthesia in EOS. Lengthenings can be performed on an outpatient basis without any anaesthesia [25, 26]. But similar biomechanical concerns are valid for MCGR because there are no apical and intermediate anchors along the main curve. Also, application of magnetically controlled telescopic rods may be problematic in deformities with severe kyphosis. In a systemic review, Thakar et al. [27] reported a more than 44% complication rate and a 33% unplanned reoperation rate for MCGR. The majority of the complications were implant related complications [27]. Magnetic rods are bulky and can cause skin problems in small children. The cost of the MCGR is significant because of the manufacturing cost of its internal magnet/actuator as compared to simpler or homemade constructs used for TGRs. Cost analysis showed that cost neutrality of MCGR to TGR was achieved over the 6-year episode. [28, 29].

GROWTH GUIDANCE SYSTEM

Recently, McCarthy et al. [30, 31] developed Shilla growth guidance system (GGS), an alternative construct for management of EOS. GGS is a new growth-sparing technology that helps provide deformity correction while allowing continued skeletal growth at the proximal and distal construct ends and obviating the need for periodic lengthening procedures. The apex of deformity is fixed with pedicle screws and fused, while the ends of the construct are instrumented with screws that are not locked to a rod. The nonlocking set screw allows the pedicle screws to slide along the rod axis during vertical growth. GGS has demonstrated clinical effectiveness in both curve correction and increasing thoracic height with similar 5-year follow-up [30, 31]. Although the GGS method resulted in a 73.4% reduction in the number of surgical procedures, the complication rate remained high (73%). GGS would be expected to reduce overall costs per patient in a similar

manner to MCGR. GGS resulted in fewer invasive surgeries and deep surgical site infections than TGR. Luhman et al. used an economic model for cost analysis to compare GGS with TGR and MCGR. GGS showed lower total costs per patient than both MCGR and TGR over a 6-year period [32]. However, this technique requires a special design instrumentation set that is expensive and more costly than a standard spine instrument set. Also fusing the apex of the deformity, which is generally located at the thoracic spine, may have a negative impact on pulmonary functions, may result in a short trunk height, and may cause sagittal alignment problems in the long-term follow-up.

To overcome problems related to distraction-based systems, we introduced a new surgical strategy called self-sliding growth guidance (SSGG) technique, which aims to provide and maintain satisfactory curve corrections on all planes, allow self growth of the spine, and preserve trunk and lung growth. We developed a dynamic fixation system instead of static fixation using distraction-based systems that can be performed with any regular spine instrumentation set. We modified the TGR technique and used apical and intermediate anchors with multisegmenter pedicle screw fixation at strategic vertebras in addition to proximal and distal anchors to provide better correction and control of the main curve in coronal, sagittal, and axial planes to prevent progression of deformity. Multiple anchors and fixation points will share and resist againts the deformitive and rotational forces, and this will eventually decrease the rate of implant-related complications. Connecting the rods using domino connectors and keeping the set screws unlocked (loosely captured) between the most proximal and the most distal fixed and fused anchors will create a dynamic fixation. This dynamic fixation will decrease the rate of spontaneous fusion, the number of repeated lenghtenings, and related complications in the long-term follow-up.

PREFERRED TECHNIQUE

After induction of anaesthesia, a traction radiograph under general anaesthesia was performed to assess curve flexibility and determine strategic vertebae. Then a Gardner-Wells tong apparatus was applied to the skull, and Steinmann pins were placed on each supracondylar femur to prepare for intraoperative skull-femoral traction that would facilitate correction during the initial procedure, provide additional flexibility, decrease the need for forceful correction maneuvers on immature the spine, and prevent possible implant failures (Figure 8f.1). Intraoperative skull-femoral traction was used only at the initial procedure to facilitate correction of the deformity. Traction was initiated with approximately 20% of the body weight of the patient in kilograms and gradually increased during the surgery. Maximum applied traction was limited to 40% of the patient's body weight in kilograms to avoid any neurological deficit resulting from excessive and sudden traction. Only initial procedures were performed under spinal monitoring. Skull-femoral traction was halted immediately if there was any signal loss that exceeded more than 20%–30% of the initial measurements.

After the skin incision, subcutaneous tissue dissection was carried out carefully without any subperiosteal dissection, and polyaxial pedicle screws were placed into the strategic vertebrae under fluoroscopic guidance with a muscle-sparing technique without exposing any posterior elements and facet joint violation. Pedicle screws were placed to the apical, end, intermediate, and transitional zone vertebrae (Figure 8f.2). To avoid any dorsal bulkiness, cervical or paediatric pedicle screw instrumentations were preferred for fixation according to patient size.

After giving proper sagittal contours, proximal and distal rods were placed, and deformity

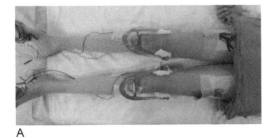

A

FIGURE 8F.1   A: Pins were placed on supracondylar femur for intraoperative traction.

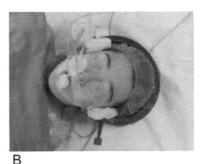

B

FIGURE 8F.1   B: Gardner-Wells tong was placed for intraoperative traction.

was corrected with cantilever correction maneuver. Proximal and distal rods were connected by a side-to-side domino connector. According to the type and magnitude of the deformity, sliding foundation (domino) connectors were placed either at proximal thoracic or lumbar spine, and self-lengthening was achieved by side-to-side domino connectors.

Then the most proximal (two levels) and most distal (two levels) screws were locked while the rest of the screws were left loose with unlocked set screws (loosely captured) at apical and intermediate regions to allow vertical growth because screw heads could slide easily over the rods in these segments (Figure 8f.3). When the domino connector was placed at the lumbar region, the distal rod was locked to the domino connector, and the proximal longer rod was kept loose in order to maintain self-sliding during growth. On the contrary, when the domino connector was placed at the proximal thoracic spine, the proximal rod was locked to the domino connector, and the distal longer rod was kept loose for self-sliding. By this, we maintain a dynamic fixation system that controls the deformity and also allows self-growth of the spine (Figure 8f.4). Spinal growth can be followed by comparing the distance between tip of the rod and the domino connector. Rod exchange procedures are planned according to available rod length at the sliding foundation.

We reviewed 25 (18 female, 7 male) patients with a mean age of 6.5 (ages 3–10) years who were managed with SSGG. Figures 8f.5 and 8f.6 show two such exemplary cases. The mean follow-up was 33.3 (26–82) months. Average main thoracic (MT) curve of 56.9° was corrected to

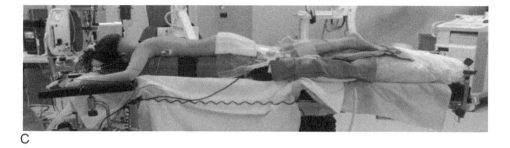

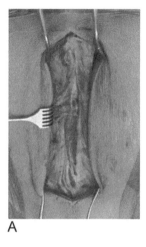

FIGURE 8F.1   C: Intraoperative skull-femoral traction during the initial procedure provides more flexibility and decreases the need for forceful correction maneuvers on the immature spine.

A

FIGURE 8F.2   A: Subcutaneous tissue dissection without any subperiosteal exposure.

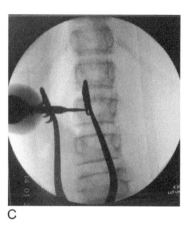

C

FIGURE 8F.2   C: The pedicle screws were placed directly under fluoroscopic guidance without exposure of posterior elements.

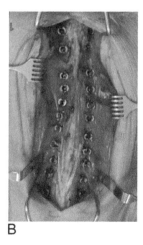

B

FIGURE 8F.2   B: The pedicle screws were placed into the strategic vertebrae with a muscle-sparing technique.

23° with a 60% correction rate. Average thoracolumbar/lumbar (TL/L) curve of 43.1° was corrected to 13.5° with a 71.7% correction rate. Preoperative thoracic kyphosis of 34.4° and lumbar lordosis of 57° was maintained at 33.4° and 56.4°, respectively. A mean increase in T1–T12 length was 0.85 mm and 1.23 mm per month in T1–S1 height. None of the patients had neurological impairment. There was no rod breakage, infection, or spontaneous fusion. Only two screws in one patient were revised for loosening. These were revised during a rod exchange procedure. The most common finding was set screw dislodgement the was found in five patients and among them only two had correction loss. This low rate of implant-related complications can be explained by the use of multiple anchors at strategic vertebrae. Stresses caused by pure distraction forces were shared among multiple anchors

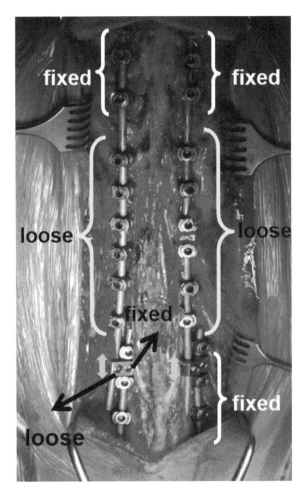

FIGURE 8F.3 The most proximal (two levels) and most distal (two levels) screws were locked, while the rest of the screws were left loose with unlocked set screws (loosely captured) at apical and intermediate regions to allow spinal growth.

and eventually decreased overall implant-related complications. SSGG prevented 79 planned lengthenings. Final fusion was performed in eight patients. When preoperative and postoperative pulmonary functions were compared, mean % predict FVC of 74,7 improved to 86 and FEV1 of 81 improved to 88,7 at final follow-up. The problem of set screws becoming dislodged can be solved easily with a small modification of the set screw design, but this may bring additional cost.

CONCLUSION

In conclusion, if EOS is left untreated, it can result in devastating and life threatening complications. Early recognition and treatment is essential for management and good outcomes. Surgical treatment of EOS is challenging and prone to high complication rates. According to the authors' experience among various surgical treatment options, SSGG offers promising and acceptable results. SSGG provides a dynamic fixation system that controls the curve progression, maintains correction on both planes, and allows self-growing of the spine. Additional apical and intermediate anchors with multisegmenter pedicle screw fixation at strategic vertebras, in addition to proximal and distal anchors to provide better correction and control of the main curve in coronal, sagittal, and axial planes and prevent progression of deformity. SSGG

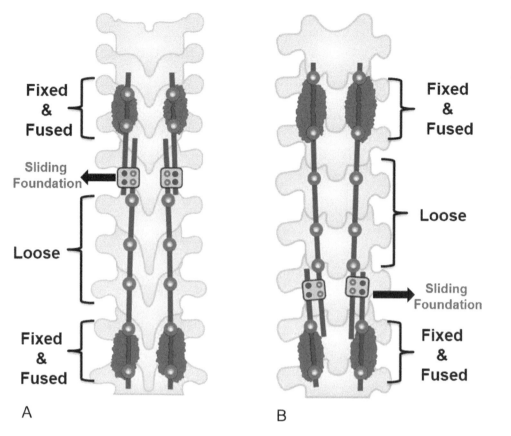

FIGURE 8F.4 A: Proximal sliding foundation located at upper thoracic spine.

FIGURE 8F.4 B: Distal sliding foundation located at thoracolumbar spine.

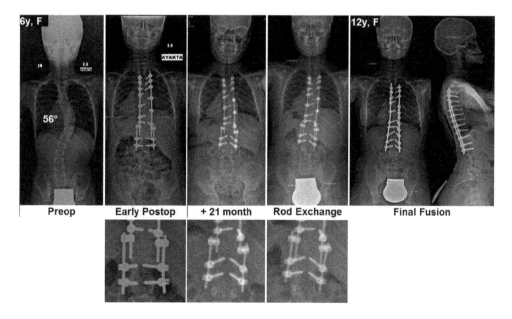

FIGURE 8F.5 6-year-old female patient with progressive EOS. Sliding foundation was located at thoracolumbar spine. Final fusion was performed after 6 years of follow-up.

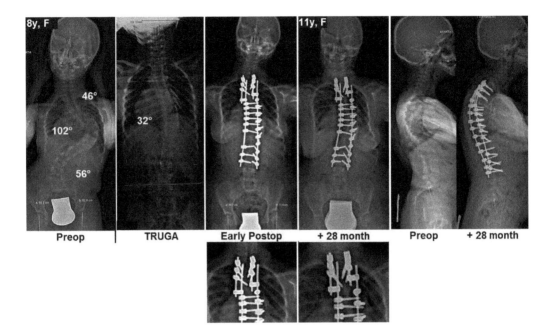

FIGURE 8F.6 8-year-old female patient with severe EOS. Traction x-ray under general anaesthesia showed more than 70% flexibility. Her flexible deformity was managed with SSGG technique. Sliding foundation was placed at upper thoracic spine. Growth of the spine was followed by the length of the sliding rods (the distance between tip of the sliding rods and the domino connector).

demonstrates low complication rates, eliminates the need for repeated lengthenings, decreases the number of planned interventions, avoids spontaneous fusion, allows spinal growth, and improves pulmonary functions. The SSGG technique does not require any special instruments and can be performed with any available spine instrumentation set without additional cost, thus offering a valid solution in resource-limited settings.

REFERENCES

1. Mundis GM, Blakemore LC, Akbarnia BA. Idiopathic early onset scoliosis. In: Akbarnia BA, Yazici M, Thompson GH, eds, *The Growing Spine: Management of Spinal Disorders in Young Children*, 2nd edition. Berlin, Heidelberg: Springer-Verlag; 2016:151–66.
2. Tis JE, Karlin LI, Akbarnia BA, et al. Early onset scoliosis: Modern treatment and results. *J Pediatr Orthop.* 2012;32(7):647–57.
3. Canavese F, Dimeglio A. Normal and abnormal spine and thoracic cage development. *World J Orthop.* 2013;4(4):167–74.
4. Dimeglio A, Canavese F. The growing spine: How spinal deformities influence normal spine and thoracic cage growth. *Eur Spine J,* 2012;21(1):64–70.
5. Campbell RM Jr, Smith MD. Thoracic insufficiency syndrome and exotic scoliosis. *J Bone Joint Surg Am.* 2007;89:108–22.
6. Vitale MG, Matsumoto H, Bye MR, et al. A retrospective cohort study of pulmonary function, radiographic measures, and quality of life in children with congenital scoliosis: An evaluation of patient outcomes after early spinal fusion. *Spine (Phila Pa 1976).* 2008;33(11):1242–49.
7. Yang S, Andras LM, Redding GJ, et al. Early-onset scoliosis: A review of history, current treatment, and future directions. *Pediatrics.* 2016;137(1):1–12.
8. Dubousset J, Herring JA, Shuffleberger H. The crankshaft phenomenon. *J Pediatr Orthop.* 1989;9(5):541–50.
9. Yang JS, McElroy MJ, Akbarnia BA, et al. Growing rods for spinal deformity: Characterizing consensus and variation in current use. *J Pediatr Orthop.* 2010;30(3):264–70.
10. Braun JT, Akyuz E, Udall H, et al. Three-dimensional analysis of 2 fusionless scoliosis treatments: A flexible ligament tether versus a rigid-shape memory alloy staple. *Spine (Phila Pa 1976).* 2006;31(3):262–68.
11. Schulz JF, Smith J, Cahill PJ, et al. The role of the vertical expandable titanium rib in the

treatment of infantile idiopathic scoliosis: Early results from a single institution. *J Pediatr Orthop.* 2010;30(7):659–63.

12. Skaggs DL, Akbarnia BA, Flynn JM, et al. A classification of growth friendly spine implants. *J Pediatr Orthop.* 2014;34(3):260–74.

13. Moe JH, Kharrat K, Winter RB, et al. Harrington instrumentation without fusion plus external orthotic support for the treatment of difficult curvature problems in young children. *Clin Orthop Relat Res.* 1984;185(185):35–45.

14. Akbarnia BA, Marks DS, Boachie-Adjei O, et al. Dual growing rod technique for the treatment of progressive early-onset scoliosis: A multicenter study. *Spine (Phila Pa 1976).* 2005;30:S46–S57.

15. Akbarnia BA, Breakwell LM, Marks DS, et al. Dual growing rod technique followed for three to eleven years until final fusion: The effect of frequency of lengthening. *Spine (Phila Pa 1976).* 2008;33(9):984–90.

16. Enercan M, Kahraman S, Erturer E, et al. Apical and intermediate anchors without fusion improve Cobb angle and thoracic kyphosis in early-onset scoliosis. *Clin Orthop Relat Res.* 2014;472(12):3902–8.

17. Xu L, Qiu Y, Chen Z, et al. A re-evaluation of the effects of dual growing rods on apical vertebral rotation in patients with early-onset scoliosis and a minimum of two lengthening procedures: A CT-based study. *J Neurosurg Pediatr.* 2018;22(3):306–12.

18. Sankar WN, Skaggs DL, Yazici M, et al. Lengthening of dual growing rods and the law of diminishing returns. *Spine (Phila Pa 1976).* 2011;36(10):806–9.

19. Cahill PJ, Marvil S, Cuddihy L, et al. Autofusion in the immature spine treated with growing rods. *Spine (Phila Pa 1976).* 2010;35(22):1199–203.

20. Hache M, Pinyavat T, Sun LS. Repetitive anesthesia concerns in early-onset scoliosis. In: Akbarnia BA, Yazici M, Thompson GH, eds, *The Growing Spine: Management of Spinal Disorders in Young Children*, 2nd edition. Berlin, Heidelberg: Springer-Verlag; 2016;873–81.

21. Akbarnia BA, Emans JB. Complications of growth-sparing surgery in early onset scoliosis. *Spine (Phila Pa 1976).* 2010;35(25):2193–204.

22. Bess S, Akbarnia BA, Thompson GH, et al. Complications of growing rod treatment for early-onset scoliosis: Analysis of one hundred and forty patients. *J Bone Joint Surg Am.* 2010;92(15):2533–43.

23. Kabirian N, Akbarnia BA, Pawelek JB, et al. Deep surgical site infection following 2344 growing-rod procedures for early-onset scoliosis: Risk factors and clinical consequences. *J Bone Joint Surg Am.* 2014;96(15):e128.

24. Upasani VV, Parvaresh KC, Pawelek JB, et al. Age at initiation and deformity magnitude influence complication rates of surgical treatment with traditional growing rods in early-onset scoliosis. *Spine Deform.* 2016;4(5):344–50.

25. Smith JT, Campbell RM Jr. Magnetically controlled growing rods for spinal deformity. *Lancet.* 2012;379(9830):1930–1.

26. Cheung KM, Cheung JP, Samartzis D, et al. Magnetically controlled growing rods for severe spinal curvature in young children: A prospective case series. *Lancet.* 2012;379(9830):1967–74.

27. Thakar C, Kieser C, Mardare M, et al. Systematic review of the complications associated with magnetically controlled growing rods for the treatment of early onset scoliosis. *Eur Spine J.* 2018;27(9):2062–71.

28. Polly DW Jr, Ackerman SJ, Schneider K, et al. Cost analysis of magnetically controlled growing rods compared with traditional growing rods for early-onset scoliosis in the US: An integrated health care delivery system perspective. *Clinicoecon Outcomes Res.* 2016;8:457–65. ecollection.

29. Akbarnia BA, Pawelek JB, Cheung KM, et al. Traditional growing rods versus magnetically controlled growing rods for the surgical treatment of early-onset scoliosis: A case-matched 2-year study. *Spine Deform.* 2014;2(6):493–97.

30. McCarthy RE, Luhmann S, Lenke L, et al. The Shilla growth guidance technique for early-onset spinal deformities at 2-year follow-up: A preliminary report. *J Pediatr Orthop.* 2014;34(1):1–7.

31. McCarthy RE, McCullough FL. Shilla growth guidance for early onset scoliosis: Results after a minimum of five years of follow-up. *J Bone Joint Surg Am.* 2015;97(19):1578–84.

32. Luhmann SJ, McCarthy RE. A comparison of Shilla growth guidance system and growing rods in the treatment of spinal deformity in children less than 10 years of age. *J Pediatr Orthop.* 2017;37(8):e567–e74.

8g Management of Spinal Tuberculosis in Young Children

S. Rajasekaran, Sri Vijay Anand KS,
Ajoy Prasad Shetty, and Rishi Mugesh Kanna

CONTENTS

INTRODUCTION

The statement, 'Children are not miniature adults', is true in spinal tuberculosis (TB) also. Spinal TB in children differs from that of adults in many ways. Children generally have a paucibacillary disease but have a higher propensity to progress from infection to disease because of their low immunity [1]. The incidence of extrapulmonary tuberculosis is higher in children (20%–25%) as compared to adults [2]. In children, a central type of lesion is more common than a paradiscal lesion, resulting in early and profound vertebral collapse. Spinal tuberculosis in children progresses faster and involves more segments, usually >3 due to its cartilaginous nature [3, 4]. The rapid destruction of immature cartilaginous vertebrae by the disease and ligamentous laxity in children frequently results in kyphotic deformity and buckling. While most deformities of spine worsen with growth, TB kyphosis tends to remain the same, progress, or correct spontaneously [5–7].

CLINICAL PRESENTATION AND DIAGNOSIS

The clinical manifestation of spinal TB depends on the duration of the disease, its severity, and associated complications. The most common clinical presentations are pain (61%), paraspinal abscess (50%), constitutional symptoms (40%), neurological deficit (23%–76%) and deformity (20%) [8, 9]. In the active stage, pain is due to vertebral destruction and inflammation, and in later stages, instability contributes to pain. While older children present with pain in the back or the neck with painful, restricted movement of the spine, the only finding in younger children and infants may be decreased playfulness and failure to thrive. Constitutional symptoms such as fever, weight loss, and loss of appetite may be present. Rarely, a child may present with stridor or dysphagia due to large prevertebral abscess in the cervical spine [10]. The predilection for anterior column involvement in spinal TB results in a kyphotic deformity, the magnitude of which depends on the amount of vertebral loss. The flexibility and immaturity of the spine in children, with its residual growth potential, can lead to a progressive deformity. A neurological deficit can occur both during the active and healed stage of the disease. Neurological deficits in the active stage are caused by 1) Mechanical pressure by necrotic debris, granulation tissue, or epidural abscess; 2) spinal instability; 3) Tuberculous myelitis or arachnoiditis; 4) spinal artery thrombosis; or 5) spinal tumour syndrome. In the healed stage, the causes include 1) stretching of the spinal cord over internal gibbus, resulting in myelomalacia, 2) instability, or 3) pachymeningitis.

A variety of investigations, including histopathological, microbiological, immunological, and imaging, are used in the diagnosis of TB; however the gold standard for confirmation of TB is the growth of mycobacterium in culture specimens obtained from infective foci.

IMAGING

Plain radiographs are usually the initial investigation in patients with suspicion of spinal TB. At least 30% of bone mineral loss must be present for a radiolucent lesion to be detected on plain radiographs. The earliest sign of TB spondylodiscitis, decreased disc space and indistinct paradiscal margin, takes a minimum of 3 weeks to appear in plain radiographs; however, as disease and vertebral destruction progress, the findings are evident. Localised osteopenia, paravertebral abscess showing typical bird-nest appearance (collection of paraspinal abscesses below D4 in the dorsal spine), and the presence of calcification within abscess are other findings that may be present. Radiographs are also helpful in the assessment of sagittal and coronal alignment of the spine, in detecting instability and quantifying kyphosis.

Magnetic resonance imaging (MRI) imaging offers the earliest possible diagnosis and has been the imaging modality of choice. MRI has an overall sensitivity and specificity of 100% and 88.2%, respectively, for tubercular infections [11]. T1-weighted images show low signal and T2-weighted and short-TI inversion recovery (STIR) images show a bright signal in infected vertebral bodies. Signal changes occur even in a very early stage. The discs are relatively preserved with the presence of intraosseous, epidural or prevertebral abscess with subligamentous spread. The advanced vertebral destruction, heterogenous focal enhancement of the vertebral body, relative preservation of the disc, thin- and smooth-walled abscesses help differentiate tubercular spondylodiscitis from pyogenic infections [12]. Screening of the whole spine must always be done for skip lesions, which may be present in around 16.3%–71.4% [13, 14]. Addition of contrast in MRI may help to identify communication between bone lesions and paraspinal abscesses [15]. The use of computerised tomography (CT) scans are limited to quantifying vertebral destruction, identifying posterior column lesions, and obtaining a targeted biopsy of the lesion [16]. Around 33%–50% of patients have an active or healed pulmonary lesion; therefore, evaluation by chest radiographs is essential [17]. However, it has to be noted that imaging findings of TB are only suggestive, and confirmation of the diagnosis is made by a histopathological examination or culture of the tissue sample.

LABORATORY INVESTIGATIONS

A spectrum of laboratory investigations is available to aid in diagnosing, confirming, and monitoring therapy with variable sensitivity and specificity. A complete blood count may show relative lymphocytosis. Markers of infection such as erythrocyte sedimentation rate (ESR) (73.2%) and C- reactive protein (CRP) (69.8%) can be elevated [18]. Though not sensitive, they are useful in monitoring therapeutic response. Other serological tests, such as the assessment of antibody titres of IgM and IgG, do not help differentiate acute, chronic infections and Bacille Calmette- Guérin (BCG) vaccinated individuals [18, 19]. Mantoux tuberculin skin testing has a high rate of producing false negatives and is limited to diagnosing latent infections.

Obtaining a tissue sample is of paramount importance, and the sample must be subjected to acid-fast bacilli (AFB) staining (Ziehl-Neelsen), histopathology, GeneXpert, AFB culture and drug-sensitivity testing (DST). Culture of mycobacteria requires only 10–100 live bacilli and is the gold standard for diagnosing TB. It has an added advantage of providing material for DST.

Spinal tuberculosis is a paucibacillary disease, hence staining and culture have low sensitivity. The reported positivity of TB culture varies in the literature between 30%–60%. The presence of caseating necrosis is the hallmark of histopathology of tuberculosis. The other common findings include epithelioid cell granulomas (90%), granular necrotic background (83%), lymphocytic infiltration (76%), and scattered multinucleated and Langhans giant cells (56%) [8]. False negatives are common and negative biopsy does not preclude a diagnosis of TB, and a decision must be made based on clinical and radiological features in such scenarios.

GeneXpert is a cartridge-based nucleic-acid amplification (NAA) test. For osteoarticular tuberculosis, the pooled sensitivity and specificity of Xpert MTB/RIF (Mycobacterium tuberculosis/resistance to rifampin) were 96% and 85%, respectively, compared to culture tests [19]. It offers several advantages, such as shorter time for results (<2 hrs), portability and ability to use at remote locations, direct use without the need for processing, less contamination, and it poses less of a biohazard. The test also detects whether the organism is resistant to rifampicin by detection of defined mutations within the core region of the RNA polymerase b (*rpoB*) gene. In the era of drug-resistant tuberculosis, Xpert MTB/RIF assay is a vital tool and is recommended by the World Health Organization (WHO) for use worldwide. Commonly used diagnostic tests are summarised in **Table 8g.1.**

MANAGEMENT

MEDICAL (MULTIDRUG CHEMOTHERAPY)

Multidrug Antitubercular chemotherapy (ATT) is the mainstay in the treatment of all cases of spinal TB. *M. tuberculosis* bacilli may be present as intracellular, extracellular, dormant, or actively multiplying in the lesion and, therefore, necessitates the use of multidrug antitubercular drugs with different properties, decreasing the chances of drug resistance. There is no consensus regarding the duration and frequency of ATT dosing to be given. The WHO recommends

TABLE 8G.1
Diagnostic Tests Used in Spinal Tuberculosis

No.	Investigation	Sensitivity	Specificity	Comments
1	Plain radiography	15%	NA	30% of bone destruction is needed for changes to be evident on plain radiographs.
2	MRI	100%	80%	Gold standard imaging technique.
3	CT	100%	NA	Identifies bone destruction.
5	ESR >20 mm	60%–90%	NA	Serial values show gradual drop after initiating treatment.
6	CRP	71%	NA	Reaches normal levels after 14 days of treatment.
7	Mantoux assay	40%–55%	75%	High false negatives. Limited use in latent infections. False positive results in BCG-vaccinated individuals.
8	Gram staining	25%–75%	99%	Ziehl-Neelsen technique—bright red bacilli; 10^4 to 10^5 bacilli/mL required.
9	Histopathology	53%–81%	NA	Epithelioid cell granulomas, Langerhans giant cells, caseous necrosis.
10	AFB culture	47%	100%	Lowenstein Jensen media; 6–8 weeks; requires 10^1 to 10^2 bacilli/mL (live bacilli).
11	BACTEC	56%	100%	4–10 days; radiometric assay
12	PCR	75%	97%	Requires only 1–10 bacilli/mL; useful in paucibacillary state.
13	Xpert MTB/RIF	96%	85%	Results <48 hours and rifampicin resistance detection.

Abbreviations: MRI, magnetic resonance imaging; CT, computed tomography; PET, positron emission tomography; ESR, erythrocyte sedimentation rate; CRP, C-reactive protein; AFB, acid-fast bacilli; PCR, polymerase chain reaction; NA, not available.

Source: Modified from Rajasekaran et al [63].

the use of a four-drug combination therapy (isoniazid, rifampicin, pyrazinamide, and ethambutol) during the initiation phase (2 months) and a three-drug regimen (isoniazid, rifampicin, and ethambutol) during the continuation phase (9–12 months). Daily regimen is currently recommended, and children should be monitored for liver function and vision on a regular basis. Optic neuritis is one of main complications of ethambutol and should be used with caution in very young children. Streptomycin should not be used as a first-line drug in children and should be reserved for multidrug-resistant cases.

The pharmacokinetics of children differ from adults. Children metabolise drugs faster, and the serum concentration of drugs is much less when compared to adults and, therefore, require higher body weight dose (mg/kg). Therefore, recent recommendations suggest 10mg/Kg of isoniazid instead of 5 mg/Kg and 10–20 mg/kg of rifampicin [20, 21]. The weight of the child should be monitored during treatment, and appropriate changes should be made to the dosage. The first line of antituberculosis drugs with dosage and safety profiles are enumerated in **Table 8g.2.**

Drug-Resistant Tuberculosis

Drug resistance is a major global threat. The prime reasons for the emergence of drug-resistant tuberculosis are inadequate and incomplete treatment, poor compliance, and spread of resistant strains. The need for prolonged treatment with second-line ATT, which is costlier, has more adverse effects, a poor success rate, and high mortality. All cases of TB are to be notified, and DST should be done in all feasible cases to diagnose resistant cases early, and all drug resistance cases should be referred to a suitable specialist. Current WHO guidelines recommend a minimum of four drugs to which the child is not exposed, including a fluoroquinolone, an injectable agent (minimum of 4–6 months after culture conversion), and at least two agents from the three remaining second-line anti-TB drug classes, including cycloserine, thioamides, and p-aminosalicylic acid, in an initial phase of at least 6 months, followed by at least three of the most active and best-tolerated drugs in a 12- to 18-month continuation phase. Second-line ATT drugs with dosage and safety profiles are enumerated in **Table 8g.3**. HIV-infected children who develop TB should be referred to a specialist for concomitant antiretroviral therapy (ART). A careful evaluation for CD4 count, viral load, and the possibility of drug interactions must be taken into account.

THE NATURAL HISTORY OF CHILDHOOD SPINAL TUBERCULOSIS AND DEFORMITY

An understanding of the natural history of a disease is essential to arrive at a suitable

TABLE 8G.2
First Line Antitubercular Drugs with Dosage and Safety Profile

Anti-Tubercular Drug	Recommended Dosage (mg/Kg)		Adverse Effects	Monitoring
	Daily Dosage	Weekly Thrice		
Isoniazid (H)	10 mg/kg (range 7–15 mg/kg); maximum dose 300 mg/day	10 (8–12)	Hepatotoxicity pyridoxine deficiency, peripheral neuropathy, rash, psychosis	Jaundice, liver enzymes
Rifampicin (R)	15 mg/kg (range 10–20 mg/kg); maximum dose 600 mg/day	10 (8–12) max. 600 mg daily	Hepatotoxicity	
Pyrazinamide (P)	35 mg/kg (range 30–40 mg/kg)	35 (30–40)	Hepatotoxicity arthralgia, rash	Jaundice, liver enzymes
Ethambutol (E)	20 mg/kg (15–25)	30 (25–35)	Optic neuritis	Vision screening
Streptomycin (S)	20 mg/kg (range 15–25 mg/kg	15 (12–18)	Auditory nerve damage	

TABLE 8G.3

Drugs Used in Treatment of Drug-Resistant Tuberculosis

Drug Group	Drug Name	Daily Paediatric Dose in mg/kg (max. dose in mg)[a]	Adverse Effects
Group 1: First-line oral drugs	Ethambutol	15	Rash, optic neuritis
	Pyrazinamide	30	Hepatotoxicity, rash
Group 2: Injectable agents			
Aminoglycosides	Amikacin(Preferred)	15-22.5 (1000)	Nephrotoxicity, hyperkalemia
	Kanamycin	15-30 (1000)	
Cyclic polypeptide	Capreomycin	15-30 (1000)	
Group 3: Fluoroquinolones	Ofloxacin	15-20 (800) 2× daily	Insomnia
	Levofloxacin(Preferred)	7.5-10 (750)	Arthralgia
	Moxifloxacin(Preferred)	7.5-10 (400)	
Group 4: Second-line oral drugs	Ethionamide (or Prothionamide)	15-20 (1000) 2× daily	Hepatotoxicity, hypothyroidism
	Cycloserine (or terizidone)	10-20 (1000) 1×/2× daily	Psychosis, convulsions, paraesthesia, depression
	p-aminosalicylic acid (PAS; 4-g sachets)	150 (12 000) 2×/3× daily	Diarrhoea, hypothyroidism
Group 5: third-line drugs of unclear efficacy (not recommended by WHO for routine use in MDR-TB patients)	High-dose Isoniazid		
	Linezolid		Myelosuppression ,Lactic acidosis, Pancreatitis
	Amoxicillin/ clavulanate		
	Clarithromycin		
	Thioacetazone		
	Imipenem/Cilastatin		
	Clofazimine		

Source: Modified from 'Guidance for National Tuberculosis Programmes on the Management of Tuberculosis in Children'. 2nd ed. WHO, 2014.

management plan. Only a few studies have evaluated the natural history and long-term outcome of spinal tuberculosis in children. Much knowledge in this subject has come from the work of Rajasekaran et al. [4] who reported the results of prospectively followed patients of spinal tuberculosis treated with ambulant chemotherapy for 15 years as part of the Medical Research Council study.

Rajasekaran [5] reported that the deformity progresses in two phases. Phase 1 or active phase, changes occur in the first 18 months, whereas in Phase 2, or the healed phase, the changes occurred after the disease was cured. While adults had an increase in deformity during the active phase and no change in deformity during the healed phase, the children had a higher deformity at presentation, a greater tendency for collapse during the active phase of the

disease, and continued and variable progression even after the disease was cured and growth was completed. Various reasons have been proposed for this increased kyphosis, including increased destruction of cartilaginous bone by the disease process, immature flexible spine, growth plate destruction, and growth modulation by the mechanical forces. In the healing phases of the disease, Rajasekaran [55] noticed that 44% of children had a reduction in kyphosis, 39% had progression of the deformity, and 17% had no change in deformity. Among these patients, he observed three patterns of changes in deformity during the growth phase (**Figure 8g.1**). A Type I curve shows continued progression after disease healing. This increase could occur continuously (Type IA) or 3–6 years after the disease was cured (Type IB). Type II curves show a reduction in kyphosis during growth either

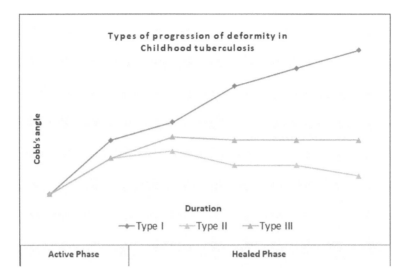

FIGURE 8G.1   Three types of progression of deformity after the active phase. Type I curves show progress of deformity after the active phase. Type II curves show a reduction in deformity, and Type III curves do not show significant change. (Redrawn from Rajasekaran [5].)

immediately after healing (Type IIA) or after 3–6 years (Type IIB). Type III shows no significant change during growth. Of these, Type IIB has most favourable prognosis, as the initial deformity and progression during the healed phase is minimal, whereas Type IB progression has the worst prognosis, as progression occurs late after the disease has healed and the patients are not in follow-up and present later with deformities of considerable magnitude emphasising the importance of following childhood spinal TB cases at least until they reach skeletal maturity [22].

This variable progression of deformity, even after the disease has healed, is unique to spinal TB. This tendency for progression also depends on various factors, including the level of the lesion, the number of vertebrae afflicted, and the age of the child. The thoracic lesions had more initial deformity but less progression and showed the most improvement with growth, whereas thoracolumbar lesions had progression during active phase as well as during healed phase. The preexistent lordosis in the lumbar spine is protective against kyphotic collapse, and more than two vertebral bodies must be destroyed before the lordosis can straighten and collapse into kyphosis [22]. Also, the rate of progression differed with age groups. Children over 10 years of age had less deformity progression

(4°) than those less than 5 years of age (10°) or between 6 and 10 years (14°) [23].

Rajasekaran [22] described that following the collapse of vertebral bodies, restabilisation occurs anteriorly by one of three methods **(Figure 8g.2):** a) When there is minimal vertebral body loss and no facetal subluxation, restabilisation occurs by wide contact; b) when there is single facetal joint subluxation, restabilisation occurs by point contact and; c) with more than two vertebral body loss, multiple facets subluxate, and restabilisation occurs by contact of the anterior vertebral body wall of superior vertebrae with superior surface of inferior vertebrae. In the absence of an intact anterior column, posterior column ligaments and facet joints are the principal stabilisers of the spine. When the kyphosis due to anterior vertebral body loss exceeds the threshold, the facet joints and posterior ligaments snap, resulting in death of the column leading to 'buckling collapse'.

Recognising the significance of the integrity of facet joints in the stability of the spine, Rajasekaran [23] proposed the 'spine at risk' signs. These signs include (a) separation of the facet joints, (b) retropulsion (c) lateral translation, and (d) toppling **(Figure 8g.3)**. These radiological signs represent spinal instability due to the facetal dislocation, and each is given a

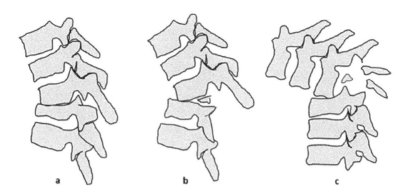

FIGURE 8G.2 'Spine at risk' signs. **a:** Facetal separation – the facet joint dislocates at the apex of the deformity, causing instability and loss of alignment. **b:** Posterior retropulsion – identified by drawing two lines along the posterior surface of the first upper and lower normal vertebrae. The diseased segments are found to be posterior to the intersection of the lines. **c:** Lateral translation – confirmed when a vertical line drawn through the middle of the pedicle of the first lower normal vertebra does not touch the pedicle of the first upper normal vertebra. **d:** Toppling sign – a line drawn along the anterior surface of the first lower normal vertebra intersects the inferior surface of the first upper normal vertebra. 'Tilt' or 'toppling' occurs when the line intersects higher than the middle of the anterior surface of the first normal upper vertebra. All these signs represent facetal dislocation and potential instability. (Redrawn from Rajasekaran [23].)

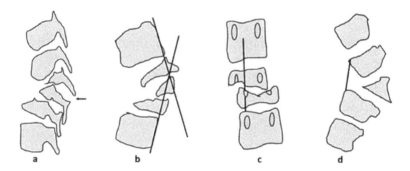

FIGURE 8G.3 Patterns of restabilisation following vertebral collapse. **a:** In the absence of significant loss of vertebral bodies or facetal subluxation, restabilisation occurs with wide contact and the progression of deformity is arrested. **b:** Restabilisation by point-contact occurs when there is single facetal subluxation following vertebral collapse. This results in a moderate deformity. **c:** In the presence of more than two vertebral body collapse and multiple facetal subluxation, the segments cranial to the lesion rotate so that anterior surface of superior vertebral body comes into contact with superior surface of inferior vertebra resulting in 'buckling collapse'. (Redrawn from Rajasekaran [22].)

score of 1. Rajasekaran also enumerated the risk factors for severe deformity progression, which are 1) an age below 10 years and loss of one or one and a half vertebral bodies 2) a pretreatment kyphosis angle of greater than 30°, especially in children 3) cervicothoracic and thoracolumbar junctional lesions, and 4) presence of 'spine at risk' radiological signs [22, 23]. While many factors influence deformity progression, an instability score of >2 is an independent 'risk' factor for progressive deformity irrespective of other factors. The integrity of facets and intact growth plates have resulted in regeneration of vertebral body and progressive improvement of deformity (Type II) after the disease has been cured. Cleveland et al. [24] followed up with 18 patients for 21 years and noted the growth of fusion mass in both sagittal and coronal planes. Moon et al. [25] performed a long-term follow-up (36 months–20 years) with 101 children and found that no change in deformity was noted in 20 children (19.8%), 14 children (13.7%) had a decrease in kyphosis, and 67 children (66.3%) had an increase in kyphosis during the follow-up period. Schulitz et al. [6] found that spontaneous correction occurred when limited debridement was done, leaving the growth plates intact. The findings of these studies suggest that the two most important factors that determine the outcome are the integrity of facet joints and intact growth plates.

SURGICAL MANAGEMENT

Spinal tuberculosis is a medically treatable disease. The indications for surgical management include 1) neurological deficits (with an acute or nonacute onset) caused by compression of the spinal cord; 2) spinal instability caused by destruction or collapse of the vertebrae, destruction of two or more vertebrae, or kyphosis of more than 30°; 3) presence of 'spine at-risk' signs; 4) no response to chemotherapeutic treatment; 5) nondiagnostic biopsy; 6) large paraspinal abscesses; and 7) intractable pain restricting mobility.

Tuli [26] observed that 38% of patients with neurological deficits improved with chemotherapy and rest while waiting for surgery and proposed his 'middle path regimen' based on these findings. However, today, any patient with a neurological deficit must be offered surgery at earliest as chances of recovery are better and faster with surgery with recovery rates of 75%–84% reported [27]. Many studies have proven that late presentation with paraplegia does not preclude surgery in spinal tuberculosis, and neurological recovery has been noted as late as 6 months [28–31]. Sai kiran et al. in his retrospective study of 48 patients, noted dramatic neurological improvement even in patients who presented late (up to 120 days) with flaccid paraplegia,gross sensory deficit,long-standing weakness, myelomalacia changes on MRI or bladder involvement.

The surgeries for spinal tuberculosis can be classified as 1) surgeries in active disease that are performed while the disease is active, and 2) surgeries for established deformity that are performed many years later after the disease has healed. Here, the patient presents with complaints of deformity and or neurological worsening.

The surgical options in spinal TB are broadly categorised as 1) biopsy; 2) stabilisation and debridement; 3) stabilisation, debridement, and anterior reconstruction; and 4) deformity correction. The choice of procedure depends on the stage of the disease, magnitude of vertebral destruction and deformity, anticipated growth remaining, presence of neurological deficit, and level of the lesion. It is mandatory to obtain tissue for biopsy, TB culture with DST, even in cases presumed to have healed, as reactivation of disease is known to occur [32]. The spine and the lesion can be accessed by various approaches, such as anterior, posterior, anterolateral, costotransversectomy, or combined approaches.

SURGERIES IN ACTIVE DISEASE

The primary aim of surgery during the active phase is to stabilise, halt, or correct the progression of kyphosis, debride the lesion, decompress, and obtain a sample for tissue diagnosis. Surgery can be done by anterior, posterior, or combined approaches. Though spinal TB is a disease of the anterior column, anterior surgeries have lost favour because of increased approach-related morbidity, difficulty in accessing long segments, and poor fixation options. Schulitz et al., Bailey et al., and Rajasekaran et al. [6, 33, 34] have attributed poor results with anterior surgery alone to aggressive debridement, leaving large defects anteriorly; therefore an anterior approach alone is considered to be unsatisfactory in thoracolumbar spinal TB for young children in terms of postoperative correction loss and is no longer recommended. However, in the cervical spine, anterior approach is routinely used and favoured. Later, combined anteroposterior approaches were used (**Figure 8g.4 and Figure 8g.5**). Such combined anteroposterior procedures have increased operating time, blood loss, morbidity, and complication rates in comparison with posterior only surgeries [35].

Due to the above concerns, the posterior approach is now favoured. Earlier sublaminar wires with Hartshill rectangles were used widely, but have lost their favour because of increased wire cut out and failures [36]. The

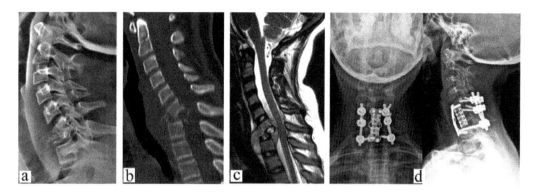

FIGURE 8G.4 **a** and **b:** 9-year-old child with C7 TB spondylitis with collapse and kyphosis (Cobb angle of 34.6°). X-rays and CT scan shows spine at risk signs. **c:** MRI shows C7 collapse with large epidural abscess indenting the cord. **d:** Patient underwent anterior debridement and Harms cage reconstruction via an anterior approach and posterior instrumentation.

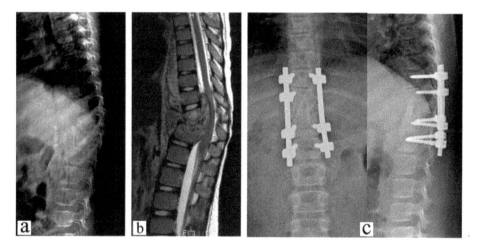

FIGURE 8G.5 **a** and **b:** 6-year-old child with T10–T11 TB spondylodisicitis with collapse of T10 vertebrae with large epidural abscess compression of the cord. **c:** Patient underwent pedicle screw instrumentation, anterior debridement, and fibular strut grafting. 2-year follow-up x-rays shows good healing and integration of graft.

pedicle screw instrumentation, with its superior stability over anterior instrumentation and the possibility of anterior debridement and reconstruction all via a single posterior approach, has shifted the paradigm toward posterior surgery. Two major concerns for the use of pedicle screw instrumentation was the fear of biofilm formation and its use in young children <5 years of age for fear of impairing normal growth. Oga et al. [37] reported that instrumentation could be safely used in spinal TB. Later Ha et al. [38] showed that the adherence and biofilm formation of *M. tuberculosis* on implants is less likely.

Many authors have reported that pedicle screw instrumentation can be used safely in children as young as 1–2 years with minimal complication rates [39–41]. Also, studies have found that instrumentation does not affect pedicle growth, the transverse plane of the vertebral body, or the spinal canal [42]. Uninstrumented surgeries in spinal TB are not recommended in children because of the potential for rapid progression of kyphosis. Wide decompression is indicated if there is a large epidural abscess/granulation tissue indenting the dura and causing secondary canal stenosis. Tissue for diagnostics and anterior debridement of disc space can be performed safely via a transpedicular approach or transfacetal approach. The disc space and adjacent infected vertebrae are debrided thoroughly until the healthy bone is reached. It is desirable to leave the vertebral growth plates intact during debridement whenever possible, as it reduces the chances of progressive kyphosis and the residual growth potential may help in spontaneous correction of the deformity [6, 7, 43]. It must be noted that radical debridement is not essential in spinal TB, unlike in pyogenic spondylodiscitis, as antituberculosis drugs can resolve the residual abscess or lesion effectively. However, the bacillary load and penetration of drugs are enhanced by a good debridement. As spinal TB affects the anterior vertebral body in most patients leaving the posterior column unaffected, it is mandatory to reconstruct the anterior column if the vertebral destruction is more with significant kyphosis >30°. Such reconstruction helps in the correction of the kyphosis and significantly reduces the chances of implant failure and complications. When there is no significant vertebral destruction noted that necessitates an anterior reconstruction, an *in situ* fixation with posterior shortening can be done. Abiliziz et al. [44] combined Smith-Peterson osteotomy with anterior debridement and allografting in 25 children with thoracolumbar tuberculosis with kyphotic deformity. He was able to achieve a correction rate of 74% from a preoperative kyphosis of 44.1°±10.8° to a postoperative value of 11.4°±3.9° [44]. Caution is required to not shorten the posterior column too much, as it might result in kinking of the spinal cord, anterior spinal artery, and result in a gross neurological deficit.

Three options exist for the reconstruction of substantial defects in the anterior column: 1) rib graft, 2) iliac strut graft, and 3) titanium mesh cage. Rib grafts were used extensively in the past; however increased complications were noted, such as subsidence, fracture of graft, resorption, and failure. Autogenous iliac crest strut graft has higher chances of incorporation than rib graft, but complications such as resorption and fracture of graft are still possible. It also has limitations such as donor site morbidity, pain, and limitation in young children with open physes. When the graft spanned more than one level, the failure rates increased [34]; therefore, it is essential to span the fixation adequately to reduce the chances of graft failure. Harms mesh cage has proven to offer better load sharing capabilities, less loss of kyphosis correction, less subsidence, and faster healing times than rib or iliac crest graft, hence its recommended for the reconstruction of the anterior column in addition to posterior instrumentation (**Figure 8g.6**) [45–47]. The bone acquired while decompression can be used to fill in titanium cages and has shown good fusion. After the placement of appropriate size cage/graft, the connecting rods need to be placed in compression to prevent dislodgement.

SURGERIES FOR HEALED TB

Surgeries for healed TB are done for severe kyphotic deformity or late-onset neurological

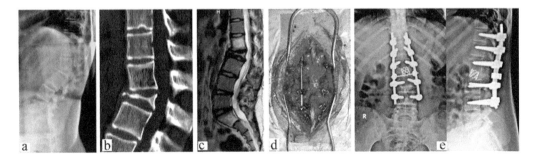

FIGURE 8G.6   **a, b**, and **c:** 13-year-old with L2 TB spondylitis with collapse and kyphosis. d. Intraoperative image showing posterior only approach with a decompressed cord and temporary stabilisation on one side. e. Patient underwent pedicle screw instrumentation and anterior reconstruction using Harms cage all via single posterior approach.

deficit. In the study by Wong et al. [32], the mean duration of presentation with late-onset neurological deficit was 26 years. Hsu et al. [48] reported a mean duration of 18 years in his study group. The neurological deficit is slowly progressive, and the usual cause is stretching and thinning of the cord over the apex of deformity. Unlike the neurological deficit occurring in active disease, the prognosis for neurological deficit in healed disease is poor despite surgery. Jain et al. [49] reported that the magnitude of thinning of the cord did not always correlate with the severity of neural deficit; however, thinning of cord in association with myelomalacia carried a worse prognosis.

Before considering any surgery, it must be recognised that this group of patients have restrictive lung disease, right heart failure, and are high-risk candidates for anaesthesia and surgery. They are also often malnourished and have poor soft tissue cover over the apex of deformity. Surgeries in this group of patients are reported to have high complication rates; therefore, it is vital to optimise the patient before surgery. Halo-gravity/halo-pelvic traction provides one such opportunity to correct the deformity gradually and optimise the patient. It has been our practise to put patients with deformity >90° in halo-gravity traction for 6 weeks in before surgery. Though the solidly fused apical segments do not show any changes with traction, it is the compensatory curves that reduce with traction, and an overall improvement in spinal alignment and balance is noted. During this period, the patient is given supervised nutrition and pulmonary physiotherapy that helps in reducing the complications and morbidity.

Although the anterior approach was initially popular, it has many disadvantages. The access to the apex of deformity is difficult in large deformities, they offer poor deformity correction, and these patients are poor candidates for anterior approach due to impaired pulmonary reserve. Combined approaches offer proper decompression and deformity correction, but increased surgical time and morbidity are the major drawbacks [50]. Improved instrumentation, neuromonitoring, and imaging have made a single posterior approach, three-column osteotomy with adequate decompression and deformity correction possible with fewer complications. Various posterior deformity correction options that have been used in post TB kyphosis include transpedicular decancellation, pedicle subtraction osteotomy (PSO), closing opening wedge osteotomy (COWO), and vertebral column resection (VCR). Each of these procedures can offer deformity correction of various magnitudes. Most of the literature on osteotomy for post TB kyphosis is on adults.

CHOICE OF THE OSTEOTOMY

A recent classification proposed by Rajasekaran et al. [51]based on column deficiency, flexibility, and curve magnitude is helpful in deciding an appropriate osteotomy for kyphosis (**Table 8g.4**). The classification includes three types: Type I – no deficiency of anterior or posterior column (Type IA – mobile discs, Type IB – fused discs with fixed deformity), Type II – deficiency of anterior (IIA) or deficiency of posterior column (IIB), an Type III- deficiency of both columns. Type III is divided into three types: Type IIIA – kyphosis <60°, Type IIIB – kyphosis >60°, and Type IIIC – buckling collapse.

Spinal TB affects the anterior column in 95% of individuals, and isolated involvement of posterior column by disease is seen in <5%. Hence, Type I deformities are not seen. In spinal TB, there is destruction and necrosis of the anterior vertebral body and intervertebral disc, rendering the anterior column defective. During the initial stages, only the anterior column is involved with intact posterior column, which is classified as Type IIA. In such cases, the deformity is resultant of partial destruction of multiple adjacent vertebrae or complete collapse of a single vertebra that results in a sharp angular kyphosis. In either case, with an intact posterior column, the deformity is seldom >60°. Such deformities with isolated anterior column deficiency can be managed by a posterior column shortening osteotomy (<30° Ponte, 30°–60° PSO, disc bone osteotomy [DBO]). Kalra et al. [65] did a pedicle subtraction osteotomy (PSO) in 15 post TB kyphosis patients with a mean age of 27 and was able to achieve a correction of 44.2° with an average blood loss of only 940 mL. Hong-Qi et al. [52] used a modified PSO to correct deformity in 26 paediatric patients

TABLE 8G.4

A guide to Choice of Osteotomy for Kyphosis Based on Classification Proposed by Rajasekaran et al.

Deformity	Ponte	Pedicle Subtraction Osteotomy	Disc Bone Osteotomy	Single Vertebrectomy	Multilevel Vertebrectomy	Anterior *In Situ* Strut Fusion	Halo + Multilevel Vertebrectomy
Type 1 A	+						
Type 1 B		+					
Type II A	+						
Type IIB		+					
Type III A			+	+			
Type III B					+		
Type III B						+	+

and achieved a correction of 40.9° with an average blood loss of 870mL. As these techniques shorten the posterior and middle column and hinge on the anterior column, reconstruction of the anterior column is not required. These techniques are useful in mild to moderate kyphotic deformities.

As the vertebral destruction progresses, the anterior column is unable to maintain the stability of the vertebral column, resulting in facetal subluxation. This results in 'functional' failure of the posterior column and leads to Type III deformities with both column deficiency. Here, the choice of osteotomy depends on the magnitude of deformity. In Type IIIA deformities with a Cobb angle <60°, posterior column shortening osteotomies, such as PSO or DBO, can be tried.

However, in severe kyphotic deformities (>60°) (Type IIIB), the anterior vertebral body loss is usually more than two. In such cases, an isolated posterior closing wedge osteotomy alone would result in kinking of cord and neurological worsening; therefore an osteotomy, that achieves correction of the deformity without altering spinal cord length is indicated. A multilevel laminectomy to decompress the cord and prevent it from compressed during deformity correction is needed along with an anterior column reconstruction. COWO or VCR techniques are employed in such deformities. Rajasekaran et al. [53, 54] used COWO to correct rigid post TB kyphosis. This a modification of the technique described by Kawahara [55]. The procedure first involves slow closing of the

wedge posteriorly until the first suggestion of kinking of the cord was evident. At that point, the closing was stopped, and the remaining gap in the anterior column was made right by a cage of appropriate size. A further correction was achieved using the cage as a fulcrum. This technique enables the achievement of excellent correction without increased risk of neurological deficit (**Figure 8g.7**). A mean correction of 56.8% ± 14.6% was achieved with an average blood loss of 820mL [53].

VCR stands at the top in the hierarchy in terms of complexity of osteotomies and correction achieved. It is technically demanding and is usually reserved for the most severe deformities. In spinal TB, it is not uncommon for patients to present with a deformity >90° requiring a major osteotomy. VCR offers a possibility of both sagittal and coronal correction with a correction rate ranging from 43%–87% [56]. Suk et al. [57] performed VCR in 25 cases of postinfection deformity and achieved a mean sagittal correction of 45.2° and reported complications in 10 patients. Lenke et al. [58] performed VCR in 35 children with severe deformities and reported improvement in global kyphosis by 55%, angular kyphosis by 58%, and kyphoscoliosis by 54%. VCR is associated with high complication rates as high as 59%. Early complications include neurological worsening, dural laceration, pleural tear, pneumothorax, haemothorax, haemorrhage, wound infection, and postoperative respiratory failure. Late complications include implant failure, pseudoarthrosis, loss of correction, adjacent

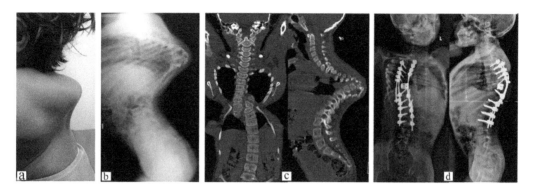

FIGURE 8G.7   a and **b**: 7-year-old child with post TB kyphosis (Cobb angle >133.4°) and buckling collapse. **c:** CT scan – coronal image shows translation of vertebral column and sharp angular kyphosis with multiple facetal subluxation and horizontalisation of vertebrae above and below. **d:** Patient underwent COWO (postoperative Cobb angle of 73.3°)

segment degeneration, proximal junctional kyphosis, and stenosis [59]. Of these, neurologic and pulmonary complications are the most common. A review article on VCR reported a neurologic complication rate of 13.3% (6.3%–15.8%) [60]. Use of neuromonitoring is strongly recommended, and up to 20% of patients show intra-operative changes in neuromonitoring [61, 62]. Maintenance of MAP >80 mmHg during osteotomy is recommended to reduce the incidence of neuromonitoring changes. Multilevel VCR is rarely indicated. A study comparing single Vs double-level VCR found no difference in deformity correction radiographically between the two; however, the operating time and neurological incidents were frequent in multilevel VCR, and it not recommended [61].

Type IIIC deformities, i.e. buckling collapse, represents the most severe deformities. They are result of multiple facetal subluxation and, ultimately, leads to translation of the vertebral column. The Cobb angle can be >120°. Here, the osteotomy is too dangerous to perform and a 4–6 week of halo-gravity traction can be applied. Halo-gravity traction slowly converts Type IIIC deformities into Type IIIB deformities for which correction can be safely attempted. In patients who are not fit for a major osteotomy or for economic constraints, a salvage procedure such as anterior *in situ* strut fusion is performed.

All the osteotomies discussed above have provided good functional outcomes. The choice of osteotomy depends on the magnitude of deformity, column deficiency, and surgeon preference. Various osteotomies performed for healed disease in spinal tuberculosis are listed in **Table 8g.5**.

CONCLUSION

Spinal TB in children differs from adults in many aspects; the most important difference is its potential for progressive kyphosis even after the disease has healed. A combination of investigations, including DST, is required for diagnosis, as no single investigation is conclusive. The potent and highly efficient multidrug antitubercular therapy has made uncomplicated spinal TB a medial disease with only a few requiring surgeries. Despite healing, all cases of childhood TB must be followed until adolescence, as the late progression of deformity after a quiescent period is known to occur. 'Spine at-risk' signs are useful in identifying such patients who are at risk of progressive kyphotic deformity. The neurological deficit, instability, progressive deformity, intractable pain, and inconclusive diagnosis remain the main indications for surgery. In the active stage, an all posterior approach with or without anterior reconstruction and pedicle screw instrumentation is the favoured procedure and offers excellent outcomes. Surgeries in healed disease for kyphotic deformity or myelopathy usually require osteotomy and are a significant undertaking with increased risk of complications. Hence, the goal of treatment in spinal TB is to achieve healing with minimal or no deformity.

TABLE 8G.5
Various Osteotomies Performed for Post TB Kyphosis and Results

S. No	Author	Technique	No. of patients	Age (years)	Preop Cobb Angle	Postop Cobb Angle	Mean Correction	Average Blood Loss	Complications
1	Basu et al. (64)	Transpedicular Decancellation	17	21(9–36)	69.3°	30.1°	38.2°	-	Nil
2	Kalra et al. (65)	Pedicle Subtraction Osteotomy	15	27(6–44)	58.8°	13.7°	44.2°	940mL	2 superficial, 1 deep infection
3	Hong-Qi et al. (52)	Modified PSO	26	11(7–16)	60.6°	19.7°	40.9°	870mL	2 dural tears, 1 deep infection
4	Rajasekaran et al. (53)	Closing Opening Wedge Osteotomy	17	18.3 ± 10.6	69.2° ± 25.1°	32.4° ± 19.5°	56.8 ± 14.6%	820mL	1 neurologic deterioration, 1 superficial infection, 1 implant revision
5	Suk et al. (57)	Vertebral Column Resection	25	27.4 (18–64)	68+/-34 (30–147)	12+/-24 (0–58)	56°	2980mL	
6	Liu et al. (59)	Vertebral Column Resection	28(5–46) years	20.8	70.7°	30.2°	40.5°	-	Dural tear, excessive haemorrhage, superficial wound infection, spinal cord or nerve root injury, and postoperative respiratory failure
7	Atici et al. (66)	Vertebral Column Resection	17 years	17.9 (9–27)	121.8°	71.5°		2280mL	4 spinal shock, 3 haemothorax, 2 postoperative infection, 2 dural laceration, 1 neurological paraplegia, 1 root injury, 2 shifted cage, 2 rod fracture

Conflict of Interest: The authors declare that they have no conflict of interest.

REFERENCES

1. Perez-Velez CM, Marais BJ. Tuberculosis in children. *N Engl J Med.* 2012;367(4):348–61.
2. Maltezou H, Spyridis P, Kafetzis D. Extrapulmonary tuberculosis in children. *Arch Dis Child.* 2000;83(4):342–6.
3. Mann TN, Schaaf HS, Dunn RN, et al. Child and adult spinal tuberculosis at tertiary hospitals in the Western Cape, South Africa: 4-year burden and trend. *Epidemiol Infect.* 2018;146(16):2107–15.
4. Rajasekaran S, Shanmugasundaram TK, Prabhakar R, et al. Tuberculous lesions of the lumbosacral region. A 15-year follow-up of patients treated by ambulant chemotherapy. *Spine.* 1998;23(10):1163–7.
5. Rajasekaran S. The problem of deformity in spinal tuberculosis. *Clin Orthop Relat Res.* 2002;398(398):85–92.
6. Schulitz K-P, Kothe R, Leong JCY, et al. Growth changes of solidly fused kyphotic bloc after surgery for tuberculosis: Comparison of four procedures. *Spine.* 1997;22(10):1150.
7. Moon M-S, Kim S-S, Lee B-J, et al. Spinal tuberculosis in children: Retrospective analysis of 124 patients. *Indian J Orthop.* 2012;46(2):150–8.
8. Garg RK, Somvanshi DS. Spinal tuberculosis: A review. *J Spinal Cord Med.* 2011;34(5):440–54.
9. Chatterjee S, Banta A. The spectrum of tuberculosis of the spine in pediatric age group: A review. *Childs Nerv Syst.* 2018;34(10):1937–45.
10. Saifi M, Kamal M, Singh MK. Tubercular prevertebral and epidural abscess presenting as stridor and dysphagia in an infant: A rare presentation of tuberculosis in infancy. *Indian J CASE Rep.* 2016:98–100.
11. Danchaivijitr N, Temram S, Thepmongkhol K, et al. Diagnostic accuracy of MR imaging in tuberculous spondylitis. *J Med Assoc Thai.* 2007;90(8):1581–9.
12. Lee KY. Comparison of pyogenic spondylitis and tuberculous spondylitis. *Asian Spine J.* 2014;8(2):216–23.
13. Polley P, Dunn R. Noncontiguous spinal tuberculosis: Incidence and management. *Eur Spine J.* 2009;18(8):1096–101.
14. Kaila R, Malhi AM, Mahmood B, et al. The incidence of multiple level noncontiguous vertebral tuberculosis detected using whole spine MRI. *J Spinal Disord Tech.* 2007;20(1):78–81.
15. Kim NH, Lee HM, Suh JS. Magnetic resonance imaging for the diagnosis of tuberculous spondylitis. *Spine.* 1994;19(21):2451–5.
16. Adapon BD, Legada BD, Lim EV, et al. CT-guided closed biopsy of the spine. *J Comput Assist Tomogr.* 1981;5(1):73–8.
17. Schirmer P, Renault CA, Holodniy M. Is spinal tuberculosis contagious? *Int J Infect Dis.* 2010;14(8):e659–666.
18. Wang H, Li C, Wang J, et al. Characteristics of patients with spinal tuberculosis: Seven-year experience of a teaching hospital in Southwest China. *Int Orthop.* 2012;36(7):1429–34.
19. Shen Y, Yu G, Zhong F, et al. Diagnostic accuracy of the Xpert MTB/RIF assay for bone and joint tuberculosis: A meta-analysis. *PLOS ONE.* 2019;14(8):e0221427.
20. World Health Organization. (2010). Rapid advice: treatment of tuberculosis in children. https://apps.who.int/iris/handle/10665/44444.
21. World Health Organization. Guidance for national tuberculosis programmes on the management of tuberculosis in children. World Health Organization; 2014.
22. Rajasekaran S. Buckling collapse of the spine in childhood spinal tuberculosis. *Clin Orthop Relat Res.* 2007;460:86–92.
23. Rajasekaran S. The natural history of post-tubercular kyphosis in children. Radiological signs which predict late increase in deformity. *J Bone Joint Surg Br.* 2001;83(7):954–62.
24. Cleveland M, Bosworth DM, Fielding JW, et al. Fusion of the spine for tuberculosis in children; a long-range follow-up study. *J Bone Joint Surg Am.* 1958;40-A(1):91–106.
25. Moon M-S, Kim S-J, Kim M-S, et al. Most reliable time in predicting residual kyphosis and stability: Pediatric spinal tuberculosis. *Asian Spine J.* 2018;12(6):1069–77.
26. Tuli SM. Results of treatment of spinal tuberculosis by "middle-path" regime. *J Bone Joint Surg Br.* 1975;57(1):13–23.
27. Jain AK, Kumar J. Tuberculosis of spine: Neurological deficit. *Eur Spine J.* 2013;22;Suppl 4:624–33.
28. Sai Kiran NAS, Vaishya S, Kale SS, et al. Surgical results in patients with tuberculosis of the spine and severe lower-extremity motor deficits: A retrospective study of 48 patients. *J Neurosurg Spine.* 2007;6(4):320–6.
29. Moon M-S, Moon J-L, Moon Y-W, et al. Pott's paraplegia in patients with severely deformed dorsal or dorsolumbar spines: Treatment and prognosis. *Spinal Cord.* 2003;41(3):164–71.
30. Moula T, Fowles JV, Kassab MT, et al. Pott's paraplegia. *Int Orthop.* 1981;5(1):23–9.
31. Chandra SP, Singh A, Goyal N, et al. Analysis of changing paradigms of management in

179 patients with spinal tuberculosis over a 12-year period and proposal of a new management algorithm. *World Neurosurg.* 2013;80(1–2):190–203.

32. Wong YW, Samartzis D, Cheung KMC, et al. Tuberculosis of the spine with severe angular kyphosis: Mean 34-year post-operative follow-up shows that prevention is better than salvage. *Bone Joint J.* 2017;99-B(10):1381–8.

33. Bailey HL, Gabriel M, Hodgson AR, et al. Tuberculosis of the spine in children. Operative findings and results in one hundred consecutive patients treated by removal of the lesion and anterior grafting. *J Bone Joint Surg Am.* 1972;54(8):1633–57.

34. Rajasekaran S, Soundarapandian S. Progression of kyphosis in tuberculosis of the spine treated by anterior arthrodesis. *J Bone Joint Surg Am.* 1989;71(9):1314–23.

35. Zhang H, Guo Q, Liu S, et al. Comparison of mid-term outcomes of posterior or postero-anterior approach using different bone grafting in children with lumbar tuberculosis. *Med (Baltim).* 2019;98(10):e14760.

36. Jain AK, Jain S. Instrumented stabilization in spinal tuberculosis. *Int Orthop.* 2012;36(2):285–92.

37. Oga M, Arizono T, Takasita M, et al. Evaluation of the risk of instrumentation as a foreign body in spinal tuberculosis. Clinical and biologic study. *Spine.* 1993;18(13):1890–4.

38. Ha K-Y, Chung Y-G, Ryoo S-J. Adherence and biofilm formation of Staphylococcus epidermidis and Mycobacterium tuberculosis on various spinal implants. *Spine.* 2005;30(1):38–43.

39. Ruf M, Harms J. Pedicle screws in 1- and 2-year-old children: Technique, complications, and effect on further growth. *Spine.* 2002;27(21):E460–466.

40. Seo HY, Yim JH, Heo JP, et al. Accuracy and safety of free-hand pedicle screw fixation in age less than 10 years. *Indian J Orthop.* 2013;47(6):559.

41. Mueller TL, Miller NH, Baulesh DM, et al. The safety of spinal pedicle screws in children ages 1 to 12. *Spine J.* 2013;13(8):894–901.

42. Olgun ZD, Demirkiran G, Ayvaz M, et al. The effect of pedicle screw insertion at a young age on pedicle and canal development. *Spine.* 2012;37(20):1778.

43. Rajasekaran S, Prasad Shetty A, Dheenadhayalan J, et al. Morphological changes during growth in healed childhood spinal tuberculosis: A 15-year prospective study of 61 children treated with ambulatory chemotherapy. *J Pediatr Orthop.* 2006;26(6):716–24.

44. Abulizi Y, Liang W-D, Maimaiti M, et al. Smith-Petersen osteotomy combined with anterior debridement and allografting for active thoracic and lumbar spinal tuberculosis with kyphotic deformity in young children: A prospective study and literature review. *Med (Baltim).* 2017;96(32):e7614.

45. Gao Y, Ou Y, Deng Q, et al. Comparison between titanium mesh and autogenous iliac bone graft to restore vertebral height through posterior approach for the treatment of thoracic and lumbar spinal tuberculosis. *PLOS ONE.* 2017;12(4):e0175567.

46. Mushkin AY, Naumov DG, Evseev VA. Multilevel spinal reconstruction in pediatric patients under 4 years old with non-congenital pathology (10-year single-center cohort study). *Eur Spine J.* 2019;28(5):1035–43.

47. Zhang H, Guo Q, Wang Y, et al. The efficiency of the posterior-only approach using shaped titanium mesh cage for the surgical treatment of spine tuberculosis in children: A preliminary study. *J Orthop Surg (Hong Kong).* 2018;26(3):2309499018806684.

48. Hsu LC, Cheng CL, Leong JC. Pott's paraplegia of late onset. The cause of compression and results after anterior decompression. *J Bone Joint Surg Br.* 1988;70(4):534–8.

49. Jain AK, Jena A, Dhammi IK. Correlation of clinical course with magnetic resonance imaging in tuberculous myelopathy. *Neurol India.* 2000;48(2):132–9.

50. Chunguang Z, Limin L, Rigao C, et al. Surgical treatment of kyphosis in children in healed stages of spinal tuberculosis. *J Pediatr Orthop.* 2010;30(3):271–6.

51. Rajasekaran S, Rajoli SR, Aiyer SN, et al. A classification for kyphosis based on column deficiency, curve magnitude, and osteotomy requirement. *J Bone Joint Surg Am.* 2018;100(13):1147–56.

52. Hong-Qi Z, Yong C, Jia H, et al. Modified pedicle subtraction osteotomies (mPSO) for thoracolumbar post-tubercular kyphosis in pediatric patients: Retrospective clinical cases and review of the literature. *Childs Nerv Syst.* 2015;31(8):1347–54.

53. Rajasekaran S, Vijay K, Shetty AP. Single-stage closing-opening wedge osteotomy of spine to correct severe post-tubercular kyphotic deformities of the spine: A 3-year follow-up of 17 patients. *Eur Spine J.* 2010;19(4):583–92.

54. Rajasekaran S, Rishi Mugesh Kanna P, Shetty AP. Closing-opening wedge osteotomy for severe, rigid, thoracolumbar post-tubercular kyphosis. *Eur Spine J.* 2011;20(3):343–8.

55. Kawahara N, Tomita K, Baba H, et al. Closing-opening wedge osteotomy to correct angular kyphotic deformity by a single posterior approach. *Spine.* 2001;26(4):391–402.

56. Zhang HQ, Li JS, Liu SH, et al. The use of posterior vertebral column resection in the management of severe posttuberculous kyphosis: A retrospective study and literature review. *Arch Orthop Trauma Surg.* 2013;133(9):1211–8.

57. Suk S-I, Kim J-H, Kim W-J, et al. Posterior vertebral column resection for severe spinal deformities. *Spine.* 2002;27(21):2374–82.

58. Lenke LG, O'Leary PT, Bridwell KH, et al. Posterior vertebral column resection for severe pediatric deformity: Minimum two-year follow-up of thirty-five consecutive patients. *Spine.* 2009;34(20):2213–21.

59. Liu C, Lin L, Wang W, et al. Long-term outcomes of vertebral column resection for kyphosis in patients with cured spinal tuberculosis: Average 8-year follow-up. *J Neurosurg Spine.* 2016;24(5):777–85.

60. Iyer S, Nemani VM, Kim HJ. A review of complications and outcomes following vertebral column resection in adults. *Asian Spine J.* 2016;10(3):601–9.

61. Hwang CJ, Lenke LG, Sides BA, et al. Comparison of single-level versus multilevel vertebral column resection surgery for pediatric patients with severe spinal deformities. *Spine.* 2019;44(11):E664–70.

62. Lenke LG, Newton PO, Sucato DJ, et al. Complications after 147 consecutive vertebral column resections for severe pediatric spinal deformity: A multicenter analysis. *Spine.* 2013;38(2):119–32.

63. Rajasekaran S, Soundararajan DCR, Shetty AP, et al. Spinal tuberculosis: Current concepts. *Glob Spine J.* 2018;8(4 Suppl):96S–108S.

64. Basu S, Rathinavelu S. Neurological recovery in patients of old healed tubercular rigid kyphosis with myelopathy treated with transpedicular decancellation osteotomy. *Eur Spine J.* 2012;21(10):2011–8.

65. Kalra KP, Dhar SB, Shetty G, et al. Pedicle subtraction osteotomy for rigid post-tuberculous kyphosis. *J Bone Joint Surg Br.* 2006;88(7):925–7.

66. Atici Y, Balioglu MB, Kargin D, et al. Analysis of complications following posterior vertebral column resection for the treatment of severe angular kyphosis greater than 100°. *Acta Orthop Traumatol Turc.* 2017;51(3):201–8.

9a Guidelines for Management in Limited-Resource Settings
Pakistan Experience

Amer Aziz and Abdullah Shah

CONTENTS

PAKISTAN INTRODUCTION

GEOPOLITICAL

Pakistan is located in South Asia encircled by Afghanistan, India, China, the Arabian Sea, and Iran. It is the 36th largest country in the world in terms of area with an area covering 881,913 km2 (340,509 sq mi) [1].

POPULATION

Pakistan is the sixth most populous country in the world, with about 216 million people, and by 2050 it will become the fourth largest populated country in the world [1].

SOCIOECONOMIC STATUS

The United Nations Development Programme (UNDP) ranked Pakistan in the Human Development Index (HDI) 146th out of 187 countries. Presently, Pakistan has a stagnant gross domestic product (GDP) of 4.71% and a Gross National Income (GNI) per capita of approximately $1550, is categorised as a low-income country, and is 65th among 102 developing countries. Currently, the literacy rate of the population is 58% [2].

HEALTHCARE SYSTEM OF PAKISTAN

Health services in Pakistan are divided purely on the public and private sectors (**Figure 9a.1**)[2].

HEALTH FINANCING

The government of Pakistan uses 3.1% of its GDP for economic, social, and community services, and 43% is used up for debt returns. About 0.8% is spent on healthcare. This spending is much less than the World Health Organization's (WHO) benchmark of a minimum of 6% spending on healthcare provision. Today, the doctor-to-patient ratio in Pakistan is 1:1300, the doctor-to-nurse ratio is 1:2.7, and the nurse-to-patient ratio is 1:20 [3]. The WHO suggests that the doctor-to-patient ratio should be 1:1000 and the doctor-to-nurse ratio 1:4 [2].

HEALTHCARE FACILITIES AND EQUIPMENT

There are 48 tertiary care hospitals in the public sector dealing with trauma and orthopaedics. All equipped with image intensifier and other necessities required for orthopaedics and spine management, but only 2 to 3 centres have the neuromonitoring apparatus needed for scoliosis surgery.

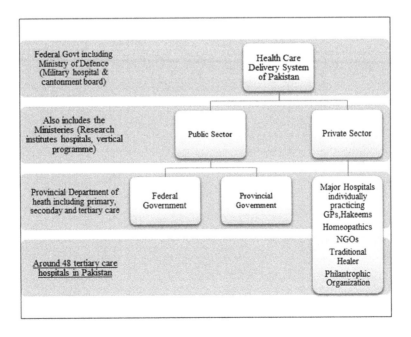

FIGURE 9A.1   Health system of Pakistan

EARLY-ONSET SCOLIOSIS

Early-onset scoliosis (EOS) is defined as a spinal deformity occurring before 10 years of age. Untreated EOS or early spinal fusion resulting in a short spine is associated with increased mortality and cardiopulmonary compromise. Because EOS is a heterogeneous condition, a uniformly accepted classification has been proposed. This includes age, aetiology (congenital, neuromuscular, syndromic, and idiopathic), significant curve, kyphosis, and progression modifier. Surgery is indicated for progressive deformities. EOS may progress rapidly and, therefore, prompt clinical diagnosis and referral to a paediatric orthopaedic unit are necessary [4].

EPIDEMIOLOGY

No large scale studies are available; there exists only regional research on congenital anomalies in the tribal area with a population of 448310. This study found 246 families with congenital anomalies and two cases of congenital scoliosis and two cases of congenital kyphosis [5]. Data from different hospitals involved in scoliosis management showed that around 20–30 patients visit out-patient departments (OPD) monthly at each tertiary care hospital with a complaint of spine deformity, including infants, juveniles, and adolescents.

SCHOOL HEALTH SERVICES/ SCOLIOSIS SCREENING

While School Health Services has been a part of the government health infrastructure since 1952, health services in schools and scoliosis screenings are still nonexistent. School health services in the private sector has evolved in the past two decades. Nongovernmental organisations (NGOs) have played a key role in implementing this programme in private schools [6].

Various local studies showed screening tests and protocols, but until now, no available research on school screening exists for scoliosis. A scoliosis-screening programme has been developed, which is quick, reproducible, and inexpensive. This involves visual observation

of the back, forward-bending test, and moiré fringe topography [7].

MODES OF PRESENTATION

Most of the patients are brought in because of cosmesis, shoulder asymmetry, pelvic asymmetry, and awkward gait. Some patients come with chest, sternum, rib cage deformity. Parents and sometimes school teachers bring in patients. Some come with pain, weakness, shortness of breath, or limb length discrepancy (LLD), and occasionally with congenital malformation/deformity evident at birth.

BELIEFS

Most people believe that this disease is from God as a response to their sins, or God wants to check their piousness and patience by giving this trouble to their children or siblings. Some also relate it to the stars, a lunar or solar eclipse, or even to evil souls.

REASONS FOR DELAY

People are afraid of going to hospitals and usually go to local spiritual healers, hakeems, bone setters, spine manipulators, and 'quacks'. By the time they come to a hospital, it is often too late and the curve has become too rigid or it has started its secondary effect on the cardiopulmonary or musculoskeletal systems.

Even general practitioners do not have sufficient knowledge regarding pathogenesis and pathophysiology of the problem and cannot guide the parents properly. Most of the time, it is said that it will be treated as a child approaches skeletal maturity (which is detrimental for EOS), or parents are frightened that surgery will cause the patient to become paralysed.

REASONS FOR REFUSAL TO RECEIVE TREATMENT

Poverty is the main reason. Illiteracy and ignorance of not recognising the future grave prognosis and fear of complications of surgery are also factors. Fear of becoming a paraplegic as told by practitioners. Limited centers in the public sector is another cause.

HEALTH PERSONNEL AND FACILITIES

NEUROSURGEONS

Around 300–350 neurosurgeons are practising in Pakistan, but only a few occasionally take on scoliosis cases on an individual basis, but there is no neurosurgical institution that regularly cares for this particular patient population.

ORTHOPAEDIC SURGEONS/SPINE SURGEONS

Few orthopaedic and spinal surgeons in the country have an interest in scoliosis management.

INSTITUTIONS CARING FOR SCOLIOSIS

- Public sector around 5–6
- Armed forces 1–2
- Private 3–5
- NGO 2–4

There are some other institutions or individuals that care for scoliosis patients, but no exact details or figures are available.

ELECTROPHYSIOLOGICAL MONITORING

Multimodality neurophysiologic intraoperative tracking appears to be the standard of care for monitoring functional integrity and reducing the risk of iatrogenic damage to the nervous system and to provide functional guidance to the surgeon. Somatosensory evoked potential (SSEP) and motor evoked potentials (MEP) should be used together for spinal cord surgeries to minimise nervous tissue insults [8, 9]. There are only six centres in Pakistan that have this neurophysiology monitoring equipment.

MANAGEMENT

The skill in managing a patient with a congenital spine deformity lies not only in the ability to perform major complex salvage surgery in patients presenting at a late stage with a severe rigid deformity but also in recognising those curves with a bad prognosis at an early stage to prevent curve progression and possible neurological complications. Meticulous management planning requires an astute knowledge of the natural history of all types of congenital spine deformity and the methods of treatment that are available. Once high-risk anomalies, such as unilateral unsegmented bars with contralateral hemivertebrae are recognised, treatment is initiated regardless of age to prevent deformity [10].

SCOLIOSIS DATA

Various local studies on adolescent idiopathic scoliosis and congenital scoliosis and their modes of treatment are available, but no significant literature on EOS could be retrieved [11].

GHURKI TRUST TEACHING HOSPITAL

- Total number of patients with scoliosis/dyphosis/khypho-scoliosis admitted at Ghurki Trust Teaching Hospital (GTTH) from 2006–19 was 948 (**Figures 9a.2a & 9a.2b, Table 9a.1).**;
- Total EOS cases = 159
- Adolescent/Adult cases = 789
- Out of 159 EOS patients, 16 were treated conservatively while 143 received different surgical procedures.
- From 2006 to 2014, most surgeries used Harrington rods and some used limited fusion *in situ* or after resection of the hemivertebrae.
- From 2015 onward, most surgeries used single or double conventional growing rods without fusion, limited fusion at the convex apex, or hemivertebrae resection.
- The above data suggest that surgical decisions are made on a case-by-case basis. However, the conventional double growing rod with and without limited fusion is a better option where resources are limited.

TREATMENT OPTIONS

CONSERVATIVE

- **Observation:** Patients with relatively stable and balanced curves that are progressing slowly are observed every 4 to 6 months.
- **Casting:** This method was attempted on some infantile cases, but the

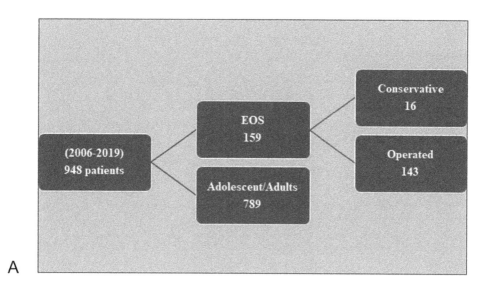

FIGURE 9A.2A Showing the distribution of patients of scoliosis/kyphosis/kypho-scoliosis admitted in GTTH from 2006–19.

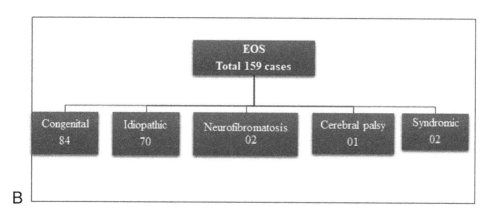

FIGURE 9A.2B Showing the distribution of EOS cases based on diagnosis done at GTTH.

compliance was very poor because of the hot and humid climate, poor housing environment, poverty, electricity failure or unavailability, and, above all, illiteracy and poor coordination and follow-up

- **Bracing:** It was found useful in very young and especially idiopathic cases to buy some time until the patient has grown enough to withstand surgical trauma and to accommodate the hardware. There are a number of patients being treated using regular bracing – Over the past 2 years, 20 EOS patients

4–10 years of age are being treated with regular follow-up at GTTH.

SURGERY

1. **Magnetically controlled growing rods (MCGR):** This is not a new technique. It is practised worldwide but mostly in developed countries, as it is very costly for a limited-resources country. Single patient treatment may cost up to $20,000, which is 15 times the annual income of a common person in Pakistan.

TABLE 9A.1

Representing the distribution of 159 procedures done on 143 patients at GTTH

Procedure	Cases
Conservative managed with bracing or unfit for surgery	16
In situ fusion with pop jacket	25
Harrington distraction rod	29
SSI with pedical screws and hooks	26
Conventional growing rods	22
Redo Harrington or exchange of Harrington to growing rod/fusion	18
Osteotomy/VCR/PSO	10
Hemivertebrae resection	5
Anterior decompression and cage stablisation	7
Galviston procedure	4
Anterior release	3
Costoplasty	3
Limited 360° fusion	2
Harrington threaded rod and rush pin fixation	5

2. **Tethering:** This is a recent technique that maintains the flexibility of the spine, yet corrects the deformity over time. This is a costly procedure.

3. **Vertical Expandable Prosthetic Titanium Rib (VEPTR):** This technique is not available

4. **SHILLA:** This technique is not attempted, as the screws are unavailable.

5. **Luque Trolly:** A technique that involves stripping a large area of the spine to achieve early fusion. This technique is used.

6. **Harrington Rods:** A lot of cases use this instrumentation without fusion with variable results, many resulting in complications, such as premature fusion, hooks cut out, rod breakage, luque wires cut out, crankshaft, and failure to stop progression, leading to failure of treatment, repeat surgeries, and sometimes worsening of the condition.

7. **Short Segment Posterior Fusion:** This has been used in a few cases of relatively mature congenital scoliosis in which parents did not want repeat surgeries.

8. **Hemiepiphysiodesis:** This technique of convex fusion and concave distraction has been used in some cases with favourable results.

1. **Resections/Hemivertebrae Resection:** This has been used on only a few cases of congenital scoliosis [12].

10. **VCR:** This techinique is used occasionally.

GTTH PROTOCOL FOR EOS

Unless a child has a tethering bony bar or uncompensated hemivertebrae, initial treatment in EOS comprises of bracing/casting. If found, the tethering bony bar or uncompensated hemivertebrae is resectioned, and the child is treated in a cast or brace.

When the child is 6–7 years old, with a Cobb angle of ~40°, a double growing rod construct is applied with pedicle screws. The growing rod is gradually distracted. When the child reaches menarche/skeletal maturity, posterior segmental spinal instrumentation is carried out (**Figure 9a.3**).

CONVENTIONAL GROWING RODS

A study conducted at a tertiary care hospital presented in a local meeting showed the result of 30 patients of EOS treated with conventional growing rods. According to this study, most patients were

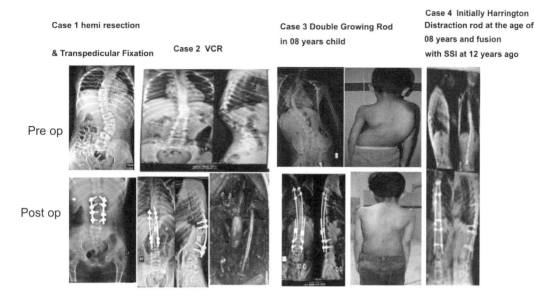

FIGURE 9A.3 Different surgical procedures, showing preoperative and postoperative radiology and other figures.

Various ways of using growing rods

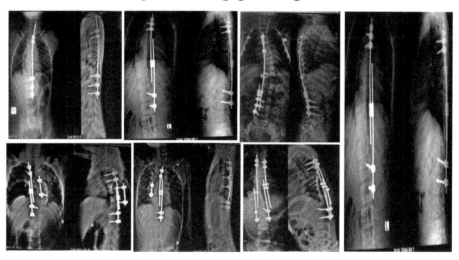

FIGURE 9A.4 Different surgical procedures of using growing rods, showing preoperative and postoperative radiology.

treated with double growing rods, showing good results and comparable complication rates with the literature (**Figures 9a.4 & 9a.5**) [13].

- Convex fusion with concave distraction using growing rods and convex hemiepiphysiodesis [14].
  - Single growing rod.
  - Double growing rod.

- **Case 1:** (upper row) hemivertebrae with mild deformity operated with *in situ* fusion at the age of 8. The patient continued to grow, and later, the implant was removed and the anterior cage was completed without posterior fusion. After 6 years, the patient developed severe kyphosis that required vertebral column resection (**Figure 9a.6**).

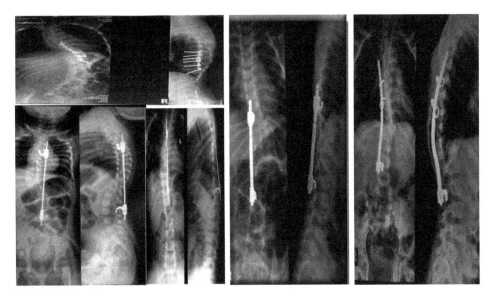

FIGURE 9A.5   Different surgical procedures using screws and wires, showing preoperative and postoperative radiology.

HOW NOT TO DO

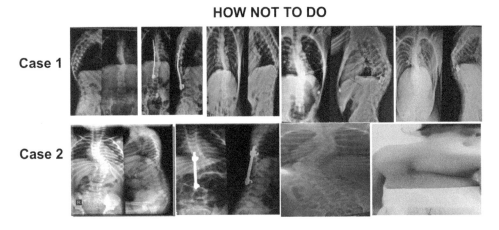

FIGURE 9A.6   Different procedures that should be avoided.

• **Case 2:** (lower row) surgery was conducted at the age of 5 with resection of diastematomyelia and *in situ* fusion, but the patient continued to grow to significant deformity and required a third surgery (**Figure 9a.6**).

Both of these cases would have been efficiently dealt with using the hemiepiphysiodesis resection and limited fusion 360° at initial surgery.

DIFFICULTIES FACED

There are various hurdles in dealing with spine surgery, especially scoliosis.

• **Politics:** Health is the least concern for government, as made evident from poor budget allocation. In the public sector, only a few centres provide spine surgery. There are many hurdles to obtain equipment, instruments, and implants from the government. A lot of the budget is used politicians for out of country treatment.

- **Spine training:** The spine is a part of the orthopaedic training programme curriculum. Still, more than 90% of teaching institutions do not treat the spine, leaving orthopaedic fellows without practical experience in the spine. There is no locally recognised diploma that specialises in the spine. The stakeholders have not agreed to launch a separate subspecialty.
- **Resources:** Because resources are limited the procedure is too costly.
- **Lack of awareness:** The general public and referring doctors and practitioners know little about the prognosis and outcome of the disease and that it is treatable if managed in time.
- **Patient factors:** These include low patient body-mass index, comorbidities, weak musculature and bones, hardware prominence or cutting out, and anaesthetic risks.
- **High cost:** Many parents are unable to afford the surgery.
- **Poverty.**
- **Fear of complications.**
- **Lack of availability of quality implants (with low profile to avoid prominence of implants after surgery).**
- **Lack of good postoperative intensive care unit (ICU) care.**
- **Lack of good follow-up.**

SOLUTIONS AND RECOMMENDATIONS

- **Political will:** Try to use your relations and authority to convince health authorities and politicians to focus on these health issues and provide funding for it.
- **Spine training:** the institutions doing spine surgeries should train doctors from other institutions who are not doing spine surgeries. There should be institutional collaboration. Practical spine training should be made compulsory by Fellow of College of Physicians and Surgeons (FCPS).
- **Resources:** Efforts should be made to raise funds and develop institutions with the help of rich, kind, and generous peoples and organisations.
- **Poverty:** Raise funds for implants for poor patients.
- **Availability of quality implants:** Use alternate implants from the local or international market that are reasonably priced and of good quality.

THE EXAMPLE OF GTTH SPINE CENTER

Established using international standards, the spine unit was developed with a cost of around $600 million. It is equipped with 10 modular theatres, a central sterile services department, 24-hour functional MRI and CT scan, rehabilitation center, image intensifier in each theatre, neuromonitoring equipment, spine endoscope, ultrasonic burr, etc. Created without government support, the spine unit provides free treatment and costs about $1.2 million annually to operate which is funded completely by local financial donors and NGOs (**Figure 9a.7**).

Community and practitioner awareness programmes dealing with the success of treatment and need for early intervention and proper referral have been created using print and electronic media, seminars held locally and in hospital settings, and information provided on television screens in waiting areas.

Patient perspective, select the right procedure for the right individual, delay the invasive process for as long as it is safe to do so to avoid complications of early fusion and also to reduce the number of lengthening procedures necessary until the patient reaches skeletal maturity, and where possible, do short segment fusion.

- Know your limitations to avoid lethal consequences.
- Use neuromonitoring where needed.
- Use proper record-keeping techniques of preoperative, intraoperative, and postoperative events.
- To publish.

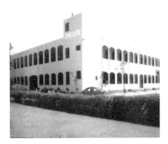
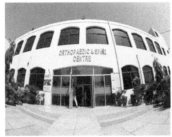
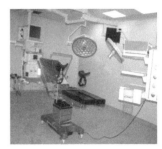
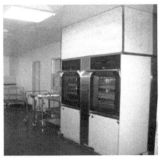
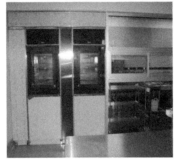
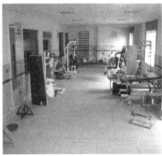

FIGURE 9A.7   Different views of internationally recognised spine centre.

CONCLUSIONS

EOS necessitates early diagnosis and prompt treatment to prevent severe and life-threatening cardiopulmonary compromise. Casting at an initial phase may cure EOS, while more severe and progressive forms of EOS typically require surgery with 'growth-friendly' techniques, such as growing rods. The development of MCGRs reduces the need for repeated surgical procedures and may reduce the risk of deep surgical site infection but is costly. Conventional double growing rods without fusion and limited fusion with or without additional distraction are reasonable approaches for countries of a low socioeconomic status.

ACKNOWLEDGMENT

We are thankful to Professor Atiquz Zaman (Department of Orthopaedic & Spine Suirgery, GTTH, Lahore) and Dr Ashfaq Ahmed (Senior Registrar, Department of Orthopaedic & Spine Suirgery, GTTH, Lahore) for their contribution and cooperation

REFERENCES

1. Wikipedia. Geography of Pakistan. 2020. https ://en.wikipedia.org/wiki/Geography_of_Pa kistan.

2. Kumar S, Bano S. Comparison and analysis of health care delivery systems: Pakistan versus Bangladesh. *Journal of Hospital and Medical Management* 2017;03(01):1–7.

3. Nishtar S. The gateway paper--preventive and promotive programs in Pakistan and health reforms in Pakistan. *Journal of the Pakistan Medical Association* 2006;56(12 Suppl 4):S51–65.

4. Helenius IJ. Treatment strategies for early-onset scoliosis. *EFORT Open Reviews* 2018;3(5):287–93.

5. Zahra Q, Shuaib M, Malik S. Epidemiology of congenital anomalies in the Kurram Tribal Agency, northwest Pakistan. *Asian Biomedicine* 2017;10(6):575–85.

6. Ahmad F, Danish SH. School health services - A neglected sphere of influence in Pakistan. *Journal of the Pakistan Medical Association* 2013;63(8):948–9.

7. Kamal SA, Sarwar M, Razzaq UA. Effective decision making for presence of scoliosis. *International Journal of Biology and Biotechnology* 2015;12(2):317–28.

8. Ali L, Iqrar A, khealani DB, et al. Utility of intraoperative neurophysiological monitering (ionm) in various surgeries at a tertery care hospital in Karachi, Pakistan. *Pakistan Journal of Neurological Sciences* 2016;11(2):13.

9. Ayoob MK, Dogar A, Hafeez A, et al. Motor and somatosensory evoked potential monitoring without wakeup test during scoliosis surgery. 2019;23(4):228–32.

10. Batra S, Ahuja S. Congenital scoliosis: Management and future directions. *Acta Orthopaedica Belgica* 2008;74(2):147–60.

11. Nadeem U, Shah A, Zaman AZ, et al. Selection of lowest instrumented vertebra in the management of thoracolumbar and lumbar adolescent idiopathic scoliosis using pedicle screw instrumentation. *Global Spine Journal* 2016;6:s-0036-1582816–s-0036-1582816.

12. Akbarnia BA, Marks DS, Boachie-Adjei O, et al. Dual growing rod technique for the treatment of progressive early-onset scoliosis: A multi-center study. *Spine* 2005;30(17S):S46–57.

13. Qureshi MA, Pasha IF, Khalique AB, et al. Outcome of hemivertebra resection in congenital thoracolumbar kyphosis and scoliosis by posterior approach. *Journal of the Pakistan Medical Association* 2015;65(11):S142–6.

14. Cheung KMC, Zhang JG, Lu DS, et al. Ten-year follow-up study of lower thoracic hemivertebrae treated by convex fusion and concave distraction. *Spine (Phila Pa 1976)* 2002.

9b China Experience

Yong Hai and Aixing Pan

CONTENTS

INTRODUCTION

Early-onset scoliosis (EOS) is defined as a curvature of the spine in children >10° with onset before the age of 10 [1], which will seriously affect the development of children's cardiopulmonary function and even mental health. According to the aetiology, EOS can be divided into congenital, idiopathic, syndromic, neuromuscular, and syndromic scoliosis. To some extent, it may be influenced by geographical circumstances, such as altitude and oxygen concentration [2].

MAIN BODY

An EOS screening system is crucial for early detection and intervention, especially in the rural and less developed areas where most cases present as severe scoliosis at their first visit. We launched the scoliosis screening and rescue public welfare action in the last decade together with many charity organisations in China. Our team has been to those remote areas, and hundreds of scoliosis patients from the high altitude and remote areas in mainland China (Tibet region) were found and brought to have treatment in our spine centre. In the meantime, we trained the local doctors and established a screening system for scoliosis that can reduce the imbalance of medical resources.

Brace and casting have proved to be effective conservative treatments for EOS [3–5]. Brace and casting could suppress scoliosis progression and delay the timing of the surgical intervention or even reduce the rate of surgery [6].

Growing-rod surgery is considered as the primary treatment for patients with progressive scoliosis when conservative treatment failed at the age of 5–10. It helps to delay the progression of deformity while maximising the growth of the spine and lungs [7]. Growing-rod lengthening surgery is performed every 12 months with 2 cm–3 cm distractions. Final correction and fusion is suggested for patients who have well-developed lung function and skeleton, Risser sign >1°, or menstruation in female patients. Hemivertebra resection and short fusion can be performed in congenital scoliosis patients who have a short, sharp curvature.

Due to the high rate of complications [8], regular follow-up visits are essential before the graduation of the treatment. X-ray film is required every 6 or 12 months, according to the patient's growth rate, to check the spinal growth, trunk balance, and surgical fixation (**Figures 9b.1- 9b.3**).

EOS, usually a systemic disease, requires a multidisciplinary consultation involving physicians from respiratory, cardiac, thoracic, anaesthesiology, and nutrition departments to complete the overall assessment. For patients with combined funnel chest deformity, thoracoplasty can be performed simultaneously with the growing rod surgery.

Medical resources and insurance policies vary greatly in different countries and regions, which is also the case in China. For patients in less developed areas of China, the help from charitable foundations plays a pivotal role. In China, there are many public welfare foundations for scoliosis, and each year hundreds of patients with scoliosis are treated with the help of the foundation (**Figure 9b.4**).

In conclusion, EOS is a disease that seriously harms the physical and mental development of

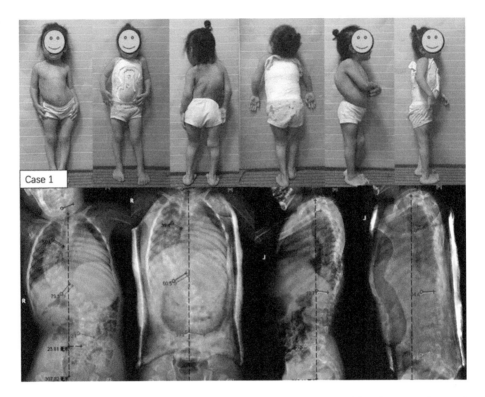

FIGURE 9B.1   Case 1 was a 3-year-old girl diagnosed with syndromic EOS. The corrective casting was made under general anaesthesia and traction. Casting and bracing can alternate every half year, between summer and winter. Conservative treatment can postpone the first growing rod operation until the age of 5 or 6, which will decrease surgical and anaesthesia complications.

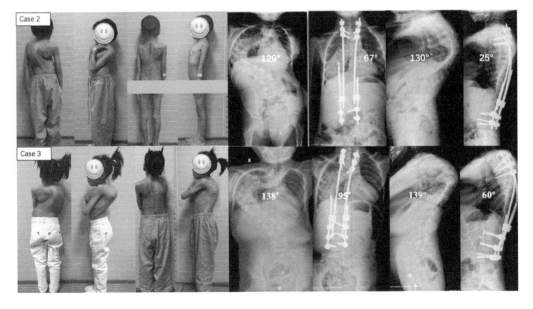

FIGURE 9B.2   Case 2 was a 7-year-old boy with EOS and a 129° left curve and 130° kyphosis. Case 3 was an 8-year-old girl with EOS and a 138° right curve and 139° kyphosis. Both patients underwent dual growing-rod surgery. The deformity was well corrected after surgery.

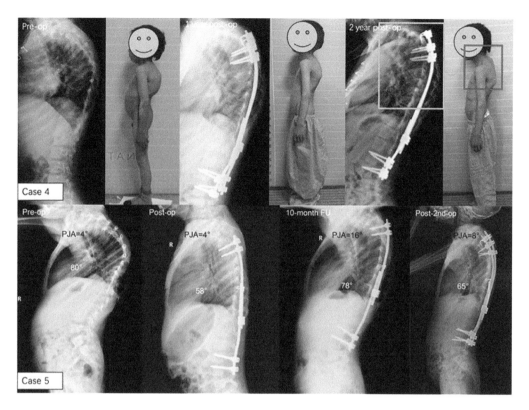

FIGURE 9B.3 Cases 4 and 5 were EOS patients who underwent dual and single growing rod surgery, respectively. During follow-up, they developed postoperative asymptomatic proximal junctional kyphosis (PJK). If the posterior ligament complex is damaged or the internal fixation becomes loose, the operative segment can be extended proximally, and Ponte osteotomy can be performed if necessary. In the meantime, proximal hook fixation can reduce the morbidity of PJK and proximal junction failure (PJF).

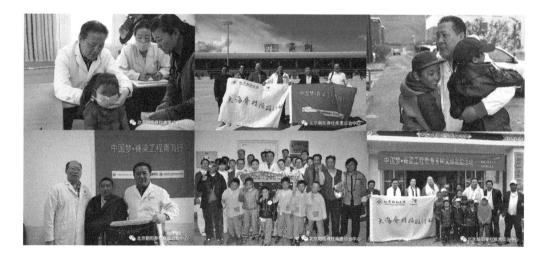

FIGURE 9B.4 We carried out scoliosis screening and rescue public welfare activities in the plateau region, southwest of China, in the last decade. Surgeons from our centre go to the remote areas two or three times a year to provide medical care to the local people. In the meantime, local medical staff has been trained and a scoliosis screening system has been established.

infants and adolescents. It is still challenging for spinal surgeons and researchers to explore the pathogenesis and develop treatment guidelines. More research and investments are needed in the future in this area.

REFERENCES

1. Skaggs David L, Guillaume Tenner, El-Hawary Ron, et al. Early onset scoliosis consensus statement, SRS Growing Spine Committee, 2015. *Spine Deform*. 2015;3(2):107–108.
2. Hou D, Kang N, Hai Y, et al. Abnormalities associated with congenital scoliosis in high-altitude geographic regions. *Int Orthop*. 2018;42(3):575–581.
3. Ballhause TM, Moritz M, Hättich A, et al. Serial casting in early onset scoliosis: Syndromic scoliosis is no contraindication. *BMC Musculoskelet Disord*. 2019;20(1):554.
4. Kawakami N, Koumoto I, Dogaki Y, et al. Clinical impact of corrective cast treatment for early onset scoliosis: Is it a worthwhile treatment option to suppress scoliosis progression Before surgical intervention? *J Pediatr Orthop*. 2018;38(10):e556–e561.
5. Thometz J Liu X-C. Serial CAD/CAM bracing: An alternative to serial casting for early onset scoliosis. *J Pediatr Orthop*. 2019;39(3):e185–e189.
6. Nanjundappa SH, Lonstein JE. Results of bracing for juvenile idiopathic scoliosis. *Spine Deform*. 2018;6(3):201–206.
7. Akbarnia BA. Management themes in early onset scoliosis. *J Bone Joint Surg Am*. 2007;89(Suppl 1):42–54.
8. Pan Aixing, Hai Yong, Yang Jincai, et al. Upper instrumented vertebrae distal to T2 leads to a higher incidence of proximal junctional kyphosis during growing-rod treatment for early onset scoliosis. *Clin Spine Surg*. 2018;31(7):E337–E341.

9c Egyptian Experience of Surgical Management of Early-Onset Scoliosis

Mohammad M. El-Sharkawi and Amer Alkot

CONTENTS

INTRODUCTION

Surgeries for early-onset scoliosis (EOS) have been practised for a very long time by several Egyptian pioneers in spine surgery in Cairo, Ain Shams, Alexandria, and Assiut universities. However, little has been published or could be traced in the literature. In recent years, sporadic reports of hemivertebrectomy [1], growing rods (GR) [2], spinal osteotomies, and fusion for complex congenital anomalies could be found in peer reviewed journals [3, 4] as well as international meetings [5, 6, 7, 8, 9, 10]. Additionally, many Egyptian surgeons have been involved in bigger series in other centres around the world [11, 12, 13, 14, 15].

In addition to the usual technical and surgical difficulties of managing EOS, the problem becomes more challenging with limited resources. To date, most major hospitals in Egypt, including ours, do not have intraoperative computerised tomography (CT) or O-Arm, neuromonitoring equipment, cell savers, or modern navigation tools. The vertical expandable prosthetic titanium rib (VEPTR) and the newly introduced magnetically controlled growing rods (MCGR) are extremely expensive and

have never been introduced in the country. To confound the issue even more, lack of family compliance with follow-up visits is customary in our region. This is probably due to unawareness of the importance and value of committing to the follow-up plans and/or the nuisances of transportation and the high costs of travelling long distances.

Historically, most children with EOS were left untreated until adulthood, which resulted in progression to a high degree of rigid curves, poor health-related quality of life, and poor body image [16, 17]. Complex reconstructive surgeries are also routinely performed in our centre for managing neglected spinal deformities [4, 18] despite the lack of the latest technologies and neuromonitoring.

More recently, however, all children in Egypt became covered by the health insurance system, which made it possible to diagnose early and properly manage an increasing number of EOS cases. In 2006, Assiut University Hospital concluded an agreement with the Health Insurance Authorities, whereby all spinal deformity cases from Upper Egypt are transferred to be managed in Assiut University Hospital rather than referring them to different hospitals in Cairo, which is 450 km away. We have also established a specialised outpatient clinic for spinal deformities, which helped to build trust and a strong bond with the patients and families. Soon after, our centre became one of the biggest centres in Egypt, treating complex spinal deformities and especially EOS. Over the years, we have treated more than 100 cases of EOS with hemivertebrectomy [8] (either isolated or combined with GRs [6]), SHILLA procedure, growing rods [10], fusion [7], and vertebral osteotomies [8].

The first time we operated using GRs in Assiut University Hospital was in 2007. Since then, we have managed more than 50 cases with GRs. Unfortunately, many of them, because of the long travel distance from all cities in Upper Egypt, did not or could not comply with the follow-up programme and did not follow the lengthening schedule. Two types of GRs have been used so far: the ISOLA system (AcroMed Corporation, United States) and the Growing Spine Profiler (GSP) (Fourth Dimension Spine, United States) (**Figure 9c.1**) which is still in use till today.

In 2009, we started a retrospective/prospective study on EOS cases treated by GRs in our institute. Inclusion criteria were: (1) any patient with EOS with a Cobb angle $\geq$ 40°, regardless of prior surgeries, and (2) the patient's age at time of first presentation was younger than 10. Exclusion criteria were: (1) the patient was older than 10, and (2) the patient's guardians refused to continue in the study.

All patients went through a thorough clinical evaluation, preoperative whole spine standing anteroposterior (AP) and lateral x-rays were made for every patient. On the AP view films, the Cobb angle of the major curve was measured; the upper and lower end vertebra as well as the apical vertebra was recorded. The T1–S1 height was measured (in mm) as the distance between the centre of T1 to that of S1 [19]. The apical vertebral distance (AVD) was measured as the distance between the centre of the apical vertebra of the major curve and the central sacral vertical line (CSVL). The space available for lung (SAL) ratio was measured as the sum of dividing the lung height in the concave side

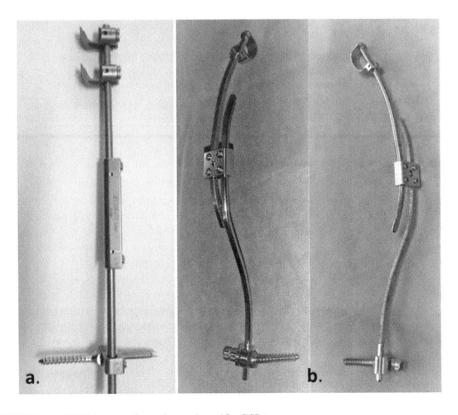

FIGURE 9C.1   **a:** ISOLA type of growing rods and **b:** GSP type.

by that in the convex side (line a by line b) [20] (Figure 9c.2). On the lateral view film, thoracic kyphosis was measured from the T5 upper end plate (or higher if visible) to the T12 lower end plate. All patients were classified according to the C-EOS classification [21].

TECHNIQUE FOR THE INDEX SURGERY

All patients received general anaesthesia and were laid prone with a soft pillow below the chest and another one below the pelvis. The skin was thoroughly sterilised, and draping was placed, keeping the whole spine and iliac crests accessible for the surgeon.

In the ISOLA group, the distal instrumented vertebra were determined with the help of C-arm fluoroscopy. Skin was incised in the midline then subcutaneous tissue and thoracolumbar fascia were dissected. The base of the transverse process was reached through a modified Wiltse approach. A small awl was used to get the entry point and then a pedicle finder was used to complete the track. A probe was used to ensure there was no cortical violation and also to measure the length of the screw, and an x-ray was taken to ensure the right trajectory. A pedicle screw of the proper size (26 mm–38 mm in length and 4 mm–6 mm in diameter) was inserted at the planned level, and the C-arm was used to ensure accurate positioning of the screws. The proper rod was inserted submuscularly and connected to the pedicle screws. Proximally, a midline incision was done over the targeted level and dissection was performed to expose the spinous process and lamina. Pedicle screws or laminar hooks were inserted in the targeted level, accurate positioning was ensured by the C-arm, and a proper rod was connected. Localised fusion around the proximal and distal foundations was routinely done. A proper size tandem was

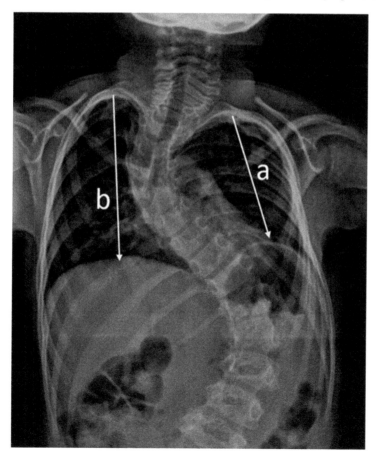

FIGURE 9C.2 Space available for the lung (SAL) ratio, **a:** concave side by **b:** convex side.

used to connect both rods in the thoracolumbar region away from thoracic kyphosis and lumbar lordosis. Initial lengthening was done, and the two locking nuts on the tandem were tightened. The wound was closed in layers after using a suction drain, and a sterile dressing was applied.

Early on in our experience, we used a single-rod technique for the sake of reducing the costs and magnitude of surgery. Later on, we converted to a dual-rod technique to minimise the complications following the recommendation of Thompson et al. [22] and Bess et al. 23]. Additionally, we also stopped using pedicle screws in the proximal foundation because of the reports of proximal pedicle screws pulling out and subsequent neurological deterioration [24, 25], and instead relied on laminar or rib hooks, keeping the pedicle screws proximally for salvage procedures only.

In the GSP group, caudal dissection was similar to that of the ISOLA group, but only one pedicle screw is inserted on each side and no fusion is performed according to the manufacturer recommendation. Proximally, a midline skin incision was done, and dissection was performed laterally creating a thick skin flap; paraspinal muscles were dissected over the planned ribs, and a suitably sized rib clamp, usually anchoring two adjacent ribs was used (16 mm or 20 mm) on each side. The two rods were contoured to mimic the thoracic kyphosis and lumbar lordosis and then connected to the rod connector (external rod assembly). After loosening the four locking nuts on the rod connector, the whole assembly is inserted under the muscle with the cranial one connected to the rib clamp and the caudal one connected to the pedicle screw. Initial lengthening was done, and the nuts were tightly locked. The wound was closed in layers after using a suction drain, and a sterile dressing was applied. According to the manufacturer recommendation, we used single rib anchor and a single-rod technique in the first three cases. Due to repeated rib breakage, rod breakage, and pulling out, we converted them to a dual-rod technique, and we used the dual-rod technique routinely in all our cases thereafter. Additionally, we always used a big rib clamp around two ribs on each side, which significantly reduced the incidence of rib fracture and proximal anchor failure.

TECHNIQUE FOR THE LENGTHENING PROCEDURES

Anaesthesia, positioning, and draping were done as in the index surgery. In the ISOLA group, skin incision was opened only over the tandem, either of the cranial or caudal nuts were released, and distraction was done between the two rods. The released nut was locked properly while maintaining distraction. The wound was closed in layers, and sterile dressing was applied.

In the GSP group, a smaller incision than that for the ISOLA group was done over the rod connector. The four locking nuts were released, and the central distraction nut was rotated clockwise or counterclockwise according to the rod configuration. After lengthening, the four locking nuts were tightened. The wound was closed in layers and dressing was used.

Distraction in both systems was controlled by feeling a strong resistance with no excessive force used at all to avoid anchor failure. The patient was transferred to his or her room. The suction drain was removed after 24 hours and antibiotics (1st generation cephalosporin) were administered according to the patient's weight. No braces or casts were used, and the patients were allowed to walk as early as they could. Stitches were removed after 10 days.

Patients were seen after 2 weeks, 2 months, and at 6 months for the next lengthening procedure, and the parents were informed to consult the surgeon at any time if they suspected anything went wrong.

RESULTS

In 2016, we reviewed all EOS patients treated in our hospital with growing rods who had a complete set of preoperative and follow-up x-rays, were compliant with the follow-up programme, and went through at least two lengthening procedures. Eight cases were excluded because of missing preoperative long films and seven cases were excluded because of noncompliance with the follow-up and lengthening protocol. An additional four cases were also excluded from this analysis because they had only the index surgery done and no lengthening (or only one lengthening) procedure had been performed yet. One case in which the patient developed a severe deep infection after the index surgery with MRSA that mandated early implant removal, was also excluded. The remaining 21 patients were included in this analysis.

Our cohort included 21 patients (13 females, 8 males); 9 syndromic (43%), 8 congenital (38%), 3 idiopathic (14%), and 1 neuromuscular (5%) scoliosis according to the C-EOS classification (Table 9c.1). All patients were younger than 5 years of age at the time of first presentation. At surgery time, their age varied between 2.5 years and 9 years.

The preoperative Cobb angle varied from 63° to 139° in the coronal plane (mean 82.33°±4.67°) and from 25° to 96° in the sagittal plane (mean 60.71°±4.53°). The ISOLA system was used in six cases, and the GSP system was used in 15 cases. All patients were neurologically free and ambulant preoperatively. Table 9c.1 shows the demographic data of our patients. In 2016, eight cases became graduate; four had undergone metal removal for various reasons and were scheduled for definitive fusion, and nine were still on the lengthening programme.

The mean scoliosis Cobb angle significantly improved from 82.33°±4.67° to 55.19°±4.89° ($p<0.001$). This equals 32.9% improvement. The AVD of the major curve significantly improved from 49.62±4.91 mm to 33.14±4.51 mm ($p<0.05$). This equals 33.2% improvement. The mean kyphosis angle significantly improved from 60.71°±4.53° to 49.38°±3.20° ($p<0.05$). This equals 18.6% improvement.

The SAL ratio improved from 69.02±2.95 to 90.57±1.78 ($p<0.05$). This equals 30.44% improvement. The T1–S1 length improved from 246.9±9.32 mm to 277.5±9.10 mm ($p<0.05$), and this equals 12.39% improvement. The mean blood loss in the index surgeries was 190.0±9.88 cc (ranging from 100 cc to 290 cc), while blood loss in lengthening surgeries was very little to be recorded or measured. The mean operative time of the index surgery was 115±10 minutes, while that for the lengthening surgeries was 25±5 minutes.

Intraoperative complications included pleural puncture in four cases (19%), but none of the patients needed an intercostal tube after consulting our cardiothoracic team. Late complications included 10 cases of superficial infection (47.6%), five cases of deep infections (23.8%),

seven cases of rod breakage (33.33%), six cases of proximal anchoring failure (28.57%), five cases of distal anchoring failure (23.8%), two cases of proximal junctional kyphosis (PJK) (9.52%), and one case of distal junctional kyphosis (DJK) (4.76%). No neurological complications were reported either early or late. The total number (40) complications was recorded in our series of 108 surgeries i.e. 0.37 per surgery.

We recorded 30 unplanned surgeries for the complicated cases. Five surgeries for debridement of deep infection (affecting proximal and distal anchoring points). Four surgeries for metal removal in deep infection after failed debridement. Six surgeries for proximal anchoring failure (4 GSP and 2 ISOLA) in which the proximal anchoring point was reinserted in a healthy one. Five surgeries for distal anchoring failure (in the GSP group) in which the pedicle screws were removed and inserted in a healthy caudal level. Seven surgeries to change the broken rods. Two surgeries for PJK (both were in the GSP group) in which the rib clamps were removed and a more cranial pedicle screws (of the same system) were inserted in T2. One surgery for DJK (in the ISOLA group); this surgery was necessary mainly because the pedicle screws were inserted in a transition zone (T11) – both screws were reinserted in a healthy caudal level.

DISCUSSION

The mean Cobb angle improved from 82° to 66° after the index surgery and to 55° ($p<0.001$) after the last follow up (33% improvement). The eight graduate cases achieved 41.5% improvement, and the nine cases who still continue on lengthening achieved 37% improvement so far. Our results are comparable to those reported by Klemme et al. [26] who achieved 30% improvement in Cobb angle at the last follow-up with traditional growing rods supplemented by bracing. They are also comparable with the 40% improvement achieved by Moe et al. [27] and the 50% improvement (in graduate cases) achieved by Akbarnia et al. [28]. Using the newer magnetically controlled growing rods, Hosseini et al. [14] reported curve improvement from 61.3° preoperatively to 34.3° (44%) after the last follow-up, which is also comparable to our results. In his comparative study, Cheung

TABLE 9C.1

Demographic Data of the Studied Patients

Case	Gender	Age (years)	Aetiology	Type C-EOS	Scoliosis°	Kyphosis°	Apical Vertebra	Shoulder Balance	Pelvic Tilt	Sagittal Balance	Coronal Balance	SAL Ratio	T1-S1 Height	UEV*	LEV**	System	Number of Lengthenings
1	Female	8	Neurofibromatosis	S-3-N	73	45	T9	Balanced	Balanced	Neutral	Balanced	71%	319	T3	L2	ISOLA	5
2	Female	6	Congenital + diastematomyelia	C-3-N	81	25	T9	Right high	Balanced	Neutral	Balanced	71%	268	T4	L1	ISOLA	6
3	Female	5	Congenital hemivertebra	C-3-+	85	63	T6	Left high	Balanced	Neutral	Balanced	65%	315	T3	T9	ISOLA	7
4	Male	8	Neurofibromatosis	S-4-N	103	51	T9	Balanced	Balanced	Neutral	Balanced	74%	285	T4	T11	ISOLA	6
5	Female	9	Congenital + unsegmented bar	C-3-+	65	77	T7	Left high	Right high	Positive	Right shift	72%	229	T3	T12	ISOLA	10
6	Male	7	Neurofibromatosis	S-3-+	95	96	T8	Balanced	Balanced	Negative	Left shift	74%	208	T5	L1	GSP	3
7	Male	6	Neurofibromatosis	S-2-N	65	41	T9	Balanced	Balanced	Neutral	Balanced	71%	330	T6	T12	ISOLA	10
8	Female	5	Congenital + Unsegmented bar	C-3-N	89	35	L1	Left high	Right high	Neutral	Right shift	66%	247	T9	L5	GSP	2
9	Male	6	Neurofibromatosis	S-4-N	139	86	T5	Balanced	Left high	Neutral	Left shift	65%	230	T2	T9	GSP	4
10	Male	4	Congenital hemivertebra	C-3-+	70	86	T8	Left high	Left high	Negative	Balanced	70%	172	T2	T11	GSP	2
11	Female	3.5	Congenital hemivertebra	C-3-+	78	55	T8	Right high	Balanced	Neutral	Balanced	77%	252	T2	T10	GSP	3
12	Female	4	Congenital hemivertebra	C-3-+	75	70	L2	Balanced	Balanced	Positive	Balanced	71%	220	T10	L5	GSP	5
13	Female	5	Idiopathic	I-3-+	70	75	L2	Right high	Balanced	Neutral	Left shift	70%	235	T11	L5	GSP	4
14	Female	6	Idiopathic	I-3-N	79	47	T7	Balanced	Balanced	Neutral	Balanced	72%	288	T4	T11	GSP	4
15	Female	3	Neuromuscular	M-3-+	87	78	T10	Balanced	Balanced	Neutral	Balanced	60%	190	T5	L1	GSP	4
16	Female	9	Neurofibromatosis	S-4-N	118	91	T9	Balanced	Balanced	Positive	Balanced	52%	230	T2	L1	GSP	3
17	Male	5	Neurofibromatosis	S-4--	100	40	T12	Left high	Right high	Negative	Right shift	69%	228	T8	L4	GSP	2
18	Female	6	Skeletal dysplasia	S-3-+	75	70	T6	Balanced	Right high	Negative	Balanced	66%	235	T2	T10	GSP	3
19	Female	2.5	Idiopathic	I-3-+	65	74	T7	Balanced	Balanced	Neutral	Right shift	70%	194	T3	T12	GSP	4
20	Male	4	Congenital hemivertebra	C-2-+	63	55	T9	Left high	Balanced	Neutral	Left shift	95%	224	T4	L1	GSP	4
21	Male	5	Neurofibromatosis	S-3-N	92	30	T9	Balanced	Balanced	Neutral	Balanced	66%	260	T7	L1	GSP	3

*UEV: Upper end vertebra **LEV: Lower end vertebra

et al. [29] reported similar improvement in the major Cobb angle between those treated with magnetically controlled rods and those with traditional rods.

The mean T1–S1 height improved from 247.9 mm to 277.5 mm (p<0.05) (average improvement of 1.1 cm per year). This is comparable to the 1.2 cm increase in T1–S1 height per year reported in a multicentre study by Akbarnia et al. [28]. Using magnetically controlled growing rods Siam et al. [30] reported increased T1–S1 height from 288 mm to 331 mm (1.5 cm per year) and Hosseini et al [14] reported increased T1–S1 height from 252.7 to 288.9 mm (1.4 cm per year).

Controversy exists in the literature about the effect of the growing-rod techniques on the sagittal profile of the patients. In our study, the mean kyphosis improved from 61° to 49° (20%). In a study conducted on a total number of 23 patients, there was initial improvement of total kyphosis from 53° preoperatively to 40° postoperatively (24%) then remained nearly unchanged with subsequent lengthening [31]. However, in another study of 21 patients (17 dual and four single), the authors showed no significant change in total kyphosis [32]. Using magnetically controlled growing rods, Thompson et al.

[33] reported increased kyphosis from 49.3° to 50.1°.

In our study, the mean SAL ratio improved from 69 to 90 (30% improvement). Very few studies in the literature had addressed this issue. Akbarnia et al. [28], in his multicentre study, showed improvement in SAL ratio from 75 to 100 (33% improvement).

The number of surgeries (both planned and unplanned) each child experiences before the final fusion is achieved is significant. In addition to the anaesthesia and surgical risks, the psychological impact on these growing children and their families from the repeated hospital admission and repeated exposure to anaesthesia and surgery cannot be overemphasised [34, 35]. Furthermore, the incidence of learning disability has been reported to almost double in children with multiple exposures to anaesthesia and surgery compared to unexposed children [36].

The introduction of MCGR was initially met with enthusiasm, but the promise of avoiding most of the complications related to the use of traditional growing rods and the problems associated with repeated invasive surgical procedures have been challenged lately. Although less frequent, proximal and distal anchoring failure, rod breakage, and infections are still occurring with MCGR

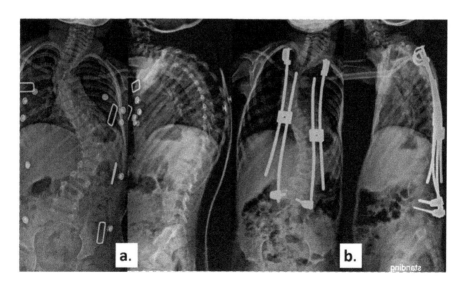

FIGURE 9C.3 Female patient, 5 years old with idiopathic EOS type (I-3-+). **a:** Preoperative AP and lateral x-rays show 70° lumbar scoliosis, 50° thoracic scoliosis, and 75° kyphosis. The T1–S1 height is 235mm, SAL ratio 70%, and AVD is 47mm. **b:** AP and lateral x-rays, after four lengthenings using the GSP, show improvement to 44° lumbar scoliosis, 40° thoracic scoliosis and 51° kyphosis. The T1–S1 height increased to 262 mm, SAL ratio improved to 96%, and AVD is reduced to 37 mm.

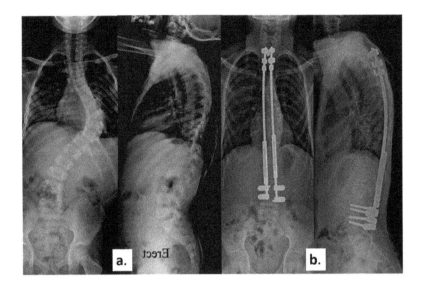

FIGURE 9C.4   Male patient, 6 years old with neurofibromatosis EOS type (S-2-N). **a:** Preoperative AP and lateral x-rays show 65° thoracic scoliosis and 41° kyphosis. The T1–S1 height is 330 mm, SAL ratio 71%, and the AVD is 57 mm. **b:** AP and lateral x-rays, after 10 lengthenings using the ISOLA GRs, show improvement to 20° scoliosis and 36° kyphosis. The T1–S1 height increased to 383 mm, SAL ratio improved to 98%, and AVD reduced to 12 mm.

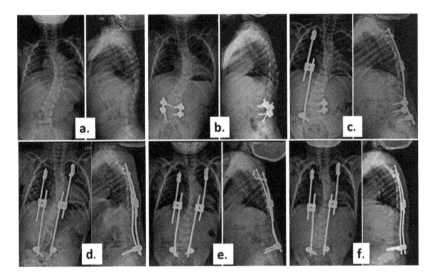

FIGURE 9C.5   A 4-year-old boy with congenital EOS type (C-2-+). **a:** Preoperative AP and lateral x-rays show L4 and T9 hemivertebrae with unsegmented bar and 55° lumbar and 63° thoracic scoliosis and 55° kyphosis. The T1–S1 height is 224 mm, SAL ratio 95%, and AVD of 43 mm. **b:** AP and lateral x-rays, after hemivertebrectomy and short segment instrumentation, show improvement of lumbar scoliosis to 34°, worsening of thoracic scoliosis to 67°, and almost unchanged kyphosis at 57°. The T1–S1 height is 222 mm, and AVD is 42 mm. **c:** AP and lateral x-rays, after single GR application, show significant improvement to 13° lumbar and 27° thoracic scoliosis, and 51° kyphosis. The T1–S1 height is 228 mm, and AVD is reduced to 21 mm. **d:** AP and lateral x-rays, after dual GRs application and lengthening, show 12° lumbar and 22° thoracic scoliosis and 49° kyphosis. The T1–S1 height is 244 mm, and AVD is further reduced to 13 mm. **e:** AP and lateral x-rays after the third lengthening show 11° lumbar and 27° thoracic scoliosis and 55° kyphosis. The T1–S1 height is 251 mm and AVD is 11 mm. **f:** AP and lateral x-rays after the fourth lengthening show 9° lumbar and 22° thoracic scoliosis and 45° kyphosis. The T1–S1 height is 258 mm and AVD reduced to 7 mm.

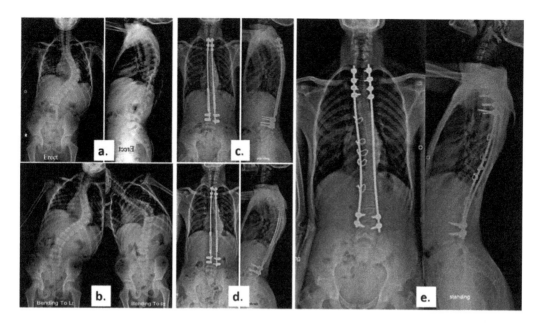

FIGURE 9C.6   Male patient, 6 years old with neurofibromatosis EOS type (S-2-N). **a:** This is the same patient in Figure 9c.4a. **b:** Preoperative AP, lateral, and bending x-rays show 65° thoracic scoliosis and 41° kyphosis. The T1–S1 height is 330 mm, SAL ratio 71%, and AVD is 57 mm. **c:** AP and lateral x-rays after 16 lengthenings show significant improvement of scoliosis from 65° to 30°. Kyphosis was maintained at 40°. The T1–S1 height significantly improved from 330 mm to 395 mm and SAL improved from 71% to 98%, and AVD improved from 57 mm to 10 mm. Because the patient was well balanced and asymptomatic, a decision was made to stop lengthening and maintain the GRs in place without doing fusion. **d:** AP and lateral x-rays 2 years later show significant progression of scoliosis to 48° and development of significant rib hump. **e:** AP and lateral x-rays 6 months after GRs removal, definitive fusion from T2–L4. Because of the significant dural ectasia and paper-thin pedicles, pedicle screws could not be inserted safely except in the most proximal and distal levels. Sublaminar wires were added in the middle segment. The T1–S1 height is 440 mm and the scoliosis was reduced to 28°.

similar to TGRs. However there is an additional peculiar complication in magnetic rods, which has not been previously reported, which is metallosis that is defined as aseptic fibrosis, local necrosis, or loosening of a device secondary to metal corrosion and release of wear debris [37].

Spinal fusion after repeated surgeries for gradual lengthening is still demanding with 20% reported reoperation rate [38] and carries higher risk of complications than *de novo* surgery, including, infection and wound dehiscence, instrumentation failure, painful or prominent instrumentation, coronal and/or sagittal deformity, pseudarthrosis, and progressive crankshaft chest wall deformity requiring a thoracoplasty [38]. Additionally, the progressive stiffness of the spine and autofusion phenomenon [39] allow for limited additional correction and increased incidence of neurologic abnormality with any

added corrective spinal osteotomy during the final spinal fusion.

Since the conclusion of our first study in 2018, many patients have already completed their lengthening procedures or suffered unsalvageable complications and had their GRs removed and final fusion done (Figures 9c.3–9c.6 show several illustrative cases). All graduates are the subject of an ongoing study now in our centre.

CONCLUSION

Despite all challenges we face in our hospital and country, the use of GRs seems to significantly help patients with EOS to improve their deformities gradually and maintain their growth potentials. The high number of surgeries per patients (both planned and unscheduled ones) is still distressing.

CONFLICT OF INTEREST

The authors certify that they have no financial conflicts of interest in connection with this article.

ACKNOWLEDGEMENTS

The authors acknowledge the generous help and advice of Dr Wael Mostafa Gad and Dr Hamdy Tammam for their help in measuring all parameters of our patients' data.

REFERENCES

1. El Banna Y, Samy S. Single-Stage Posterior Hemivertebra Resection with Transpedicular Instrumented Fusion for Correction of Congenital Scoliosis Egy. *Spine J.* 2016;19:35–47.
2. ElMiligui Y, ElSebaie H, Koptan W, et al. Growing Rods in Neurofibromatosis Scoliosis. *The 2nd ICEOS (International Congress on Early Onset Scoliosis and Growing Spine)*, 2007; Madrid, Spain.
3. ElSebaie H, ElMiligui Y, Koptan W. Single Stage Osteotomy for Congenital Lumbar Spine Deformities. *Egypt Orthop J.* 2004;39(2):283–289.
4. El-Sharkawi M, Koptan W, ElMiligui Y, et al. Pedicle Subtraction Osteotomies for Correcting Sagittal Imbalance. *Egypt Spine J.* 2012; 2(1):20–29.
5. ElSebaie H, ElMiligui Y, Koptan W. Surgical Correction of Established Congenital Spinal Deformities. *The 11th IMAST (International Meeting on Advanced Spine Techniques)*, 2004; Bermuda.
6. El-Sharkawi M, Koptan W, ElMiligui Y. Treatment of Congenital Spinal Deformities Associated with Intra-Spinal Anomalies by Growing-Rods. *The 78th AAOS Annual Meeting*, 2010; San Diego, California.
7. ElMiligui Y, Koptan W, El-Sharkawi M, et al. Correction of Neglected Congenital Spinal Deformities Associated with Intraspinal Anomalies. Is It Safe? *The 18th IMAST Meeting*, 2011; Copenhagen, Denmark.
8. El-Sharkawi M, Soliman O, Koptan W, et al. Single Stage Vertebral Column Resection of Hemivertebrae in Children under the Age of 10 Years. *The 46th Annual SRS Meeting*, 2011; Louisville, Kentucky.
9. El-Sharkawi M, Koptan W, Alkot A, et al. Posterior Vertebral Column Resection (PVCR) in Early Onset Spinal Deformities (EOSD). *Global Spine Congress & World Forum for Spine Research*, 2016; Dubai, UAE.
10. El-Sharkawi M, Koptan W, Alkot A, et al. Management of Early Onset Scoliosis Using Growing Spine Profiler (GSP). *Global Spine Congress & World Forum for Spine Research*, 2016; Dubai, UAE.
11. Elsebaie H, Koptan W, El Miligui Y, et al. Anterior Instrumentation and Correction of Congenital Spinal Deformities under Age of Four without Hemivertebrectomy. *Spine.* 2010;35(6):E218–E222.
12. Akbarnia BA, Pawelek JB, Cheung KM, et al. Traditional Growing Rods Versus Magnetically Controlled Growing Rods for the Surgical Treatment of Early-Onset Scoliosis: A Case-Matched 2-Year Study. *Spine Deform.* 2014;2(6):493–497.
13. Abol Oyoun N, Stuecker R. Bilateral Rib-to-Pelvis Eiffel Tower VEPTR Construct for Children with Neuromuscular Scoliosis: A Preliminary Report. *Spine J.* 2014;14(7):1183–1191.
14. Hosseini P, Pawelek J, Mundis GM, et al. Magnetically Controlled Growing Rods for Early-Onset Scoliosis: A Multicenter Study of 23 Cases with Minimum 2 Years Follow-Up. *Spine (Phila Pa 1976).* 2016;41(18):1456–1462.
15. ElBromboly Y, Hurry J, Padhye K, et al. Distraction-Based Surgeries Increase Spine Length for Patients with Nonidiopathic Early-Onset Scoliosis—5-Year Follow-Up. *Spine Deform.* 2019;7(5):822–828.
16. Soliman H. Health-Related Quality of Life and Body Image Disturbance of Adolescents with Severe Untreated Idiopathic Early-Onset Scoliosis in a Developing Country. *Spine.* 2018;43(22):1566–1571.
17. Soliman H. Health-Related Quality of Life of Adolescents with Severe Untreated Congenital Kyphosis and Kyphoscoliosis in a Developing Country. *Spine.* 2018;43(16):E942–E948.
18. Elnady B, Shawky Abdelgawaad A, El-Meshtawy M. Anterior Instrumentation through Posterior Approach in Neglected Congenital Kyphosis: A Novel Technique and Case Series. *Eur Spine J.* 2019;28(8):1767–1774.
19. O'Brien M, Timothy R, Kathy M, et al. *Radiographic Measurement Manual*, 2008. Medtronic Sofamor Danek USA.
20. Campbell R, Smith M, Mayes T, et al. The Characteristics of Thoracic Insufficiency Syndrome Associated with Fused Ribs and Congenital Scoliosis. *J Bone Joint Surg Am.* 2003;85-A(3):399–408.
21. Williams B, Matsumoto H, McCalla D, et al. Development and Initial Validation of the Classification of Early-Onset

Scoliosis (C-EOS). *J Bone Joint Surg Am.* 2014;96(16):1359–1367.

22. Thompson GH, Akbarnia BA, Kostial P, et al. Comparison of Single and Dual Growing Rod Techniques Followed through Definitive Surgery: A Preliminary Study. *Spine (Phila Pa 1976).* 2005;30(18):2039–2044.

23. Bess S, Akbarnia BA, Thompson GH, et al. Complications of Growing-Rod Treatment for Early-Onset Scoliosis: Analysis of One Hundred and Forty Patients. *J Bone Joint Surg Am* 2010;92(15):2533–2543.

24. Skaggs KF, Brasher AE, Johnston CE, et al. Upper Thoracic Pedicle Screw Loss of Fixation Causing Spinal Cord Injury: A Review of the Literature and Multicenter Case Series. *J Pediatr Orthop.* 2013;33(1):75–79.

25. Bekmez S, Kocyigit A, Olgun ZD, et al. Pull-Out of Upper Thoracic Pedicle Screws Can Cause Spinal Canal Encroachment in Growing Rod Treatment. *J Pediatr Orthop.* 2018;38(7):e399–e403.

26. Klemme W, Denis F, Winter R, et al. Spinal Instrumentation without Fusion for Progressive Scoliosis in Young Children. *J Pediatr Orthop.* 1997;17(6):734–742.

27. Moe J, Kharrat K, Winter R, et al. Harrington Instrumentation without Fusion plus External Orthotic Support for the Treatment of Difficult Curvature Problems in Young Children. *Clin Orthop Relat Res.* 1984;5(185):35–45.

28. Akbarnia B, Marks D, Boachie-Adjei O, et al. Dual Growing Rod Technique for the Treatment of Progressive Early-Onset Scoliosis: A Multicenter Study. *Spine.* 2005;30(17):S46–S57.

29. Cheung K, Cheung J, Samartzis D, et al. Magnetically Controlled Growing Rods for Severe Spinal Curvature in Young Children: A Prospective Case Series. *Lancet.* 2012;379(9830):1967–1974.

30. Siam A, Shaheen E, Mohamad-Ali N, et al. Preliminary Results of Treatment of Early Onset Scoliosis Using Magnetic Growing Rods. *Glob Spine J.* 2016;6(1):21–23.

31. Atici Y, Akman Y, Erdogan S, et al. The Effect of Growing Rod Lengthening Technique on the Sagittal Spinal and the Spinopelvic Parameters. *Eur Spine J.* 2015;24(6):1148–1157.

32. Chen Z, Qiu Y, Zhu Z, et al. How Does Hyperkyphotic Early-Onset Scoliosis Respond to Growing Rod Treatment? *J Pediatr Orthop.* 2017;37(8):e593–e598.

33. Thompson W, Thakar C, Wilson J, et al. The Use of Magnetically-Controlled Growing Rods to Treat Children with Early-Onset Scoliosis. *Bone Joint J.* 2016;98-B(9):1240–1247.

34. Bakri MH, Ismail EA, Ali MS, et al. Behavioral and Emotional Effects of Repeated General Anesthesia in Young Children. *Saudi J Anaesth.* 2015;9(2):161–166.

35. Haché M, Pinyavat T, Sun LS. Repetitive Anesthesia Concerns in Early-Onset Scoliosis. In: Akbarnia B., Yazici M., Thompson G. (eds) *The Growing Spine.* Springer, Berlin, Heidelberg, 2016.

36. Wilder RT, Flick RP, Sprung J, et al. Early Exposure to Anesthesia and Learning Disabilities in a Population-Based Birth Cohort. *Anesthesiology.* 2009;110(4):796–804.

37. Teoh K, von Ruhland C, Evans S, et al. Metallosis Following Implantation of Magnetically Controlled Growing Rods in the Treatment of Scoliosis: A Case Series. *Bone Joint J.* 2016;98-B(12):1662–1667.

38. Poe-Kochert C, Shannon C, Pawelek J, et al. Final Fusion after Growing-Rod Treatment for Early Onset Scoliosis. *J Bone Joint Surg.* 2016;98(22):1913–1917.

39. Sankar WN, Skaggs DL, Yazici M, et al. Lengthening of Dual Growing Rods and the Law of Diminishing Returns. *Spine.* 2011;36(10):806–809.

9d Mozambique Experience

Alaaeldin Azmi Ahmad

CONTENTS

INTRODUCTION

In this chapter, we will describe the challenges dealt with during the implementation of an early-onset scoliosis (EOS) service in Mozambique, which aims to give similar guidelines for implementing this service in sub-Saharan region.

The idea of implementing this service came in 2017 through collaboration between the Palestine International Cooperation Agency (PICA) and the Ministry of Health (MOH) in Mozambique. In Mozambique, there were no spine deformity services due to the lack of necessary implants and experienced people in this field. Previously, the country had scattered missions that came infrequently, performing cases with a lack of follow-up. The head of the orthopaedic department in Maputo Central Hospital (MCH) was interested in implementing a paediatric spine deformity service through regular missions aiming to build the necessary local manpower that can continue this service in the future.

During the 2017 meeting of the College of Surgeons of East, Central and Southern Africa (COSECSA), we spoke with the minister of health about establishing paediatric spine services at MCH, with full support of the head of the orthopaedic department in Mozambique and the executive hospital manager. The collaboration between PICA and the MOH in Mozambique began in 2018 through a Memorandum of Agreement (MOA) signed by both sides.

BACKGROUND

In 2017, the population of Mozambique was 30 million [1] with 100,000 assumed cases of scoliosis that needed clinical attention (extrapolated prevalence). Healthcare providers that would implement this service include the Ministry of Health (MOH) hospitals, university hospitals, and nongovernmental organisation (NGO) hospitals. Paediatric orthopaedic care with a special focus on spinal deformity surgery was chosen for the following reasons:

1. Unfortunately, there is a severe lack of manpower for this service in southeastern region of Africa, with no local facility in the whole region providing this service.
2. It is a highly demanding field that needs a long, sustainable programme to promote local doctors to be qualified to do this service.
3. There is already an orthopaedic training programme established by COSECSA, in which Mozambique is involved. It is the second largest surgical training institution in sub-Saharan Africa, but they do not have the spinal deformity training service. By implementing this service in Mozambique, it can spread through this established programme to many countries in the region.

4. There are a lot of projects through many organisations in Africa, but they mainly depend on volunteerism by short-term missions that are resource intensive with limited follow-up and provide minimal teaching. This programme aims to establish a new model focussing mainly on sustainable partnerships with significant involvement from academic institutions, including research, training, and capacity building.
5. It will be a good base to collaborate with many other global institutions working in low- and middle-income countries (LMICs) to avoid duplications.
6. It is an opportunity to provide a model for implementing a highly advanced service on a regional level that continuously strives to provide 'appropriate treatment' and high-quality services in an appropriate setting that will improve the health of the patient in the most cost-effective manner given the society (appropriate care is society-centred).

The Goals

The short- and medium-term goals for this programme were:

1. Adding paediatric spine service as a part of the paediatric orthopaedic services in MCH with the support of Dr Antonio Costa, head of orthopaedic services in Mozambique, a fellow of the orthopaedic college of Mozambique, and Fellowship of the College of Surgeons (FCS) COSECSA.
2. Establishing scientific cooperation with highly experienced paediatric spine surgeons who come on a regular basis, aiming to improve surgical services, screening, tracking, and follow-up protocols.
3. Getting funds for a 3-year programme aiming primarily at local capacity building through teaching and direct clinical service in the field of paediatric orthopaedic including paediatric spine surgery.

The long-term strategy for this programme was:

1. Helping local healthcare workers to help themselves in the long run, using what is available locally.
2. Building capacity and developing country-specific training programmes in the COSECSA region.

Methods and Results

From previous experiences with paediatric spine programmes, we know that the first mission is crucial, especially when beginning from scratch. The first mission can be looked at with skepticism from the local health professionals with a big question of 'can this be done here?', especially if they are already adapted to a pathway that was satisfactory, e.g. sending patients to India or South Africa for these surgeries. Considering the complications from these complex spine surgeries, any mistake might cause catastrophic results that would close the programme, and it will be extremely hard to convince the health authorities to continue with it

From the beginning, Dr Antonio Costa's help was used to arrange a multidisciplinary team. Meetings with the head of paediatrics, the intensive care unit (ICU), radiology, and anaesthesia departments discussed paediatric spine surgery and the needs from these departments preoperatively and postoperatively. The deficiencies faced were discussed, mainly the inability to do MRI in the hospital because the machine is not working, which led to an arrangement to do the MRI outside of the hospital, with the financial support of a private radiology centre for selected cases, mainly the EOS cases.

Additionally, the anaesthesia department asked to have an experienced anaesthetist because they did not have experience in this field. There was also a lack of tranexamic acid, and we needed to work without it.

Our first mission included a finding a paediatric spine surgeon, an anaesthetist experienced in dealing with scoliosis surgeries, a neuromonitoring technician highly experienced in intraoperative neuromonitoring, and a staff nurse who is competent in the operating room (OR) (**Figure 9d.1**). Our aim was to help establish a team in which each one of the team members

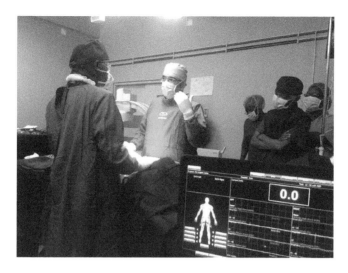

FIGURE 9D.1   The neuromonitor in the operative room run by our neuromonitoring technician.

would train a local health worker during the surgeries, while maintaining optimum safety conditions

We did five scoliosis cases, two EOS cases were performed using the apex active correction (APC) technique. The APC technique is a modification of the SHILLA technique and has advantages in decreasing complications, particularly in LMICs. All cases were done with the active participation of two local orthopaedic surgeons nominated by the head of the MCH orthopaedic department to be the future paediatric spine surgeons (**Figure 9d.2**).

A C-arm of good quality was available. The surgical implants and instruments were available as a generous donation from a company that manufactures spinal surgical equipment. The OR table used was a not a table designed for spinal surgery, so pillows were placed at the upper chest and pelvis with the patient in the prone position to remove any pressure on the abdomen.

The surgeon needs to look at every detail, such as avoiding pressure on bony prominences and ulnar and femoral nerves, be sure that antibiotics are given 30 minutes before incision, and try to avoid crowding in the OR

Because tranexamic acid and cell savers were not available, specific precautions were taken to minimise the bleeding by doing careful dissection and placing the incisions in harmony with the anchor sites. Usually, I begin with a

small proximal incision to install the proximal anchors, extend the incision to the apex to install the tethering screws, and then extend the incision to install the distal anchors.

Both cases were transferred postoperatively to the ICU with all postoperative details written out to ensure that everything was done according to the protocol and to answer any questions related to the patient details. We try to get the patient out of bed on the first or, at most, second postoperative day so that the Foley catheter can be removed and the patient can regain bowel sounds with the ability to take food orally and stop IV fluids. We needed to be sure that the patients would have the ability to move comfortably within 5 days after surgery before they went back home, as both patients lived far from the capital, and it was hard for the child and the family to come frequently. We utilised internet and smart phone technologies to follow-up on the patient pictures, x-rays, and lab investigations regarding general conditions through the local doctors who participated in the surgery

With the success of the first mission, everybody was enthusiastic in implementing this technique, including the health authorities in Mozambique, the sponsoring company, and of course our team. The second mission was done in 2019, with four cases of scoliosis, two of which were EOS cases done with the same technique as the previous mission. The difference during the second mission was clear in

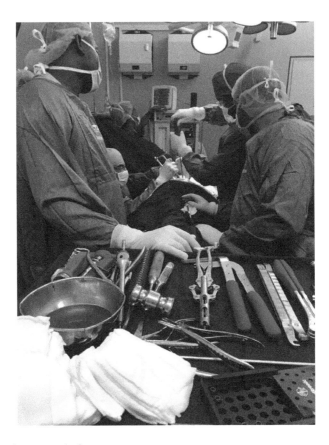

FIGURE 9D.2   Local surgeon placing screws.

the mood of the local OR workers being more relaxed and confident. The surgeons contributed more in the placement of the screws, there was more participation by the local OR nurse, and the ICU managed the cases better.

Our successful experience in implementing EOS services in a LMIC was due to:

1. Implementing within the context by:
   a. Having clear support from the MOH and the head of the MCH orthopaedic department to do this programme through a MOA with a clear timetable. This is of great importance because, in most LMICs, the MOH has most of the health resources, and the only way to do complicated cases is by doing them in the central governmental or university hospitals.
   b. Doing these surgeries in a hospital that all people can access for free because these surgeries

are expensive for most people in LMICs.
   c. Giving sustainability for this programme by acknowledging the local multidisciplinary team and engaging them in the programme. After all, it is not only surgery.
   d. Giving the local health professionals space to be engaged and understand that, at the end of this programme, they will be able to comfortably do most of the cases.
   e. Using regular implants that make it easier for the government to buy cost-effective implants that can do the work.
   f. Doing the surgeries in accordance with the appropriate basis but with adjustments that will work within the context, e.g. techniques to minimise bleeding; doing the surgery with accepted universal techniques, such as posterior tethering;

and avoiding risky procedures such as osteotomies.

2. Using the APC technique.

APC is a relatively new technique and one that is considered a modification of the SHILLA technique. This is essentially a nonfusion SHILLA procedure that is performed by placing pedicle screws on the convex side, above and below the wedged vertebrae. The pedicle screws are compressed before final tightening to create an artificial compensatory pressure on the vertebral body, gradually allowing its remodulation (reverse modulation) and reduction in the wedging over time. In contrast to the conventional SHILLA approach, the addition of APC could reduce future loss of correction, and eliminate the complications related to the need for osteotomies as a byproduct. This is because no screw is required at the concave side of the apex (**Figure 9d.3** and **9d.4**).

We did a study comparing the results of 20 cases done with the APC technique and 26 cases with the traditional growing rod [2]. The APC was performed to modulate the apical vertebra. The sliding of the rods was done through connecting the tethered rod with proximal and distal rods, thereby permitting spine growth without the need of distraction under general anaesthesia (**Figure 9d.5**). The study suggested clinical equivalency of correction between the APC and traditional growth rod systems but sound that growth rod procedures displayed higher complications rates than APC.

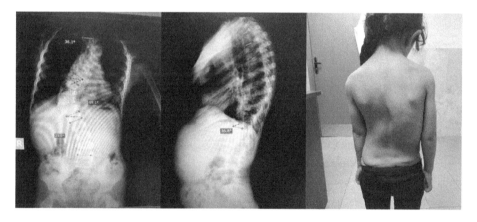

FIGURE 9D.3   Preoperative infantile idiopathic scoliosis for a 4-year-old child.

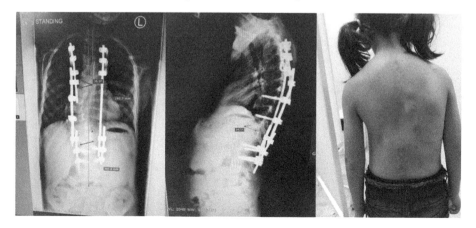

FIGURE 9D.4   Postoperative active apex correction (APC) technique.

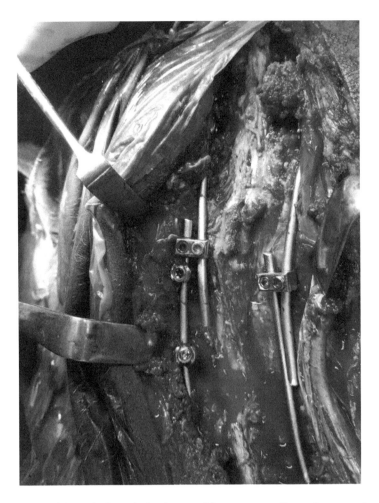

FIGURE 9D.5   Sliding of the rods through dominos avoiding recurrent distraction surgeries under GA.

Advantages of the APC technique include:

1. Tethering effect through posterior approach, which is the popular approach of most spine surgeons.
2. Fixation of the rod in the centre of the deformity without fusion will improve the rigid fixation.
3. The distance from the rod to the apex of the spinal deformity is minimal, which will give more efficiency to compression.
4. No direct compression on the intervertebral disc.
5. Rod fixation goes with the structural geometry of the spine.
6. Neurocentral synchondroses is not affected by this technique.

The APC technique is easy to implement in LMICs because:

1. The technique is done using posterior approach, which is a popular approach for most spine surgeons.
2. There is no need for any special implants. The procedure can be done with regular spinal implants produced from any company with no need for specific expensive implants.
3. The technique can be done with hybrid fixation in case there is no navigation or good quality digital C-arm.
4. The technique overcomes the lack of regular follow up and the need for frequent distractions every 6 months because the rods will slide up to 4 cm.

To make this programme sustainable, we need to:

1. Arrange for a budget to get good quality and more cost-effective implants than what we used before and an intraoperative neuromonitor.
2. Involve the local community in funding these projects.
3. Make this programme regional by merging it with the educational COSECSA programmes for orthopaedic and neurosurgery residency and paediatric orthopaedic fellowship.
4. Increase the role of online educational activities such as webinars and blended learning.

CONCLUSION

Paediatric spine surgery, including EOS, is a service with high priority, as the timely management of this condition is considered a life-saving measure (**Figure 9d.6**). Part of the management can be conservative with casting under general anaesthesia, which can be therapeutic in infantile idiopathic scoliosis cases and would also work as a delaying technique for surgery for other EOS cases.

Implementing the programme in LMICs needs to begin with the clear vision that most health services come through the MOH. In these complex surgeries, a MOA with the MOH is mandatory, as well as critical support from the head of the orthopaedic and/or neurosurgery departments, that in our case we were very lucky to have. Making these programmes regional helps to decrease the financial burden, with consistency in multicentre educational and research activities. Get motivated health workers who will lobby MOH officials to improve the service in the future.

Surgery, which plays big role in managing these cases, can be done in these areas within the health and financial context by applying techniques that can overcome excessive intraoperative bleeding, expensive implant usage, and a malfunctioning follow-up system, as well as avoiding the risk of doing complicated procedures such as osteotomies or putting screws in severely deformed pedicles. One of these techniques is the APC technique that we used safely for the complicated cases we did in MCH. There are many other techniques, e.g. the Miladi technique [4], that would benefit the surgeon by not bearing big risks in doing these surgeries and can be done with regular spine implants purchased from many companies

One of the most important factors in establishing a sustainable programme for these complicated surgeries is the relationship between the expert and the local surgeons [5]. The relationship needs to be based on adding knowledge and getting the local surgeons more involved through hands-on guided learning. This involves appropriate mentoring, supervision, guidance, assessment, feedback, and must be planned on a timescale that is long enough to sufficiently

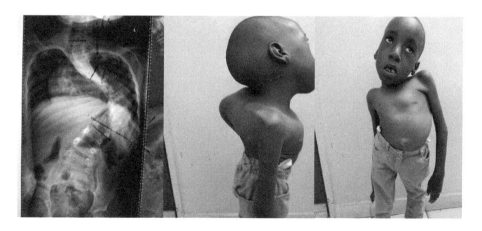

FIGURE 9D.6   Neglected case of congenital kyphoscoliosis affecting the pulmonary function.

enable learning from experience and from trial and error.

Such a collaborative approach would require a dose of humility and an understanding of the expert's role in perspective, including what they do not know and what they rely on the local surgeon for help with. Doing so will encourage innovation by adapting existing technologies to best fit a complex local context.

REFERENCES

1. *Mozambique Poverty Assessment - World Bank Documents- World Bank Group.*
2. Agarwal A, Aker L, Ahmad AA. Active apex correction (modified SHILLA technique) versus distraction-based growth rod fixation: What do the correction parameters say? *Spine Surgery and Related Research.* 2019.
3. Agarwal A, Aker L, Ahmad AA. Active apex correction with guided growth technique for controlling spinal deformity in growing children: A modified SHILLA technique. *Global Spine Journal.* 2020;10(4):438–42.
4. Miladi L, Mousny M. A novel technique for treatment of progressive scoliosis in young children using a 3-hook and 2-screw construct (H3S2) on a single sub-muscular growing rod: Surgical technique. *European Spine Journal.* 2014;23(4):432–7.
5. Ahmad AA. What's important: Recognizing local power in global surgery. *Bone and Joint Surgery.* 2019;101(21):1974–5.

9e Chile Experience

Samuel Pantoja

CONTENTS

INTRODUCTION

Early-onset scoliosis (EOS) represents a subgroup of spine deformity patients in the paediatric population in which management challenges can be significant. Dealing with this condition, even in a setting with substantial resources available, can be very difficult, depending on the particulars of the affected patients and the nature and severity of their conditions. This situation will naturally become even more complex in a setting where resources are limited.

In this chapter we will describe some of the aforementioned challenges. Also, how these have been addressed in Chile, a country with relatively good health indicators and in the middle ground in the scale of socioeconomic development, but with limited resources in this area of tertiary health provision. In this matter, it is representative of a number of countries, particularly in the Latin America, Eastern European, Middle Eastern, and some regions of Asia.

HEALTH PROVISION ORGANISATION

In keeping with a majority of countries in the region mentioned above, Chile has a health system that combines provision from public medicine and private insurers, with corresponding public and private hospitals. Here, we will concentrate on public health service provision by the state, both because it represents the greater challenge from the volume of patients and complexity of cases and because the provision from private insurance varies greatly and is difficult to encompass in one single representative group.

The management of paediatric spinal deformity can vary greatly in its complexity and in the resources required. In the case of EOS in particular, it is not infrequent that these challenges are far greater than in those of a patient representative of an average case of adolescent idiopathic scoliosis; managing a young child with a severe and complex deformity, with the frequent addition of significant comorbidities and that will probably require various surgical interventions starting at an early age can quite significantly stress the health system [1, 2]. As an example, a brief list of typically required resources may include:

- Assessment by a paediatric spine deformity specialist requiring multiple visits, frequently for patients who will have to travel from sometimes distant regions to a tertiary health provision location.
- Assessment by other medical specialists, such as anaesthesiology, cardiology, respiratory medicine, genetics, and others. Again, this usually requires repeated travel to a tertiary provider for many patients and their family.
- Magnetic resonance imaging (MRI) for spinal canal evaluation that must

usually be performed under general anaesthesia.

- Computerised tomography (CT) scans for anatomical details that require significant radiation exposure for some patients.
- The use of serial casting methods that again will frequently require general anaesthesia and repeated visits to the tertiary provider centre.
- The use of growth-friendly implants for deformity correction. These are often costly and may represent a substantial proportion of the financial burden of treating patients with EOS.
- The potential need for replacing a growth-friendly system for a definitive scoliosis correction system at a later date.

The above list succinctly represents some of the difficulties, both financial and administrative, associated with treating patients with EOS. In this chapter, we will detail some of the adaptations, both from the administrative and the medical aspects, that we have utilised in our setting when approaching this condition.

ADMINISTRATIVE ORGANISATION

As mentioned above, there are substantial costs involved in treating this condition. Historically, even in a public health system aiming for universal coverage, as is provided in Chile, the proportion of the cost of implants in particular and the opportunity for receiving the required treatments (usually in the form of obtaining a slot in the operating theatre waiting list for surgery) were transferred to the patient and their families. Many times, patients were required to either provide the funds or even directly acquire the implants, and it was also commonly observed that a slot in theatre was only obtained after repeated insistence from the patient's family to the designated hospital authorities. An enormous breakthrough resulted from a law reform that was adopted in 2005; this was initially named the AUGE and is now known as the GES (explicit health warranty) law. This law was focussed on assigning both a timing (opportunity), a competent provider (quality), and the required resources (financial protection) for treating a list of pathologies, which includes spinal deformity. In particular, for spinal deformity it was determined that patients of up to 23 years old who required surgery for their condition should be treated within a year from surgical indication. Also, in keeping with its complexity, the public health ministry assigned the responsibility for surgical treatment of the condition to only a few hospitals. It was the responsibility of the hospitals to provide both the technical expertise and the required resources, implants included, for surgical treatment. For this purpose, the health ministry assigned funds that were considered adequate for covering the cost of treating each case. Since its introduction, this law has allowed patients and their families to be treated in a timely manner, with a reasonably equivalent level of expertise in certified hospitals. The law has been modified since it's introduction; for example, inclusion of neural monitoring, which was not initially covered; the maximum time allowed from surgical indication to the actual surgical intervention was reduced from 12 to 9 months; and better financial coverage was specifically introduced for neuromuscular scoliosis, accounting for the usually greater resource expenditure required for treating patients with this condition.

This author is not an expert in public health and, as such, cannot be a judge of this aspect of the health reform mentioned. The above information is provided as an example of the enormous impact that changes in health organisation can have in treatment in this complex area of spine surgery, both for patients and their families and health providers. It is the belief of this author that, in Chile, the introduction of this law has put the interest of the patients first and resulted in a vast improvement in the management of those affected.

EOS TREATMENT

EPIDEMIOLOGY

The true prevalence of EOS is difficult to determine, mainly because it encompasses a variety of inhomogeneous diagnoses [1, 3]. As an indicator, in our institution, patients who were treated with either a growing system or subject to focal surgery for congenital scoliosis in the undeveloped spine (an indication commonly contemplated for patients under 7 years of age in our institution) accounted for 1.6% of the population of patients subject to surgery. Thus, in keeping with most reports, EOS accounts for roughly 1.5%–2.0% of the paediatric spine deformity population [1].

An additional problem, for both reviewing the results of treatment and planning for resource allocation in the public health system in our region is that we lack a centralised database for these patients. Again, with the GES law, there is some advance in this matter, as the prevalence of spine deformity in general in the Chilean population is now clear to the ministry of health.

EOS presents multiple additional challenges to the treatment of the spinal deformity itself. The Scoliosis Research Society guidelines on EOS provide focus on the obvious need to consider the potential sequelae of limitation in both the growth of the spine and the thorax, the presence of additional diseases that can influence treatment, and the possibility of requiring multiple surgeries for the same patient are just some of these [4].

One of the key concepts to consider when treating this group of patients is that if surgical intervention cannot be avoided, it should be delayed for as long as it is possible to allow for the maximum period of spinal growth. Besides surgery, the only treatment that has been demonstrated to be effective in avoiding progression of deformity is the use of bracing and/or casting techniques [5]. Sequential casting under anaesthesia is a method that has been used for a few years in our setting. This is a preferred method for patients who present a noncongenital deformity that is at least moderately flexible. In our unit, the procedure usually involves two or three instances of a cast brace, which is modelled under general anaesthesia. The consecutive episodes of cast bracing allow for a moderate but progressive initial correction and are separated usually 3 weeks after the final cast bracing. This is finally replaced for a thermoplastic removable brace that is frequently used by the child for 6 to 8 months before it requires replacement,

depending on body growth. The patient receives instructions on constant use of the brace (23 hours to allow for hygiene) and is reviewed every 6 months, both clinically and with an x-ray that is obtained with the brace removed for at least 4 hours prior to obtaining the image. Treatment is considered successful is the curve is maintained within 5° of the Cobb angle compared to the previous image. Treatment adhesion can be a problem, particularly during the warm weather. The patient's family is encouraged to maximise time of usage, but patients are usually allowed to remove the brace during short periods for swimming or other forms of exercise that may stimulate trunk mobility. With the notable exception of a majority of patients with congenital deformity, a trial of casting and/or bracing is almost always considered for EOS of greater that 30° in our institution. As mentioned, this can be effective for curve magnitude reduction in some patients and as a time gaining procedure to allow for spinal growth before surgery in others.

SURGICAL MANAGEMENT

Although every effort is made to avoid surgery in small children, should the curve increase during brace treatment, the patient should be considered for growth-friendly surgical intervention. The problem associated with early surgical intervention in these patients is twofold: early fusion will limit thoracic cage volume, which can have a deleterious effect on respiratory capacity, and, as a sequela, it may render the patient with a relatively short trunk respective of his or her lower extremities.

The available options for surgical management in EOS have changed significantly in recent years [2, 6, 7]. Of note, more recent advances include rib-based distraction systems that use ribs or a combination of rib and spinal or pelvic anchoring points for distraction (such as the vertebral expansion titanium rib device; VEPTR) and magnetically controlled growing rods (MCGR) that allow for elongation without repeated surgical intervention, and nonmagnetic systems that are small-size specific and may incorporate sliding implants specifically designed for elongation [8]. The VEPTR device has been used in the public setting in our region, and its concept has been adapted to include rib anchoring points obtained using more traditional laminar hooks applied as rib hooks, mainly because of cost containment. Although MCGR systems are available in Chile, it serves as an example of how the elevated cost results in a gap when the system is not provided for in public hospitals. The methods almost exclusively used in public hospitals in Chile consist of a variety of nonmagnetic distraction systems for repeated elongation. Literature suggests elongation should occur usually every 6 months, but the 9-month period of elongation modality is also accepted and is frequently used in our unit, mainly because it reduces the pressure on surgical theater time from patient waiting lists for surgery, which is a constant limitation in public hospitals. The method preferred consists of two or three level fixations in the extremes of the curve, using either pedicle screws, hooks, or a combination thereof. We perform a fusion of these points of fixation, attempting to reduce the frequent complication of implant dislodgment associated with this technique. Longitudinal rods are fitted with an elongation system and are inserted under the fascia, aiming to minimise soft tissue disruption close to the section of the spine that will be elongated, as this tends to produce spontaneous fusion, particularly in younger children (Figures 9e.1– 9e.3). For cases in which the main curve is particularly rigid and combines with a kyphotic component, we sometimes elect to include a convex growth-arrest by adding three or four points of pedicle screw insertion in the convexity, using a small additional incision (Figure 9e.4). As with every distraction technique, the law of the diminishing returns applies, and this will result in less effective elongation after consecutive attempts. Because of this, it is not frequent for us to go beyond a fourth or fifth elongation procedure.

Growth-friendly instrumentation may be considered conceptually as a temporising procedure that should ultimately be replaced with a definitive instrumentation and fusion. The indication for this may be from the patient attaining final trunk growth or because of recurrence of spinal deformity after the initial correction obtained (a phenomenon not infrequently observed during the increased peak growth velocity of the

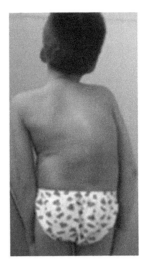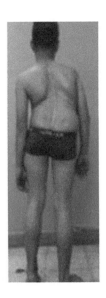

FIGURE 9E.1 A sequelae of short trunk relative to lower extremities in a 16-year-old boy who had a posterior spinal fusion for severe infantile idiopathic scoliosis at age 5.

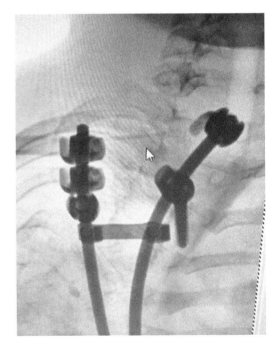

FIGURE 9E.2 An example of a proximal rib-based anchor using laminar hooks, used, in this case, for the revision of a patient who presented proximal implant pull-out and resulting poor bone stock.

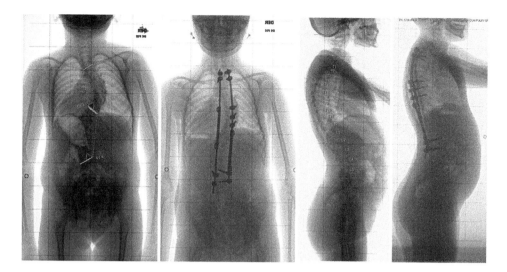

FIGURE 9E.3 A 7-year-old girl with significant kyphoscoliosis and a distraction system combining convex growth-arrest at the apex of the thoracic curve. The aim in this case is to combine convex growth-arrest with improved implant protection from pull-out. The potential drawback is reduced growth potential when compared to fixation and fusion limited to the proximal and distal anchor points.

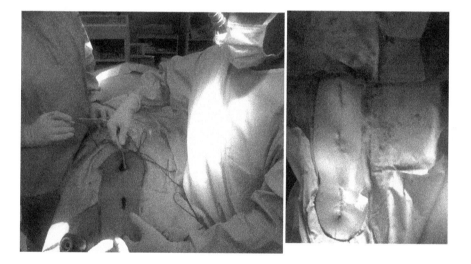

FIGURE 9E.4 Operative view of the technique of mini-open installation of a posterior distraction system.

preadolescent and adolescent period). However, it is fairly common to observe that patients who had growth-friendly instrumentation installed maintain an adequate control of their spinal deformity with no significant symptoms years after the procedure. For this reason, an indication to replace it for a definitive, adult-size scoliosis instrumentation system is only affected in roughly 25% of patients.

The management of EOS may sometimes be particularly challenging. Because of difficulties such as those related to patient's early age at initial surgery, the surgical technique or type of implants employed, the development of complications during treatment, and occasionally because of an unforeseen effect of body growth, tertiary reference centres occasionally have to deal with failed EOS surgery patients that constitute a particularly complex patient population. In our region, it is in this setting that on very particular situations, the public health system may require and provide the required funding to

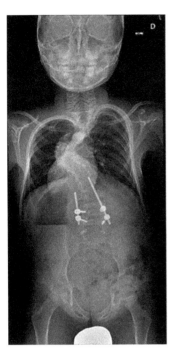
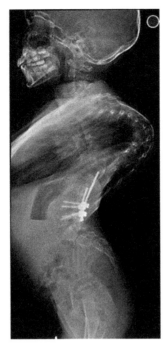
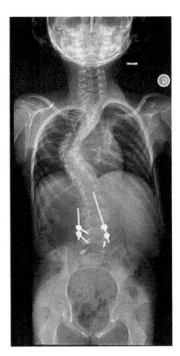

FIGURE 9E.5 A 9-year-old child with a history of five prior surgeries for congenital scoliosis, the index surgery at age 3, followed by various attempts at correcting complications The latest intervention was 2 years prior to his consultation and included partial implant removal with development of progressive kyphoscoliosis. The three figures show the standing anteroposterior and lateral views and an anteroposterior view in decubitus under traction.

a private hospital specialist team to participate in the treatment of these highly complicated cases. This frequently occurs because the private hospital can, on occasion, offer a form of advanced technology that is not available in the public hospital and that may make a substantial difference in dealing with these particularly complex cases. As an example of this situation, we include the case of a patient (Figures 9e.5–9e.6) with a very severe case of progressive kyphoscoliosis after multiple previous surgical attempts, that was managed with a period of halo-gravity traction, had surgical planning aided with a 3D printer model of his CT images and was subject to surgery with navigation and intraoperative CT control. In situations such as the one described, it becomes apparent that, albeit a small one, there exists a gap in technological developments available in some private institutions when compared to public hospitals. It also shows that, in justified cases, in our country, the public health provider will act symbiotically for the benefit of the patient.

CONCLUSION

EOS constitutes a small proportion of the paediatric spinal deformity populations subject to treatment. Complexities originating from the spinal deformity itself, the patient's medical comorbidities, and limited available resources and administrative and geographical challenges result in this area of spine deformity treatment presenting a more substantial proportion of resource expenditure. In Chile, public health initiatives that have improved organisation have designated a limited number of highly specialised centres for treatment provision and many times the incorporation of adaptations of the currently available technical methods have allowed for adequate treatment of very complex cases and, together with the growing experience of surgical teams, improved the treatment of these patients for their benefit and that of their families. This is of course a dynamic situation, and the incorporation of new techniques and implants that have a proven benefit remains a responsibility for the health provider.

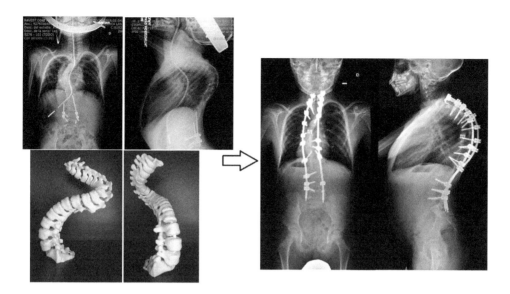

FIGURE 9E.6 A 9-year-old child with a history of five prior surgeries for congenital scoliosis, the index surgery at age 3, followed by various attempts at correcting complications. The latest intervention was 2 years prior to his consultation and included partial implant removal with development of progressive kyphoscoliosis. Top left figures show slight correction after 3 weeks of halo-gravity traction. A duodenal catheter for hypernutrition in preparation for surgery is visible. Bottom left shows images of a 3D impression based on CT, obtained for surgical planning. Figures on the right present his status after revision by proximal and distal extension, T9 vertebral body resection, and titanium cage insertion from the posterior approach.

REFERENCES

1. Yang S, Andras LM, Redding GJ, et al. Early-onset scoliosis: A review of history, current treatment, and future directions. *Pediatrics.* 2016;137(1):e20150709.
2. Hardesty CK, Huang RP, El-Hawary R, et al. Early-onset scoliosis: Updated treatment techniques and results. *Spine Deformity.* 2018;6(4):467–72.
3. Thompson GH, Lenke LG, Akbarnia BA, et al. Early onset scoliosis: Future directions. *Bone & Joint Surgery.* 2007;89:163–6.
4. Skaggs DL, Guillaume T, El-Hawary R, et al. Early onset scoliosis consensus statement, SRS Growing Spine Committee, 2015. *Spine Deformity.* 2015;3(2):107.
5. D'Astous JL, Sanders JO. Casting and traction treatment methods for scoliosis. *Orthopedic Clinics of North America.* 2007;38(4):477–84.
6. Yang JS, McElroy MJ, Akbarnia BA, et al. Growing rods for spinal deformity: Characterizing consensus and variation in current use. *Journal of Pediatric Orthopaedics.* 2010;30(3):264–70.
7. Lampe LP, Bövingloh AS, Gosheger G, et al. Magnetically controlled growing rods in treatment of early-onset scoliosis: A single center study with a minimum of 2-year-follow up and preliminary results after converting surgery. *Spine.* 2019;44(17):1201–10.
8. Cunin V. Early-onset scoliosis–current treatment. *Orthopaedics & Traumatology: Surgery & Research.* 2015;101(1):S109–18.

9f Evolution of Experience and Practise in Two Nations

Ujjwal Kanti Debnath,

CONTENTS

INTRODUCTION

Thirty years ago, I was apprenticing with the first scoliosis surgeon in India, Dr R. N. Mitra in the early 1990s. He was trained by Dr Walter P. Blount at Milwaukee and later with Dr John E. Hall in Toronto. He had been treating children with spinal deformity since the 1960s in Kolkata, India. During these 4 years of training with him, I first came across few children between 2–8 years of age with scoliosis (infantile or juvenile idiopathic types). I observed that many of these children had resolution of the spinal deformity over a period of time. Since the days of Hippocrates, orthopaedic surgeons were taught that infantile scoliosis worsens with growth [1]. Scott and Morgan [2] noted two patterns of curve behaviour: progressive and resolving. However, when left untreated, the condition can get worse, leading to back pain; impaired cardiorespiratory function; and physical, psychological, and social disability [3,4].

India-born Dr Mehta had the pioneering idea of casting babies with progressive curves and introduced rib-vertebral angle deformity (RVAD) [5, 6]. I was trained to apply casting on these children followed by bracing. Children with proximal thoracic curves required the use of a Milwaukee Brace, which is usually not well-tolerated (Figure 9f.1) [7–9]. My conscious effort to find a solution for those children with infantile or juvenile scoliosis started building. I scripted the first monograph on scoliosis in India, *Scoliosis – Facts, Figures & Follow-Up for Clinical Research* [7]. This book included contributions from Dr John Hall, Dr Alf Nachemson, Dr John Kostuik, Dr Robert Winter, and Dr Yves Cotrel

The concept of early-onset scoliosis (EOS) was just evolving after Prof Dickson from Leeds coined the term in the early 1990s [10, 11]. This classification was based on the functional abilities of the child connected with their lung and thorax growth [12]. There is an increase in the alveolar growth and number in the first year of life that reaches its maximum by the age of 8 years [13]. The use of growing instrumentation may delay definitive fusion and may help to maintain pulmonary health [14].

Currently, EOS includes all forms of scoliosis in children below the age of 10 who have spinal curvature more than $10°$ [15]. A higher rate of comorbid disorders is associated with infantile and juvenile scoliosis [16, 17]. In the long

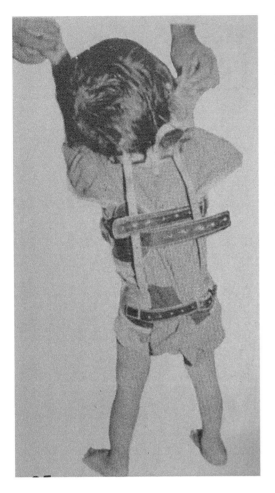

FIGURE 9F.1   Photograph of a 2-year-old girl with EOS treated with Milwaukee bracing in 1972 (from monograph by Mitra and Debnath, 1995).

term, infantile and juvenile scoliosis have high mortality [18].

My pursuit for further knowledge and skill to understand the disease led me to the British Isles. I spent a few years in Ireland, where I had tried to set up a school screening programme to detect children with EOS in a county hospital, but this failed due to lack of funding. Later, I passed the Fellowship of the Royal Colleges of Surgeons exam (FRCS) and went to the United Kingdom.

NOTTINGHAM, 1999

In the first few months at Queens Medical Centre (QMC), Nottingham, it was difficult to keep pace with the scoliosis world. Dr John Webb, legendary spine surgeon, had enormous experience in treating difficult spinal problems. It was difficult in those days to be in his surgical theatre because there was a significantly high number of surgeons converging to train here from around the world. I spent most of my time in the clinic seeing as many patients with spinal deformity. This improved my knowledge about the different indications for surgery in each patient, and I kept my notes for my future reference. I observed many postoperative follow up patients who had unilateral growth arrest, segmental posterior instrumentation without fusion (Luque Trolley with or without convex epiphysiodesis) [19]. Convex epiphysiodesis alone did not prevent deformity progression and the addition of instrumentation could slow progression but did not reverse it [20]. The initial results of treatment of progressive EOS with Luque Trolley alone at this centre were disappointing, so an apical convex epiphysiodesis was added. I realised that convex epiphysiodesis has a tethering effect on growth phenomenon and should be avoided when growth guided instrumentation is used.

In Luque Trolley, initially called 'L' rods, were used with the straight ends being left long to allow for spinal growth. The 'L' portion is secured to the laminae of the end-vertebrae (Figure 9f.2). Subsequently, 'U' rods were used (Figure 9f.3a & b). The Luque Trolley acts as a brace for the spine against curve progression. The curve correction by this method was predicted by two factors, i.e. less upper end vertebral tilt and concave rib droop [21]. The results of Klemme et al. [22] suggest that progressive scoliosis can be controlled in many children while allowing normalised growth of instrumented spinal segments. The progressive structural changes alter the curve response to incremental distraction. These changes determine the treatment duration and ultimate gain in spinal length.

I had met many spinal fellows at Nottingham from around the world who remain great friends; most notable was Dr J. R. McConnell from Allentown, Pennsylvania. My interaction with them had updated my knowledge on surgical management of EOS. Subsequently, I joined as a specialist trainee in orthopaedics in Cardiff in 2002.

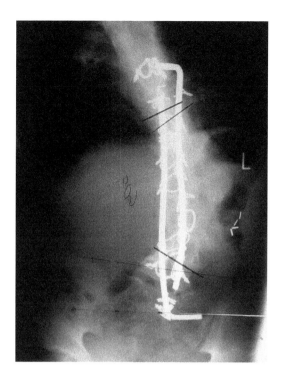

FIGURE 9F.2 Postoperative AP view x-rays of a 9-year-old boy with EOS and Luque Trolley in 'L' configuration.

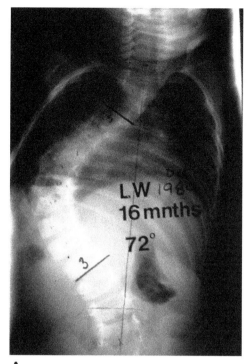

A

FIGURE 9F.3A AP view x-ray of a 16-month-old girl with EOS.

CARDIFF, 2005

During my training in Cardiff, I had developed the first web-based scoliosis registry and database for the spinal unit at University Hospital of Wales (UHW) with help from Dr John Howes, Consultant Spine Surgeon. He had invited Dr Robert Campbell from the United States who had developed VEPTR (vertical expandable titanium prosthetic rods). He demonstrated the technique of application in children with thoracic insufficiency syndrome [23, 24] [Figure 9f.4]. This technique indirectly fixes scoliosis without fusion. VEPTR treatment has demonstrated continued spinal growth with serial expansion improving the coronal curves [25]. Over the next few years, a hybrid technique using growing rods with VEPTR was introduced to reduce the complications. The hybrid technique incorporates the VEPTR concept by using ribs as proximal anchor sites but also uses pedicle screws for distal anchors [26, 27].

NOTTINGHAM, 2007

I returned to QMC, Nottingham, to do my spinal fellowship programme. I now had the opportunity to do surgeries alongside Dr J. K. Webb, Dr S. M. H. Mehdian, Dr M. P. Grevitt, and Dr B. J. C. Freeman. These surgeons had wide clinical and surgical acumen. The most notable experience was with Dr Webb, who I consider my mentor in spine surgery (spine guru) (Figure 9f.5). I had done many complex surgeries independently with his guidance with or without him. I devoted most of my time on spinal clinics, surgery, and research in the unit. I was reviewing the EOS cases performed here. The growth-rod concept had evolved in Nottingham, like elsewhere, in the last 5 years. The idea behind growth rods in treating EOS is to correct spinal curvature and permit skeletal growth. Luque Trolley was abandoned due to high incidence of complications, spontaneous fusion, and inadequate spinal growth. This technique was replaced by dual growth rods and sublaminar wiring (Figure 9f.6a–b). We

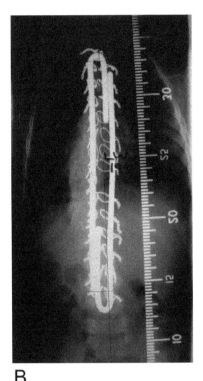

B

FIGURE 9F.3B 5 years postoperative AP view x-ray at 7 years of age with Luque Trolley in 'U' configuration.

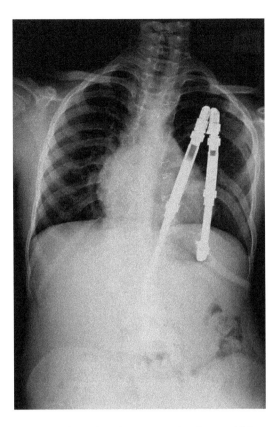

FIGURE 9F.4 AP view x-ray of a 6-year-old boy with EOS and thoracic insufficiency syndrome treated with VEPTR.

used proximal (hooks or screws) and distal pedicle screws as anchors. The two titanium rods placed side by side anchored with sublaminar wires. In our experience, proximal fixation was obtained over three levels with at least five fixation points. We performed lengthening every 6 to 12 months, depending on the age. It has been shown that frequent lengthening (≤6 months) may have greater curve correction and overall increased spinal growth [28, 29]. Ouellet et al. [30] published five patients treated with a modern Luque Trolley technique in which the proximal and distal ends of the construct were instrumented and fused. I worked with Dr Mehdian, an innovative surgeon with whom I have published many papers. He showed me the use of an H bar construct (Figure 9f.7) for EOS neuromuscular scoliosis (spinal muscular atrophy, Duchenne muscular atrophy, and cerebral palsy) [31, 32].

In the flurry of surgeries and my ongoing thesis work on lumbar spondylolysis, I was

studying the timing of definitive fusion for these EOS children who had grown as adolescents (the research question that had intrigued me 7 years ago). I presented a paper in Scoliosis Research Society (SRS) meeting at Salt Lake City, Utah [33]. During this meeting, I learnt a lot through presentations by many surgeons who were engaged in different types of research with EOS. Most surgeons were discussing the distraction-based strategies, and only a few spoke on growth-guided strategies for the treatment of EOS (Figure 9f.8). Notable papers did imprint an image of the various kinds of EOS treatment based on multiple surgical experiences, e.g. Dr Flynn on VEPTR [34], Dr Akbarnia on congenital scoliosis (posterior resection and growing rods) [35] and SHILLA procedure by Dr McCarthy. McCarthy et al. [36] developed the SHILLA growth guidance system (SGGS), which included short segment posterior fixation and fusion at the apex of the deformity. The rods

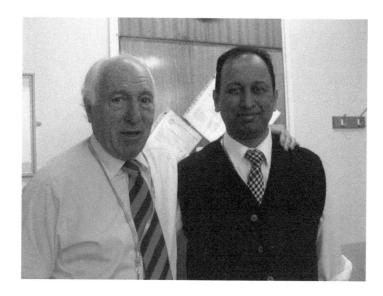

FIGURE 9F.5 Dr John Webb (spine guru) and Dr U. K. Debnath at QMC, Nottingham, 2007.

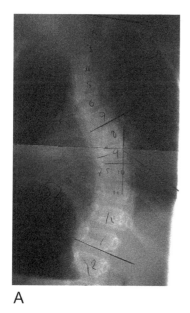

A

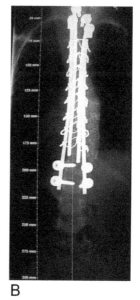

B

FIGURE 9F.6A AP view x-ray of a 7-year-old boy with EOS.

FIGURE 9F.6B Postoperative AP view x-ray showing posterior hybrid Luque fixation in the same boy.

can slide across the proximal and distal anchor points. The complications of rod breakage were reported up to 30% of patients [36].

Tsuji et al. from Nagoya, Japan, presented a casting technique to reinforce conservative treatment in EOS until growing rod surgery could be performed [37]. The need for

repeated surgeries under general anaesthesia is a major drawback in growth-rod surgery. High incidence of anaesthetic and wound complications were reported [38, 39]. Patients who were younger at the time of initial surgery had higher complication rates, as I observed in a 10-year-old boy who had multiple surgical debridements

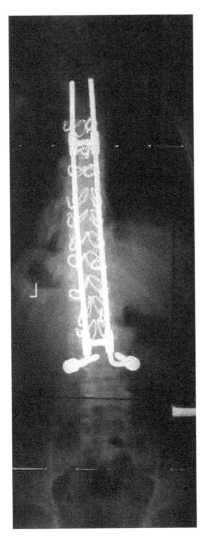

FIGURE 9F.7 AP view x-ray of 9-year-old boy with neuromuscular EOS treated with Luque Trolley with H bar.

for ongoing infection following growth rods at 6 years of age.

During this period of my fellowship, I had learnt significantly through interactions with a multidisciplinary team that included a spinal clinical nurse specialist, clinical psychologist, paediatrician, radiologists, anaesthetists, physiotherapists, and of course the theatre staff. The tertiary care UK hospitals have a well-tuned multidisciplinary team for delivering children's spine surgery. This group of clinicians meets to review the proposed benefit and risk of spinal surgery for the child. The parent and families are provided with all the necessary information

at their preoperative visit by the nurse who comprehensively reinforces the procedure and plan. Clinical photography forms an essential part of the management. As part of the team, we all were responsible for providing compassionate, high-quality, safe care whilst working in an acute fast-paced environment.

I successfully performed many operations to correct the spinal deformities in children and my 1-year fellowship ran out before I realised. During this time, I was supported by all my co-fellows, who were incidentally neurosurgeons, and became great friends for life.

OPERATION STRAIGHT SPINE (OSS), KOLKATA

'Operation Straight Spine', a transatlantic collaboration between the two surgeons for treating spinal problems in the underprivileged children in India, was taking shape. In November 2006, Dr J. R. McConnell, a consultant spine surgeon and I embarked on this journey with a team to perform a spinal surgical workshop at a charitable teaching hospital in Kolkata (Figure 9f.9). This required a tireless, organised effort in an uncharted sea. Following the success of the first surgical workshop in 2006, I was travelling between India and UK to establish this annual programme doing at least 10 spinal operations. At this time, we treated few children with EOS. Many of them underwent simple traditional dual growing rods (TGR) with dominos in which the rod slides.

KOLKATA, 2011

I relocated from London to Kolkata in 2011 and started to practise spine surgery at a private hospital. But my engagement with spinal patients of OSS continued in a more organised fashion in the charitable sector. The annual workshops continued to support the cause. EOS cases were evaluated in a weekly clinic. Our work was gradually recognised by SRS who endorsed the programme as the first global outreach programme (GOP) for spinal surgery site in India. We were honored at an SRS meeting at Anchorage, Alaska, in September 2014 for 'Operation Straight Spine'.

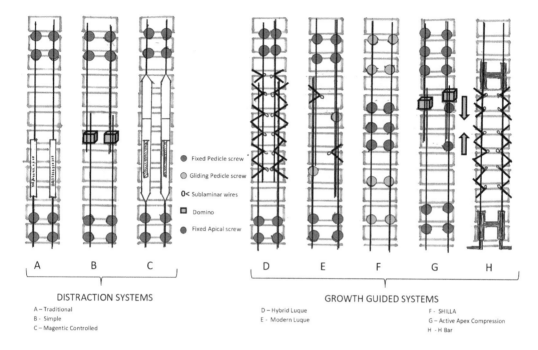

FIGURE 9F.8 Schematic diagram of growing rod techniques.

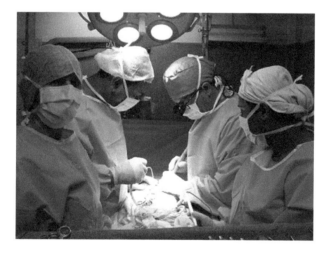

FIGURE 9F.9 Dr J. R. McConnell (Allentown, Pennsylvania) and sister Marian Barry (London) with Dr U. K. Debnath during OSS 2010 at surgery in Kolkata, India.

LONDON, 2015

I returned to the UK for a short fellowship at Great Ormond Street Hospital, London. I reviewed many children with EOS who were idiopathic, congenital, neuromuscular, or syndromic. I was introduced to magnetically controlled growing rods (MCGRs) here, and I did

many implantation, removal, exchanges, and revisions for EOS children. The MCGR procedure can be safely and effectively used in outpatient settings minimising psychological distress and improved quality of life [40, 41].

I was part of an audit on 46 EOS patients treated in past 3 years who had undergone MCGR. The mean age was 6.8 ± 1.9 years at the time of primary surgery. The major coronal curve magnitude improved from a mean Cobb angle of 70° (preoperative) to 34° (postoperative) in primary cases. Device failure occurred in 16 children (28%), leading to a decision for operative revision in 14 cases. It was observed that four patients developed a superficial wound infection. In the dual rod group, two patients had pull-out of proximal hook and another had prominent metalwork. Six patients had a rod breakage.

The MCGR consists of a titanium spinal distractible rod with an enlarged midportion containing a rotating mechanism (thickened actuator portion that houses the magnet) (Figure 9f.10a and b). Dual rods have been shown to produce increased distraction forces and to allow for differential correction [41]. The maximum length distractible is 4.8 cm. During outpatient distraction visits, patients were positioned prone, and a skin marker was used to mark the internal magnet. A hand-held magnetic external remote controller (ERC) was placed on the patient's back. Once the magnetic field was applied, the rod lengthens thus distracting the spine. Although MCGR has reduced the number of planned surgeries for distraction, there are incidences of unplanned visits to the operation theatre [42]. A skill well learnt could not be transferred to the patients in my practice due to the enormous costs [43].

The National Health Services' (NHS) machinery of a multidisciplinary team was more established in this hospital. The surgical team (nurse in-charge, scrub nurses, and scrub technicians) prepared the environment and the necessary instruments and equipments in readiness for an anaesthetic, surgery, or recovery of patients. Patient safety and good practice depends on an effective surgical team working along with a highly skilled surgeon. The whole team enhances the performance of the team and

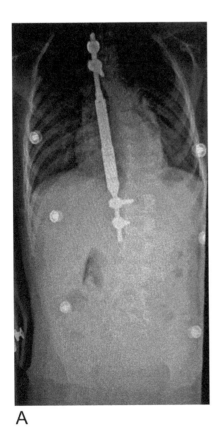

A

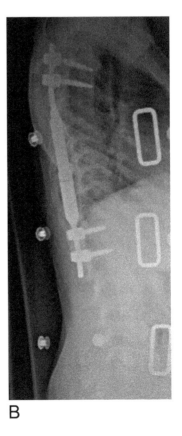

B

FIGURE 9F.10A Postoperative AP view x-rays of a 6-year-old with single MAGEC rod.

FIGURE 9F.10B Postoperative lat view x-ray of the same boy.

results in good patient outcomes. This organised facility was lacking in my practice in India.

SRS GOLDEN JUBILEE MEETING, MINNEAPOLIS, MINNESOTA, 2015

The SRS committee awarded me with a scholarship to attend the 50th annual meeting in Minneapolis, Minnesota, in October 2015. I attended the precourse meeting on EOS, which updated my ongoing learning. There was still no consensus on ideal age, threshold Cobb angle, and lengthening interval

Instrumentation for EOS is based on either distraction, guided-growth, or compression-based strategies (Figure 9f.8). Most surgeons were using distraction-based growth rods (submuscular insertion) for EOS between 4–10 years of age with a curve over 70° [44]. Dr Akbarnia reported 46% complications (mostly implant failures and infection) and a spinal growth of 1.8 cm/yr [28]. Compression-based techniques have gained attention with the development of anterior vertebral body tethering, e.g. stapling [45]. SGGS had fewer surgeries (2.8) compared with growth rods (7.4) but had high rates of complication [46]. The TGR group had more surgeries, but SGGS patients had more unplanned procedures [47].

KOLKATA 2016–20

I continued to deliver the OSS programme supported by the team from the United States and UK. We had a good team of paediatric anaesthetist and nurses led by Dr Neena Seth, Dr Meera Kurup, Dr Priya Krishnan and Dr Caroline Davies from St. Thomas' hospital, London, who has always provided support for all the scoliosis patients during OSS. We continued doing the TGRs with dominos. The phenomenon of decreasing gains in spinal lengthening was reported [48]. This 'law of diminishing returns' was observed in our patients as well.

Although MCGR was advantageous in many respects, e.g. noninvasive outpatient lengthening, reduced risk of infection, avoiding multiple surgeries, and improved patient satisfaction, the disadvantages were complications and technical issues [49,50]. After gaining knowledge on distraction-based systems, my inclination toward

growth-guided techniques were influenced recently by a new classification of EOS [51]. This was deemed valid and demonstrated its potential use in guiding decision-making [52].

I had organised the OSS '20 programme recently. We had successfully treated eight scoliosis patients. This time Dr Alaaeldin Ahmad, a paediatric spine surgeon from Palestine, joined us for the workshop on my invitation. He was discussing his new technique of guided-growth implantation, called Active Apex Correction (APC) technique. There were few unique aspects in this construct [53,54]. In this modified technique, the most wedged vertebra was selected followed by insertion of pedicle screws in the convex side of the vertebrae above and below the wedged one. Instead of apical fusion, apex compression was applied at the wedged vertebra (Figure 9f.8g). The procedure was more economical (using two screws instead of six at the apex of the curve) for underprivileged patients globally [53].

During this programme, Dr Ahmad performed the APC technique in three children with EOS with my assistance (Figure 9f.11). One 13-year-old girl had surgery on four previous occasions. Now, the girl has grown tall, but there was a progressive curve decompensating at L2/L3 vertebral disc on radiographs. Due to a lack of surgeries for growth modulation for last 3 years, she developed a crankshaft phenomenon. She underwent APC technique of dual growing rods (Figure 9f.12a–g).

'Children diagnosed with EOS can lead healthy active lives if detected early and advised treatment in right direction' [55]. This dictum holds true for many of my patients. One 14-year-old boy with EOS had simple growing rods (with dominoes) when he was just 6 years old. He had good correction achieved through the previous lengthening procedures. The growth rods were removed this year. This gives me the utmost satisfaction when such children say 'my scoliosis surgery changed me and my life for the better, because my back is now straighter and I don't have any physical restrictions'. However, recent evidence indicates that the removal of implants without fusion is an unacceptable treatment strategy that leads to poor outcomes [56, 57].

In my experience, patients with repeated surgery in EOS demonstrated some psychosocial

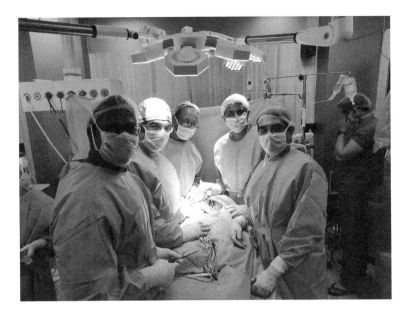

FIGURE 9F.11   Dr Alaaeldin Ahmad (Palestine), Dr U. K. Debnath (Kolkata, India), Dr Shah Alam (Dacca, Bangladesh) and spinal fellows at surgery during OSS '20 at Institute of Post-Graduate Medical Education and Research,Kolkata.

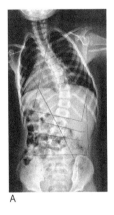

A

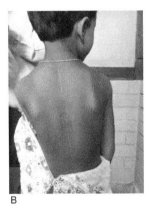

B

FIGURE 9F.12A   AP view x-rays of a 5-year-old girl with EOS treated during OSS 2012.

FIGURE 9F.12B   2 months postoperative photograph of the 5-year-old girl with EOS treated with simple growing rods.

issues. The children are anxious and depressed when they introspect on the multiple invasive procedures. It has been reported that in EOS children, there is abnormal psychosocial scores with a positive correlation between behavioural problems and the number of repeat surgeries [58].

There is no multidisciplinary team to discuss regarding the patient's surgical and emotional needs in India. There are major gaps and healthcare inefficiencies and inequalities in India.

The surgeon, for his own interest, builds up a dedicated team for a successful campaign for children's spine surgery. Above all, the burden of caregiving, decision-making, parent counselling, surgery, and postoperative follow-up is handled singularly by the surgeon. A dedicated team of spinal surgical nurses and scrub technicians have been shown to improve surgical outcomes [59]. Constant surveillance and continuous improvement of the quality and safety

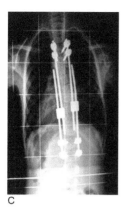

FIGURE 9F.12C   AP view x-rays of the same girl with EOS showing dual growing rods.

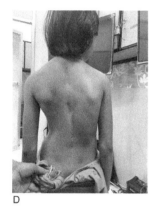

FIGURE 9F.12D   Photograph of the same girl at 13 years old showing curve progression.

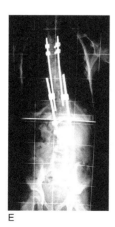

FIGURE 9F.12E   AP view x-rays of the same girl showing decompensation at L1 vertebrae.

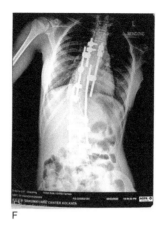

FIGURE 9F.12F   AP x-rays of the same girl showing active apex compression (APC) technique of growth rods.

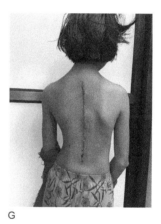

FIGURE 9F.12G   Postoperative photograph of the same girl showing curve correction during OSS 2020.

of spine treatments is imperative in modern healthcare where the responsibility needs to be shared [60].

CONCLUSION

Although there are various cultural and social differences that exist between the UK and India, the UK's NHS presents an excellent working environment in which aspiring surgeons from India or other nations are able to significantly progress their careers. The broad training and experiences from numerous excellent centres under many legends, enabled me to give my EOS patients and their parents a decision, a treatment plan, and a prognostic idea. In India, surgeons constantly adjust treatment based not on accepted 'best' treatment modalities, but on what is 'appropriate' for a particular individual. In fact, decisions regarding management are based on how much a patient or their families can afford.

The wide experience of two nations has certainly made me wiser. Multiple treatment options for EOS are available to us, and each has its advantages and disadvantages. 'Choosing wisely' enables us to provide the best care [61]. Therefore, I choose techniques that are tailored to the individual patient's needs to achieve the best long-term functional outcome. Amongst all these differences, practising in India is much more satisfying because most patients are still inordinately grateful. It is a little more gratifying to apply the skill and knowledge gained from training in the NHS in treating such complex spinal problems.

REFERENCES

1. Marketos SG, Skiadas P. Hippocrates. The father of spine surgery. *Spine (Phila Pa 1976)* 1999;24(13):1381–1387.
2. Scott JC, Morgan TH. The natural history and prognosis of infantile idiopathic scoliosis. *J Bone Joint Surg Br* 1955;37(3):400–413.
3. Choi JH, Oh EG, Lee HJ. Comparisons of postural habits, body image, and peer attachment for adolescents with idiopathic scoliosis and healthy adolescents. *J Korean Acad Child Health Nurs* 2011;17(3):167–173.
4. Kontodimopoulosa N, Damianoua K, Stamatopouloub E, et al. Children's and parents' perspectives of health-related quality of life in newly diagnosed adolescent idiopathic scoliosis. *J Orthop* 2018;15(2):319–323.
5. Mehta MH. The natural history of infantile idiopathic scoliosis. In: Zorab PA, *Scoliosis*: *Proceedings of a 5th Symposium*. Academic Press, London, 1977: 103–122.
6. Mehta MH. The rib-vertebra angle in the early diagnosis between resolving and progressive infantile scoliosis. *J Bone Joint Surg* 1972;54(2):230–243.
7. Mitra RN, Debnath UK. *Scoliosis – Facts, Figures & Follow-Up for Clinical Research*. Monograph. Academic Publications, Kolkata, 1995; 1st ed: 1–122.
8. Hopper WC Jr., Lovell WW. Progressive infantile idiopathic scoliosis. *Clin Orthop Relat Res* 1977;126(126):26–32.
9. McMaster MJ, Macnicol MF. The management of progressive Infantile idiopathic scoliosis. *J Bone Joint Surg Br* 1979;61(1):36–42.
10. Dickson RA. *Early Onset Idiopahic Scoliosis*, vol. 1. Raven, New York, 1994.
11. Dickson RA. Idiopathic scoliosis. *BMJ* 1989;298(6678):906–907.
12. Latalski M, Fatyga M, Starobrat G, et al. Strategies in early-onset scoliosis treatment. *J Spinal Stud Surg* 2017;1:45–50.
13. Emery JK, Mithal A. The number of alveoli in the terminal respiratory unit of man during late intrauterine life and childhood. *Arch Dis Child* 1960;35:544–547.
14. Karol LA. The natural history of early onset scoliosis. *J Pediatr Orthop* 2019;39(6):S38–43.
15. El-Hawary R, Akbarnia BA. Early onset scoliosis - Time for consensus. *Spine Deform* 2015;3(2):105–106.
16. Jarvis J, Garbedian S, Swamy G. Juvenile idiopathic scoliosis: The effectiveness of part-time bracing. *Spine* 2008;33(10):1074–1078.
17. Horan MP, Milbrandt TA. Scoliosis in pediatric patients: Comorbid disorders and screening. *Pediatr Health* 2009;3(5):451–546.
18. Pehrsson K, Larsson S, Oden A, et al. Long-term follow up of patients with untreated scoliosis: A study of mortality, causes of death, and symptoms. *Spine (Phila Pa 1976)* 1992;17(9):1091–1096.
19. Patterson JF, Webb JK, Burwell RG. The operative treatment of progressive early onset scoliosis. A preliminary report. *Spine (Phila Pa 1976)* 1990;15(8):809–815.
20. Marks DS, Iqbal MJ, Thompson AG. Convex Spinal epiphysiodesis in the management of progressive infantile idiopathic scoliosis. *Spine (Phila Pa 1976)* 1996;21(16):1884–1888.
21. Pratt RK, Burwell RG, Cummings SL, et al. Luque trolley and convex epiphysiodesis in the treatment of infantile and juvenile idiopathic scoliosis. *Spine* 1999;24(15):1538–1547.
22. Klemme WR, Denis F, Winter RB, et al. Spinal instrumentation without fusion for progressive scoliosis in young children. *J Pediatr Orthop* 1997;17(6):734–742.
23. Campbell RM Jr., Smith MD, Mayes TC, et al. The effect of opening wedge thoracostomy on thoracic insufficiency syndrome associated with fused ribs and congenital scoliosis. *J Bone Joint Surg* 2004;86-A(8):1659–1674.
24. Campbell RM Jr. VEPTR: Past experience and the future of VEPTR principles. *Eur Spine J* 2013;22 (Suppl 2):S106–117.
25. Schulz JF, Smith J, Cahill PJ, et al. The role of the vertical expandable titanium rib in the treatment of infantile idiopathic scoliosis: Early results from a single institution. *J Pediatr Orthop* 2010;30(7):659–663.

26. Evans N, Moideen A, Davies PR, et al. The operative management of early onset scoliosis using VEPTR: The complete patient journey. *Spine J* 2017;17(11):S331.

27. Yamaguchi KT Jr., Skaggs DL, Mansour S, et al. Are rib versus spine anchors protective against breakage of growing rods? *Spine Deform* 2014;2(6):489–492.

28. Akbarnia BA, Breakwell LM, Marks DS, et al. Dual growing rod technique followed for three to eleven years until final fusion. *Spine* 2008;33(9):984–990.

29. Thompson GH, Akbarnia BA, Campbell RM Jr. Growing rod techniques in early onset scoliosis. *J Pediatr Orthop* 2007;27(3):354–361.

30. Ouellet J. Surgical technique: Modern Luqué trolley, a self-growing rod technique. *Clin Orthop Relat Res* 2011;469(5):1356–1367.

31. Mehdian H, Stokes OM. Growing rod construct for the treatment of early-onset scoliosis. *Eur Spine J* 2015;24:647–651.

32. Mehdian H, Arealis G, Quraishi NA, et al. Segmental self-growing rod constructs in the management of early onset neuromuscular scoliosis. *Spine J* 2013;13(9):S135.

33. Debnath UK, Harshavardhana NS, Burwell GR, et al. Timing of definitive fusion in early onset scoliosis (EOS) treated by growing rods (GR) – A long term follow-up study. *Scoliosis Research Society Annual Meeting*, Salt Lake City, 2008.

34. Flynn J, St. Hilaire T, Emans J, et al. An analysis of the 39 "VEPTR graduates". *Scoliosis Research Society Annual Meeting*, Salt Lake City, 2008.

35. Akbarnia BA. When and how to use osteotomy for congenital spine deformity (Risser 0). *Scoliosis Research Society Annual Meeting*, Salt Lake City, 2008.

36. McCarthy RE, Luhmann S, Lenke L, et al. The Shilla growth guidance technique for early-onset spinal deformities at 2-year follow-up: A preliminary report. *J Pediatr Orthop* 2014;34(1):1–7.

37. Tsuji T, Kawakami N, Miyasaka K, et al. Clinical significance of a corrective cast/brace in the era of non-fusion surgery – Treatment of early onset scoliosis. *Scoliosis Research Society Annual Meeting*, Salt Lake City, 2008.

38. Akbarnia BA, Emans JB. Complications of growth-sparing surgery in early onset scoliosis. *Spine (Phila Pa 1976)* 2010;35(25):2193–2204.

39. Bess S, Akbarnia BA, Thompson GH, et al. Complications of growing-rod treatment for early-onset scoliosis: Analysis of one hundred and forty patients. *J Bone Joint Surg Am* 2010;92-A(15):2533–2543.

40. Tsirikos AI, Roberts SB. Magnetic controlled growth rods in the treatment of scoliosis: Safety, efficacy and patient Selection. *Med Devices Auckl* 2020;13:75–85.

41. Cheung KM, Cheung JP, Samartzis D, et al. Magnetically controlled growing rods for severe spinal curvature in young children: A prospective case series. *Lancet* 2012;379(9830):1967–1974.

42. Johari AN, Nemade AS. Growing spine deformities: Are magnetic rods the final answer? *World J Orthop* 2017;8(4):295–300.

43. Harshavardhana NS, Noordeen MHH, Dormans JP. Cost analysis of magnet driven growing rods for early onset scoliosis at 5years. *Spine (Phila Pa 1976)* 2019;44(1):60–67.

44. Fletcher ND. Current treatment preferences for early onset scoliosis: A survey of POSNA members. *J Pediatr Orthop* 2011;31(3):326–330.

45. Theologis A, Cahill P, Auriemma M, et al. Vertebral body stapling in children younger than 10 years with idiopathic scoliosis with curve magnitude of 30° to 39°. *Spine (Phila Pa 1976)* 2013;38(25):E1583–1588.

46. McCarthy RE, McCullough FL. Shilla growth guidance for early-onset scoliosis: Results after a minimum of five years of follow-up. *J Bone Joint Surg Am* 2015;97(19):1578–1584.

47. Andras LM, Joiner ER, McCarthy RE, et al. Growing rods vs. Shilla growth guidance: Better Cobb angle correction and T1–S1 length increase but more surgeries. *Spine Deform* 2015;3(3):246–252.

48. Sankar WN, Skaggs DL, Yazici M, et al. Lengthening of dual growing rods and the law of diminishing returns. *Spine (Phila Pa 1976)* 2011;36(10):806–809.

49. Thakar C, Kieser DC, Mardare M, et al. Systematic review of the complications associated with magnetically controlled growing rods for the treatment of early onset scoliosis. *Eur Spine J* 2018;27(9):2062–2071.

50. Cheung JPY, Cheung KMC. Current status of the magnetically controlled growing rod in the treatment of early onset scoliosis: What we know after a decade of experience. *J Orthop Surg* 2019;27(3):1–10.

51. Williams BA, McCalla D, Matsumoto H, et al. Development and initial validation of the classification of early-onset scoliosis (C-EOS). *J Bone Joint Surg Am* 2014;96(16):1359–1367.

52. Park HY, Matsumoto H, Feinberg N, et al. The classification for early-onset scoliosis (C-EOS) correlates with the speed of vertical expandable prosthetic titanium rib (VEPTR) proximal anchor failure. *J Pediatr Orthop* 2017;37(6):381–386.

53. Agarwal A, Aker L, Ahmad AA. Active apex correction (modified SHILLA technique) versus distraction-based growth rod fixation: What do the correction parameters say? *Spine Surg Relat Res* 2019;16(4(1)):31–36.

54. Ahmad AA. Early onset scoliosis and current treatment methods. *J Clin Orthop Trauma* 2020;11(2):184–190.

55. Yang S, Andras LM, Redding GJ, et al. Early-onset scoliosis: A review of history, current treatment, and future directions. *Pediatrics* 2016;137(1):1.

56. Kocyigit IA, Olgun ZD, Demirkiran HG, et al. Graduation protocol after growing-rod treatment: Removal of implants without new instrumentation is not a realistic approach. *J Bone Joint Surg Am* 2017;99(18):1554–1564.

57. Shen TS, Schairer W, Widdman R. In patients with early-onset scoliosis, can growing rods be removed without further instrumentation? An evidenced-based review. *HSS J* 2019;15(2):201–204.

58. Matsumoto H, Williams BA, Corona J, et al. Psychosocial effects of repetitive surgeries in children with early-onset scoliosis: Are we putting them at risk? *J Pediatr Orthop* 2014;34(2):172–178.

59. Murgai RR, Andras LM, Nielsen E, et al. Dedicated spine nurses and scrub technicians improve intraoperative efficiency of surgery for adolescent idiopathic scoliosis. *Spine Deform* 2020;8(2):171–176.

60. Jiang F, Wilson JRF, Badhiwala JH, et al. Quality and safety improvement in spine surgery. *Glob Spine J* 2020;10(1S):17S–28S.

61. Lavelle-Jones M. Choosing wisely in surgery – A perspective from the UK. *Indian J Surg* 2018;80(1):1–4.

9g Experience of EOS Management in Two Worlds-II

*Fernando Rios, Behrooz A. Akbarnia,
and Gregory M. Mundis, Jr.*

CONTENTS

INTRODUCTION

The lack of care for surgically treatable conditions takes a serious human and economic toll and can lead to acute, life-threatening complications, resulting in chronic disabilities that make productive employment impossible and impose a burden on family members and society. This failure to appreciate the role of surgery in addressing important public health problems is the main cause of disparities in surgical care worldwide. Approximately 2 billion people lack access to essential surgical care [7] and 28% of the global burden of disease is amenable to surgical intervention, a proportion that is higher in the developing world [6]. It is now clear that inequities in surgical delivery have resulted in vast numbers of the population in low- and middle-income countries (LMICs) being denied access to care for potentially treatable surgical diseases. To illustrate this point, 74% of all the surgical interventions worldwide are performed in the wealthiest third of the world's population, whereas only 3.5% are performed on the poorest third [4]. These numbers may be underestimated when it comes to the delivery of spine care to LMICs, as the availability of expensive implants needed to treat the patients frequently does not exist.

PLATFORMS THAT DELIVER CARE IN LMICS

A major problem in LMICs is the lack of financial support for those who need healthcare, deterring service use and burdening household budgets [20]. Regardless of the funding source, contribution mechanisms, and collection agents within a health system, most LMICs share the same main healthcare platforms, all of which the authors of this chapter have been closely exposed to in several LMICs: private medicine, or 'out-of-pocket'; private health insurance, or prepaid plans; and public health, or social security insurance. Unfortunately, the availability of healthcare professionals with the appropriate training to treat early-onset scoliosis (EOS) in LMICs is very limited. To illustrate this point, the Scoliosis Research Society (SRS) has 489 registered members in the United States, as opposed to seven members in Mexico, three in Poland, and one in Colombia [21].

On average, almost 50% of healthcare financing in low-income countries comes from out-of-pocket payments, as compared with 30% in middle-income countries and 14% in high-income countries [19]. Furthermore, the unaffordable hospital bills, expensive costs of the appropriate instruments and implants, and elevated surgeon fees make the accessibility of EOS treatment in the private sector nearly unreachable to most of the population in said areas.

One of the most commonly encountered shortcomings in private health insurances is coverage, and most paediatric spinal deformity conditions are frequently not included. If and when they are covered, unlike out-of-pocket surgeries, healthcare providers are usually limited to operate with a preauthorised list of implants that are not always the most appropriate or of the best quality and do not include the necessary instruments and technology to safely execute the surgeries. Considering that only 1% of the population in low-income and 2%–9% of middle-income countries have private health insurance, expected expenses of private health insurance plans (i.e. copays, coinsurance, and deductibles) lowers accessibility to EOS treatment even more. This is assuming that the appropriately trained surgeon is within the insurance's network, otherwise EOS surgery, from the patients' perspective, results in being practically an out-of-pocket treatment.

A third platform commonly found in developing countries is the public health system, or social security insurances. With variable demand amongst different LMICs, the common limitations on the different modalities of public health systems are long waiting lists, availability of only a handful of institutions that specialise in treating specific and complicated conditions such as EOS, limited resources (e.g. operating rooms, sutures, implants, surgeons, imaging, etc.), and much like private health insurance, the struggle to operate with a preauthorised list of implants of questionable quality and outdated technology. These limitations ultimately result in a lower opportunity of achieving the best possible outcomes.

Unfortunately, due to the high costs involved, the availability of properly trained healthcare providers, and the appropriate infrastructure, the treatment of EOS in LMICs is fairly limited in almost every platform available in these areas. Luckily, there is a fourth platform to deliver care for paediatric spinal deformities that is rarely mentioned: the charitable platforms.

The literature suggests that charitable organisations deliver surgery in two basic ways: by establishing specialty surgical hospitals, or by focussing on more temporary platforms [1]. Temporary surgical platforms are by far the most common and can be further classified into short-term surgical mission (STSM) trips and self-contained surgical platforms (SCSPs). STSMs send healthcare professionals along with surgical instrumentation and technology into LMICs' hospitals and clinics for short periods of time. These often perform a restricted set of surgeries, relying on local physicians for follow-up. SCSPs are significantly rarer and often spend longer in-country (months to years) than STSMs and carry their infrastructure with them. Organisations such as Mercy Ships are an example [1]. In contrast, specialty surgical hospitals establish an entire physical structure dedicated to the treatment of one or a few related surgical conditions. Organisations such as Shriners Hospitals for Children fit this model.

Surgical volunteerism has become an increasingly popular means for surgeons to exercise their generosity, share their knowledge, establish new friendships, and bridge cultural gaps. Many nonprofit organisations (NPO) exist with the purpose of providing medical and surgical care to children and adults in LMICs, and the most common way that surgeons donate their time and talent is through STSMs [1]. The charitable sector of STSMs has been growing at a pace surpassing the US GDP by 20% [2]. Johns Hopkins University and the United Nations collaborated on a study and found what most people already suspected: NPOs and volunteering constitute a massive economic force [3]. A note on terminology: although some NPOs providing surgery in LMICs are faith-based, not all are. The word *mission* does not refer only to faith-based organisations. Similarly, the word *charitable* is usually limited to missions and organisations that are, at least in part, funded by private donations [1].

GLOBAL SPINE OUTREACH

Our experience with EOS in areas of limited resources has been primarily through a NPO in the form of a STSM platform: Global Spine Outreach (GSO). GSO is a 501(c)(3) NPO that was founded in 2013. The mission of this organisation is to provide surgery free of charge by collaborating with local medical communities to build self-sustaining spine centers by engaging surgeons through hands-on training and education from leading spine surgeons from around the world. To accomplish GSO's mission, it was essential to develop protocols to evaluate a site for the appropriateness and safe execution of surgical care for children with spinal deformities. GSO was founded with the desire to have a turn-key operation for initiation of a STSM. GSO's STSMs have been occurring every 6 months with each mission lasting 8 days: two days for travel, one dedicated day in clinic and 5 consecutive days in the operating room (OR), most commonly utilising 2 ORs per day. Follow-up has been established with the local surgeons for a 1- and 3-month follow-up time points and all subsequent follow-ups are arranged based on the return visit of GSO every 6 months. Standard follow-up continues at 6-months postoperatively, 1 year, 2 years, 3–5 years, and 5–10 years.

CHALLENGES WITH EOS AND STSMS IN LMICS

There have been many reports including four systematic reviews regarding STSMs focussing on the safety, quality, and reproducibility [1, 2, 5, 14]. In all four reports, the shortcomings of STSMs are highlighted and include: difficulty with follow-up; higher mortality and complication rates; the inherent difficulty of establishing a multidisciplinary approach in STSMs; detrimental cost-effectiveness when the condition can be treated by other platforms; inability to meet the large burden of unmet need as a result of the fragmentation in delivery due to the treatment of the same conditions that are otherwise treated in local hospitals; and lastly, disrupting local infrastructure, even after the team's departure. Given the risk of a potentially negative effect that STSMs could have, the need for a standardised protocol to initiate, maintain, and grow a safe and sustainable STSM trip is of the outmost importance.

There are presently no published reports that unify the safe delivery of paediatric spine surgical care in LMICs. The SRS has made tremendous efforts to provide common ground for various volunteer organisations to collaborate and provide education. The global outreach committee exists to help with the collaboration, basic data collection, education at their annual meeting, and ultimately provide credibility to the volunteer organisations as either recognised or endorsed sites based on the sites' ability to report data and maintain a good standing with the SRS. At the present time, there are four endorsed sites and 18 recognised sites by the SRS [8].

The STSM model anecdotally appeared to have a relatively limited role in the delivery of surgical care [1]. Given the potentially unsatisfactory results, detrimental effects on health-seeking behaviour, and stress on the local infrastructure, the short-term stand-alone surgical mission, when other options exist, has been thought to be inefficient [1]. On the other hand, STSMs can provide meaningful care in the lives of patients who may otherwise not have access and a rich educational environment for the medical professionals and staff, allowing physicians and different healthcare providers to find a meaningful way to offer their services outside of their own practices sharing their time and talent with others in need. In an attempt to standardise sustainable care provided for children with scoliosis and spinal deformities in LMICs, GSO has provided a framework (available on globalspineoutreach.org) for the planning and execution of a STSM, from its inception to its establishment as a sustainable site, that includes prework, site visitation, pre-STSM clinic visit, initial STSM, and recurring STSM, using a model that has 7 years of experience and 30 STSMs successfully completed.

SUCCESS OR FAILURE?

Since its foundation, GSO has executed 30 STSMs, evaluated 1,545 patients, performed 358 surgeries and launched four additional sites, now having a total of five sites in three countries on two continents: Poznan and

Otwock in Poland, Chihuahua and Monterrey in Mexico, and Cali in Colombia. One site was moved, including its patients, for 2 years, from Chihuahua to Monterrey, as there was no local surgeon to maintain the site at that time. GSO has brought 16 different US surgeons on the STSMs; eight surgeons have been on more than one STSM and six surgeons on four or more STSMs. Since 2013, 17 local attending surgeons have been engaged in an STSM, and all have participated in more than one mission (this does not include the various fellows and residents that have participated). There have been 106 different volunteers on the 30 STSMs, 70 of whom were involved in at least two trips, 32 on three trips, and 17 on more than three trips. On these trips, five different industry partners have been engaged to donate implants for the STSMs, and four have partnered with GSO on two or more trips.

OVERCOMING CHALLENGES

Over the past decade several authors have raised concerns regarding STSMs in LMICs, particularly as it relates to the lack of follow-up care, the safety of patients, the reproducibility and sustainability, serving in parts of the world where the services provided are not wanted or needed, failure to match technology to the local needs and capabilities, and leaving a mess behind after the STSM is over. The model proposed by GSO does not entirely address all these concerns, and as with many living organisations, their current model is continually undergoing change. As their experience grows, the feedback becomes more mature, and the model is revised based on the quality assurance process.

By holding frequent and consistent conferences with the host hospitals, administrative staff, local NPOs and surgeons, GSO has been able to not only ensure that patients receive their follow-up visits on the preestablished timepoints, but also to promote a comfortable environment for open feedback, creating opportunities to improve their model. This continuous interaction has also opened the opportunity to build bridges between cultures, strengthen relationships, and allow for a better delivery of care. Organisers of different STSMs often reflect on the importance of establishing continuous and mutual relationships in order to have the most impact [15].

The concern for safety is paramount to lower mortality and complication rates on any successful STSM, particularly as it relates to EOS. Strong evidence exists for an association between surgical volume and outcomes in North America [12]. Poilleux and Lobry [11] reviewed 114 surgical missions over two decades that performed more than 17,000 operations in sub-Saharan Africa and found an overall mortality of 3.3%, which is 20 times higher than in high-income countries (HIC). Maine et al. [10] reported a rate of oronasal fistula after cleft palate repair more than twentyfold higher in STSMs than in HIC. In their study, cases performed by experienced local and North American surgeons on a surgical mission to Ecuador were compared with cases performed by similar surgeons at an American tertiary hospital. All surgeons showed this twentyfold increase in complication rates, and no differences were found between the local and North American surgeons. These findings lead to the belief that mission volume has potentially more impact than surgeon experience. For this reason, GSO has stayed consistent in regard to: 1) the number or volume of surgeries per STSM, 2) the duration of the STSMs, 3) the timing of the STSMs, and 4) the protocols that limit variability (e.g. establishing checklists to determine if a site meets the requirements for a GSO STSM, preoperative protocols, preanaesthesia checklists, blood-loss management protocols, intraoperative neurologic deficit protocols, etc.). Limiting variables is one of the cornerstones for reproducibility, as consistency is to sustainability.

SURGEON SKILL AND LMIC FACILITY MISMATCH

It is quite common for there to be a mismatch between surgeon skills and host facility. Many skilled surgeons volunteer their time and make plans to execute surgical procedures appropriate for their practice within an HIC and its infrastructure, and do not fully take into consideration the differences in practices between the LMICs and an HIC. Simple assumptions, such as the availability of blood products, neuromonitoring, haemostatic agents, or an ICU bed, can have devastating consequences if the appropriate measures are not taken with anticipation.

IMPROVISING OR STAYING CREATIVE?

As mentioned, local surgeons in LMICs are often exposed to deficiencies in regard to availability of quality implants, incomplete set of instruments (e.g. one reduction tower per paediatric spinal deformity tray, no paediatric pedicle probes, sets with no *in situ* benders, etc.), 'hybrid' set of implants (pedicle screws with different company set-screws), limited number of screws per surgery regardless of degree of deformity, unavailability of bipolar cautery or bone cutting burrs, just to mention a few. These deficiencies can force the surgeon to improvise in the middle of a procedure and thus run into trouble, but it can also create room for creativity. Figure 9g.1 shows a common wheelchair adapted by the patient's father, in collaboration

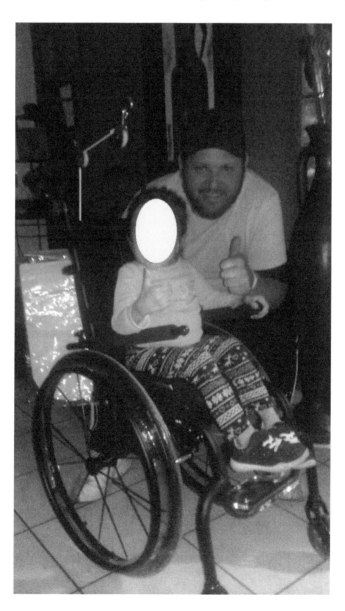

FIGURE 9G.1 Picture of a common wheelchair adapted by the patient's father in collaboration with the surgeon.

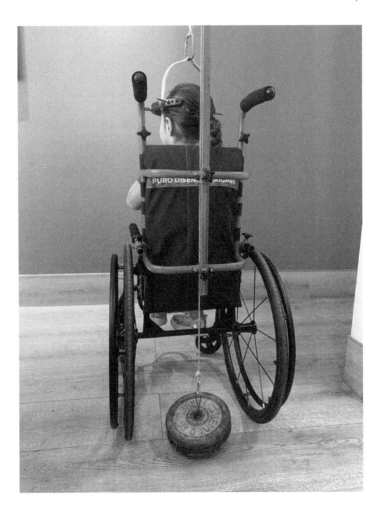

FIGURE 9G.2   The same wheelchair seen in Figure 9g.1, being used for halo-gravity traction with 50% of the patient's body weight.

with his surgeon, in order to treat the child with preoperative halo-gravity traction; the same wheelchair is shown in Figure 9g.2 being used by the patient using 50% of her bodyweight for traction. Figure 9g.3 shows a GSO volunteer surgeon casting a patient hanging from the operating room's ceiling, as a Mehta casting table was not available. Figure 9g.4 is a concrete screwed hook installed on a patient's home to allow the patient to be under halo-gravity traction as many hours a day as possible.

THE ROLE OF OUTREACH IN TRAINING

Referring back to the lack of appropriately trained surgeons as being one of the main

limitations to treat EOS in developing countries, many authors laud the salutary role that STSMs have in the education of surgical trainees in HIC [1]. But apart from Vargas' study [16], which documented an increase in more complex surgeries performed by the local surgeons after repeated missions, no other studies have reported the impact of short-term missions in training. Through the evolution of GSO's first site, they have been able to see the impact that a sustainable STSM can have on the local surgeons' team. As this site matured, the complexity of the surgeries performed also increased. Initially, the surgeries performed were mainly simpler forms of deformity including traditional growing rods (TGR). As a result of this progressive training, the local

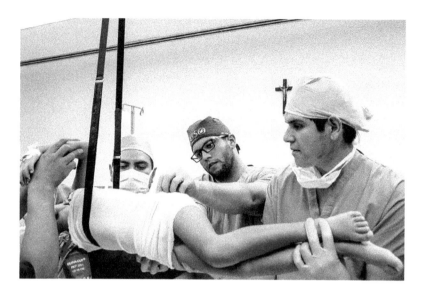

FIGURE 9G.3 Casting technique used by a GSO volunteer surgeon when Mehta casting tables were not available. The patient is suspended, under sedation, in a lateral decubitus position by a smooth-surfaced one-inch width material, positioned at the ribs that correspond to the apex of the major curve, while two assistants aid to hold the head and extremities in a neutral position.

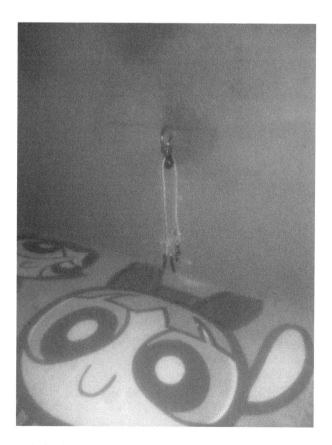

FIGURE 9G.4 Picture of a hook screwed to a concrete wall installed by the patient's father in a bedroom to accomplish the daily targeted time for halo-gravity traction.

surgeon team that started with two members has grown to four members, and they are now performing more than 150 deformity cases a year without GSO present (187 complex spinal surgeries done in 2019) only after 13 STSMs at that site, demonstrating the impact that STMSs can have in training.

CONCLUSION

Treating EOS in areas of limited resources implies a great deal of shortcomings, regardless of the platform of care delivery. It is firstly limited by the availability of human resources – paediatric spinal deformity trained surgeons – followed by the quality instruments and implants, and lastly the economic resources. These limitations make the treatment of EOS and its access more challenging than it already is. The authors have been exposed to all platforms of care in developing countries and found that the best and safest environment to treat EOS is LMICs is through outreach. The demand for STSMs focussed on paediatric deformity in LMICs is anecdotally very high. Despite the concerns regarding STSMs in LMICs, NPOs, such as GSO, have implemented solutions to overcome these shortcomings. As a result, GSO has been approached to launch new sites, and the successful launch and sustainability of their first site was the impetus to develop a protocol that can be used to safely initiate and maintain a paediatric spinal deformity STSM to promote a lasting impact on the local community, showing that when no other platform can treat these conditions adequately in a timely manner, surgical missions may be the only hope for these patients.

REFERENCES

1. Shrime M, Sleemi A, Ravilla T. Charitable Platforms in Global Surgery: A Systematic Review of Their Effectiveness, Cost-Effectiveness, Sustainability, and Role Training. *World J Surg.* 2015;39(1):10–20.
2. Casey K. The Global Impact of Surgical Volunteerism. *Surg Clin North Am.* 2007;87(4):949–960, ix.
3. Salamon L. Putting the Civil Society Sector on the Economic Map of the World. *Ann Public Coop Econ.* 2010;81(2):167–210.
4. Weiser T, Regenbogen S, Thompson K, et al. An Estimation of the Global Volume of Surgery: A Modelling Strategy Based on Available Data. *Lancet.* 2008;372(9633):139–144.
5. Fisher Q, Fisher G. The Case for Collaboration among Humanitarian Surgical Programs in Low Resource Countries. *Anesth Analg.* 2014;118(2):448–453.
6. Institute of Health Metrics and Evaluation. *Global Burden of Disease.* 2010.
7. Funk L, Weiser T, Berry W, et al. Global Operating Theatre Distribution and Pulse Oximetry Supply: An Estimation on Reported Data. *Lancet.* 2010;376(9746):1055–1061.
8. Scoliosis Research Society. Global Outreach Program. https://www.srs.org/professionals/global-outreach-program/srs-endorsed-programs (accessed 04/01/2020).
9. Wang X, Lenke L, Thuet E, et al. Deformity Angular Ratio Describes the Severity of Spinal Deformity and Predicts the Risk of Neurologic Deficit in Posterior Vertebral Column Resection Surgery. *Spine (Phila Pa 1976).* 2016;41(18):1477–1455.
10. Maine R, Hoffman W, Palacios-Martinez J, et al. Comparison of Fistula Rates after Palatoplasty for International and Local Surgeons on Surgical Missions in Ecuador with Rates at a Craniofacial Center in the United States. *Plast Reconstr Surg.* 2012;129(2):319e–326e.
11. Poilleaux J, Lobry P. Surgical Humanitarian Missions. An Experience Over 18 Years. *Chirugie.* 1991;117(8):602–606.
12. Birkmeyer J, Siewers A, Finlayson E, et al. Hospital Volume and Surgical Mortality in the United States. *N Engl J Med.* 2002;346(15):1128–1137.
13. Mitchell K, Balumuka D, Kotecha V, et al. Short-Term Surgical Missions: Joining Hands with Local Providers to Ensure Sustainability. *S Afr J Surg.* 2012;50(1):2.
14. Roche S, Ketheeswaran P, Wirtz V. International Short-Term Medical Missions: A Systematic Review of Recommended Practices. *Int J Public Health.* 2017;62(1):31–42.
15. Catholic Health Association of the United States. Short-Term Medical Mission Trips: Phase I Research Findings. Practices & Perspectives of U.S. *Partners.* 2014.
16. Vargas G, Price R, Sergelen O, et al. A Successful Model for Laparoscopic Training in Mongolia. *Int Surg.* 2012;97(4):363–371.
17. Donkor P, Bankas D, Agbenorku P, et al. Cleft Lip and Palate Surgery in Kumasi, Ghana: 2001–2005. *J Craniofac Surg.* 2007;18(6):1376–1379.
18. Fletcher A, Donoghue M, Devavaram J, et al. Low Uptake of Eye Services in Rural India: A

Challenge for Programs of Blindess Prevention. *Arch Ophthalmol*. 1999;117(10):1393–1399.

19. Global Health Expenditure Database. Table of Regional Averages for Key Indicatiors. https://apps.who.int/nha/database/Regional_Averages/Index/en (accessed 04-18-2020).

20. Mills A. Health Care Systems in Low- and Middle-Income Countries. *N Engl J Med*. 2014;370(6):552–557.

21. Scoliosis Research Society. Find a Specialist. https://www.srs.org/find/index.php (accessed 04/17/2020).

9h Cross-Border Spine Surgical Treatment: Issues to Consider

Harwant Singh

CONTENTS

INTRODUCTION

In this modern age of an increasingly interconnected world, many patients travel across borders for surgical treatment, and many surgeons travel across borders to deliver surgical treatment. This situation raises many issues about the care that is delivered, and it is appropriate to discuss the rights of the patients and the protection of surgeons who deliver such care, and the consent for spine surgery in such situations. This chapter is not meant to be a text on surgical ethics and law but to introduce some concepts in consideration of cross-border surgical treatment, especially patients' rights, surgeon protection, and informed consents. As this is a developing area, the suggestions in this chapter may change over time.

Categories of Cross-Border Treatments

Cross-border treatments are most pronounced in broadly two categories: medical tourism and outreach/teaching. Medical Tourism is defined as the process in which a patient travels outside his or her usual residence for the purpose of medical or surgical treatment [1]. This may be from a lesser developed region to a more developed region for the purposes of receiving technically complex procedures or, conversely,

from a more developed, more expensive region to a less costly region for procedures that cost considerably less. The more common conditions for this type of travel for treatment are plastic/cosmetic surgery and transplant surgery [2].

Medical tourism in the latter category is usually more common and are usually located in the emerging economies where more up-to-date health infrastructure exist and have the capacity to care for patients. This has a large revenue generating capacity for the economies concerned and sometimes are advertised formally. The major characteristic in this healthcare delivery is that the patient travels to the surgeon for treatment. The main driver for this type of medical tourism are patients seeking substantially lower costs abroad [3].

Outreach or teaching programmes are usually when surgeons travel to the patient to deliver specific or complex care that is not available in the host region. There is also a significant teaching component in delivering this complex care at the host institutes. Many professional surgical societies organise such training programmes as a social and educational responsibility. An example would be the Global Outreach programme [4] of the Scoliosis Research Society. The main driver for outreach and teaching programmes are the altruistic behaviour of surgeons and surgical societies in the interest of raising the standard of surgical care for the less fortunate.

HISTORICAL PERSPECTIVE

Medical responsibility is a concept that has been around for at least 3,700 years. The Code of Hammurabi (6th Babylonian King reigning from 1792 to 1750 BC in Mesopotamia) had already enacted laws to that effect. The key development is the concept of holding the medical professionals accountable for deaths or injuries that could have been reasonably prevented. The Romans subsequently developed the legal foundation for compensation for medical injuries, which qualified the injuries as intentional and nonintentional [5]. Of course, medical mishaps are really unintentional injuries.

The wide adoption of Roman Laws in the European continent up to the Middle Ages led to the development of this concept in English Common Law and, subsequently, in the 1800s, greatly influenced the development of medical law and compensation in the American legal system [5]. Key to the development and implementation of a working system to help adjudicate medical injuries are the concepts of an *expert witness* to ascertain the quality and appropriateness of treatment in question and the concept of *standard of care.*

BASIC CONSIDERATIONS

In the evolution of modern surgical ethics and consent to surgical treatment, the legal standard has shifted from what was defined as the 'community professional standard - where a body of surgeons determine what to disclose to a recipient of surgical care' to 'the reasonable person standard - where the reasonable patient decides on what treatment he or she wants, based on all material risk disclosures and the outcome if the condition is not treated'. This is also known as 'informed consent', and is the standard seen in almost all legal jurisdictions in the world, as patient autonomy is increasingly the standard adopted [6].

The concept of 'informed consent' is primarily a development of surgical ethics and not initially a development of law, as most legal advocates would suggest. John Gregory, a Scottish physician and ethicist (1724–1773), is to be credited for the first concepts of a patient's right to decide on the treatment proposed for him or her and the right to refuse treatment [7]. However, when it is the surgical procedure that has an unexpected or unsatisfactory outcome, legal authorities rely on the concept of medical evidence provided by an expert witness who will assist a court to determine if the standard of care was maintained in the treatment received by the patient.

Therefore, a framework of the ethical considerations should be in place when there is cross-border spine surgical treatment being contemplated. What is being discussed is just a suggestion. This is new territory, and the concepts are evolving. At the time of writing, the world is experiencing an unprecedented viral pandemic with major travel restrictions, and its impact on cross-border surgical treatments is yet to be seen.

ETHICAL CONSIDERATIONS OF PATIENTS RECEIVING CROSS-BORDER HEALTH CARE

In deciding the rights of patients in cross-border healthcare, the ethical considerations can be viewed in four convenient sections [8].

1. **Autonomy:** This is the capacity of the patient to think, decide, and act on the basis of such thought and decision, freely and independently. The health professionals and the carers must help the patient come to their own decision by facilitation or provision of important information about the surgery being planned. Also, it is important to respect and allow the patient to follow that decision, even if the health professional may not agree with it.

2. **Beneficence:** This is the moral importance of doing good to the patient. This principle means doing what is best for the patient. The difficulty is in deciding who has the power to make decisions on what is best for the patient.

An objective, relevant health professional may determine what is in the best interest of a patient, however, the patient may choose a course of action that is not in his or her best interest. There must be a mechanism that allows for the resolution of such conflicts. It is fortunate that in the vast majority of situations, autonomy and beneficence are congruent.

3. **Nonmaleficence:** This is the concept of avoiding harm. It is logical that medical professionals actively work not to harm patients. Surgical treatments have a small but real chance of an unexpected outcome that may be more harmful than beneficial. It is not that such treatments are to be totally avoided in the belief that avoiding harming a patient should take priority over doing good; however, the risk/benefit probability must be evaluated, deciding on what is in the best interest for the patient overall. In society, we have a duty not to harm anyone, whereas in clinical practise, we owe a duty of beneficence to our patients.

4. **Justice:** Allocation of resources in effecting the best possible treatment can be a major issue when such resources are not available. This may be clinical expertise, health infrastructure or finance issues and may be the reason for the cross-border healthcare whether for medical tourism or for outreach/teaching programmes. The principle of justice should be considered in two ways – patients with the same clinical condition should have access to the same level of care, and allocation of resources must be equal for all patients with the same clinical condition, for example, time, money, expertise, and infrastructure.

SPECIFIC RISKS IN MEDICAL TOURISM

- **Funding for travel:** In deciding that treatment will be done at another geographical location, finance becomes a major consideration. Although such trips are taken because the care at the host country is less costly, there are considerations such as transportation, hotel, and hospital costs besides treatment costs. The postsurgical treatment costs also must be considered, such as costs for repatriation and any special preparations thereof. There should be provision for funds to be available for this. These funds may be made available from local authorities or charities who deem that travelling for treatment is appropriate.

- **Postoperative care/conflict in continuity of care:** The surgery itself is only one component of the patients total and comprehensive care. The other elements include presurgical consultations, nonsurgical treatment, preoperative educational programmes, rehabilitation and long-term continued care after surgery [9]. It has been suggested that some domestic health professionals (from the patient's country of origin) believe that cross-border healthcare compromises continuity of care [10], as there might be disruption or an incomplete flow of information. A meaningful discussion allowing the individual to make an informed decision is a major prerequisite prior to travel; however, the domestic health professional may not be in a position to advise or help if they are not part of the caregiving team. Also, it may be that the domestic health professional may prefer not to take any significant responsibility in the decision-making process so that they avoid fiduciary duty that brings an element of responsibility should an adverse event occur [11]. Domestic health professionals insulate themselves from liability should an adverse event occur by not having any interaction with the patient before and after the surgical intervention. This provides protection from liability, especially if there have been no referrals, no advice, no recommendations, and no involvement in presurgical or postsurgical care. This leads to a breakdown in the patient's total care. In this situation, the cross-border surgery only becomes an isolated component of the patient's total care that is not desirable. Interestingly, the more interaction a domestic health professional has with the patient, the higher the risk of liability, but it increases the quality of total care for the patient [11]

- **Revision surgery for poor outcome:** Risks of surgical complications are real, and no matter how low the probability, they do occur. An unexpected outcome is a disappointment both for the patient and the surgeon. It is more pronounced when complications occur during a patient's return trip home. This may entail unexpected costs that were not planned for beforehand. Other than the unexpected surgical outcomes, complications such as postsurgical wound infections, postsurgical venous thromboembolism during return travel, and a host of other complications may occur when patients have no healthcare professional looking after them. This is the 'blind spot' in cross-border healthcare. Should there be other postsurgical complications that occur on the return of the patient's return home, the difficulty of getting another surgeon to continue care may be a problem. This has been seen in cosmetic and transplant surgeries. The revision surgery will add to the cost and can be substantial in some instances and often underestimated by the patients [12].

- **Recovery for surgical injury:** Many centres that provide cross-border healthcare have built-in waiver clauses, that must be signed as a prerequisite to care, that state that there will be no opportunity for recovery of surgical damage should it occur [13]. This is a prudent step to reduce financial liability of the healthcare professional and hospital. Should there be an unsatisfactory outcome after the surgical treatment abroad, recovery for the loss is subject to jurisdictional control. Normally, a claim for recovery should be filed in the country where the treatment was performed. This requires the physical presence of the complainant in the country of treatment. If the surgical injury is as a result of negligence, the standard under ordinary negligence in tort entails the following be satisfied [14].

- There is a duty of care by the treating surgeon to the patient.
- There is failure to meet the standard of care (breach of the duty).
- There is injury resulting from the failure to meet the standard of care.

SPECIFIC RISKS IN OUTREACH/TEACHING PROGRAMMES

The risks inherent to patients who are receiving outreach or care in teaching programmes are essentially similar to those who travel for medical tourism.

- **Postoperative care/conflict in continuity of care:** When a surgeon has travelled to a host country for the purpose of providing surgical care or imparting clinical knowledge that involves surgical care, several issues may arise. Among these are the subsequent care for the patient who has received surgical care. It is always the practise to provide advice for postsurgical care, especially if the host facility is not familiar with the care provided by the visiting surgeon, or if there is no expertise to give continuing care. To this end, usually a carefully constructed postsurgical care plan is provided. A list of possible complications that may develop after the visiting surgeon has departed should also be discussed and contingency plans made. There should also be a line of communication from the patient to the visiting surgeon should it be required. Should the patient wish to continue care with the visiting surgeon, there should be provision for this, too. Again, funds for travel and care at the surgeon's facility may be an issue

- **Revision surgery:** Usually the surgery performed by the visiting surgeons are exemplary, and they are excellent for teaching the hosts; however, unexpected complications can and do occur. This may be immediate or after the visiting surgeon has returned to his home facility. The complication should be managed satisfactorily at the host facility with the least delay. This also adds a dimension of extra cost. Again, there should be provision for the extra finances required to manage the complications. These could range from infections to revision surgery should it be needed.

- **Recovery for surgical injury:** If there is an unexpected outcome that has led to a claim for surgical damages, the claim will be filed in the country where the surgery had occurred. The operating surgeon, the team, and the centre where the surgery was conducted may the subject of legal action. Issues such as the validity of the consent, the patient's understanding the surgical procedure, the conduct of the procedure, and many more will be the focus of the action. The local host surgeon and facility may be the target of the action if the operating surgeon is not available. The delegation and limits of legal responsibilities must be clear by everyone on the surgical team before the onset on treatment. Should the outcome of the legal challenge not be satisfactory for the treating team, provisions for the restitution of the damages should be provided for, usually by the treating team's indemnity insurance and the healthcare facility insurance that protects for vicarious liability.

A SUGGESTED EXAMPLE OF A PATIENTS' CHARTER IN CROSS-BORDER HEALTH CARE

It is essential to have a framework of rights in the form of a patients' charter in both types of cross-border spine surgical treatments [15].

- **Health protection:** the right to have services that promote health and well-being, prevent disease, support, and empower those with chronic illnesses to actively participate in self-care. This includes the right to receive all information to best manage the existing problem, and to know if cross-border surgical treatment is the best option.

- **Access:** the right to access healthcare services according to individual health needs and requirements. This includes the right to a specialist care plan where available and, where not available, access to appropriate cross-border treatment.

- **Information:** the right to give and receive information about their condition that requires surgical treatment. This includes care options, risks, and prognosis. The discussions should be in a language that the patient fully understands. There should be additional information provided should it be asked for. If a second opinion is requested, it should be provided by an independent specialist healthcare provider who agrees that cross-border health care is appropriate.

- **Participation and informed consent:** the right to participate in the collaborative process of decision-making related to the condition needing treatment and to make informed consent about the proposed treatment and care. This includes all information related to risks, benefits, and consequences of refusal of any treatment or care: to be able to make an informed choice. The patient who is a minor or incapable of making an informed decision must have the next of kin be able to participate in the decision for surgical treatment. Healthcare professionals should refrain from participating in such decisions unless in exceptional cases in which care is urgent or time sensitive. The appropriateness of cross-border treatment also must be discussed. Should the cross-border treatment involve clinical research, it should be disclosed to the patient.

- **Privacy and confidentiality:** To expect one's privacy is respected when receiving cross-border healthcare. To be able to refuse information or photography for use in teaching, especially for those whose surgery has been arranged under an outreach programme. To be able to access one's own medical records in accordance with the protocols existing at the facility delivering the surgical treatment.

- **Dignity and respect:** the right to be treated as an individual with dignity, patience, empathy, tolerance, and courtesy. Also, the right to be given time to decide about any examination or treatment without coercion from the healthcare providers, especially in teaching programmes.
- **Safe health care:** the right to safe and effective care. There must be access to health treatments and services that meet adequate safety standards. Also, the right to expect that the care received will be free from harm resulting from the poor functioning of cross-border facilities, medical malpractise, and medical error. There must be proper handover of care so that a seamless and safe continuity of care between services in the cross-border situation is ensured. The cross-border care must be delivered by properly qualified and experienced staff.
- **Comments and complaints:** the right to comment on cross-border care received and provide constructive criticism and complaints. There must be a mechanism to facilitate this aspect of outcome assessment without any fear of retribution, compromise, or quality of care. This includes feedback, suggestions, and raising of concerns or complaints as deemed necessary. This should also include the significant others or carers of the patients who received cross-border care.

PROTECTION OF THE SURGEON

As discussed previously, despite delivering the best care by the treating team, a treating surgeon can be the focus of a legal action should there be an unsatisfactory, unexpected outcome. The outcome can fall into one of three categories: 1) successful defence of the claim, 2) unsuccessful defence of the claim for which there are damages to settle, and 3) A mutual agreement to settle without going through a legal proceeding. There would be a requirement for legal representation of the treating surgeon, other members of the treating team, and the healthcare facility. For these to be optimal (or regularised - to be regular) the following conditions must be satisfied:

- **Registration to practise surgery at the location where the surgery was performed:** For medical tourism, this is not an issue, as the surgeon is already registered in his or her jurisdiction; however, it may be an issue in an outreach/teaching situation in which the visiting surgeon should be registered to practise medicine and surgery through temporary registration at the time the surgery is performed. Other requirements to be satisfied include entry into the specialist's registry, and credentialling at the facility the surgery is to be performed.
- **Indemnity:** This is also a prerequisite for performance of surgery. Again, this is not an issue for surgeons performing surgery in home territory, but it may pose an issue for visiting surgeons. The indemnity could be worldwide or in the host country for a fixed period of time when the surgery is performed. This gives the financial and legal protection to the surgeon should there be a legal challenge to the surgical treatment done.
- **Informed consent:** The documentation of a proper informed consent is essential and acts as protection for the treating surgeons in both medical tourism and outreach/teaching programmes. The informed consent should be complete, comprehensive, and well understood by the patient in a language intelligible to him or her. Ideally the consent should be obtained by the surgeon performing the surgery.

ISSUES TO CONSIDER WHEN CONSENTING TO CROSS-BORDER SURGICAL TREATMENTS

Informed consent is a process that ideally begins long before the surgical procedure and not at the immediate moment before the surgery. There should be adequate time for the patient to understand all issues pertaining to the surgery. This informed consent process should include the following [16]:

- **Identify and authorise surgeon:** The surgeon performing the procedure should be named, and it should include a statement authorising the surgeon to perform said procedure.
- **Document condition to be treated:** The diagnosis and the condition to be treated should be clearly documented. If there is more than a single diagnosis, this should be indicated, too.
- **Document procedure to be done:** The procedure to be performed has to be clearly and completely documented. If there are several procedures to be done at the same time, this must be clearly indicated.
- **Document expected benefits:** There must be a statement or indication of the benefits to be expected from the surgical procedure as well as some indication of the probability of success. This may be defined as a functional improvement or an improvement in pain. An objective appraisal is desired so that there is no ambiguity in the expected outcome.
- **Explain possible complications:** This is important in an informed consent process. The material risks must be disclosed so that the patient is able to make an informed decision. It is prudent for the surgeon to discuss all the material complications him- or herself and not delegate this to a member of the team.
- **Documentation that all alternatives have been discussed:** For an informed consent to be appropriate, there should be a statement that the patient has been given information of other treatments or alternatives. The patient must acknowledge that all alternatives have been presented to him prior to deciding on the surgery.
- **Explanation that tissue may be removed for study:** Sometimes tissues may be removed for histological or microbiological evaluation or study. If the tissue is to be used for educational purposes at a future date, this also should be indicated.
- **Presence of trainees for purposes of learning and/or medical equipment representatives:** An indication should be made regarding the people who may be present during the surgical procedure other than the surgeon and the treating team. Usually this will include surgical trainees or representatives/vendors of the surgical equipment used.
- **Consent understood with or without interpreter:** If the patient does not understand the language of the consent, ideally an interpreter familiar with the patient's ethnic group or language should be present to explain the details of the procedure to the patient. There should be direct contact between the surgeon, interpreter, and patient face to face.
- **Anaesthetic consent and complications:** An appraisal of the anaesthetic risks should be discussed, possibly in a separate consent by the anaesthetist who would be present. Again, this should not be delegated to another member of the anaesthetic team, but the anaesthetist who would be conducting the procedure.
- **Processes for continued care:** If the patient has travelled for the expressed purpose of receiving treatment in a medical tourism situation, there should be a statement regarding the continuity of care so that conflict in the post-surgical care is avoided. A referral to the patient's home country should be provided with all the material information regarding the treatment performed. Ideally there should be a process

whereby there is a facility identified in the home country prior to travel. In the situation of an outreach/teaching situation, a statement regarding who or which facility will continue the care after the visiting surgeon returns home. In the rare situation that the patient wants to follow with the visiting surgeon for subsequent care, this should be discussed and documented so there is clear delegation of legal responsibilities.

- **Signature of patient, surgeon, guardian, witness, interpreter:** In the conclusion of the informed consent process, all those present – patient, surgeon, guardian, witness and interpreter – should attest that the consent is true and proper with a signature. Completing the process correctly prevents any issue of ambiguity should it arise postsurgery.

CONCLUSION

The modern interconnected world has witnessed the advent of cross-border surgical treatments seen in two main forms: medical tourism and outreach/teaching care. Both of these types of cross-border surgical treatments have inherent risks. The best method to minimise these risks is to have processes in place that protect the patient and the surgeon. These include a high standard of ethics, a patients' charter, an appraisal of the risks inherent in both types of cross-border surgical treatment, an informed consent of a high standard, and a statement of continuity of care so that ambiguity is reduced. With the adoption of these suggestions, it is hoped that the process of cross-border surgical treatments can be formalised safely with a very high standard of care for the patient and sufficient protection for the surgeon providing the care.

REFERENCES

1. Lunt N, Smith R, Exworthy M, et al. *Medical Tourism: Treatments, Markets and Health System Implications: A Scoping Review.* Directorate for Employment, Labour and Social Affairs. Paris: OECD, 2011.
2. Chin JL, Campbell AV. Transplant tourism or international transplant medicine? A case for making the distinction. *Am J Transplant.* 2012;12(7):700–707.
3. Underwood HR, Makadon HJ. Medical Tourism: Game-changing innovation or passing fad? *Health Financ Manag.* 2010;64(9):112–114.
4. Scoliosis Research Society. *Global Outreach Program.* https://www.srs.org/professionals/global-outreach-program (cited on 18 May 2020).
5. Bal BS. An introduction to medical malpractice in the United States. *Clin Orthop Relat Res.* 2009;467(2):339–347.
6. McCullough LB, Jones JW, Brody BA. Informed consent: Autonomous decision making of the surgical patient. In: McCullough LB, Jones JW, Brody BA (eds.) *Surgical Ethics.* New York: Oxford University Press, 1998: 15–37.
7. McCullough LB. *John Gregory's Invention of Professional Medical Ethics and the Profession of Medicine.* Dordrecht, The Netherlands: Kluwer Academic Publishers, 1998.
8. Beauchamp TL, Childress JF. *Principles of Biomedical Ethics.* 5th ed. New York: Oxford University Press, 2001.
9. Cheung IK, Wilson A. Arthroplasty tourism. *Med J Aust.* 2007;187(11):666–667.
10. Johnston R, Crooks VA, Snyder J, et al. What is known about the effects of medical tourism in destination and departure countries? A scoping review. *Int J Equity Health.* 2010;9:24. doi: 10.1186/1475-9276-9-24.
11. Cheung IK, Wilson A. Arthroplasty tourism. *Med J Aust.* 2007;187(11):667.
12. Boyle KA. A permanent vacation: Evaluating medical tourism's place in the United States healthcare system. *Health Lawyer.* 2008;20(5):45.
13. Steklof CD. Medical tourism and the legal impediments to recovery in cases of medical malpractice. *Wash Univ Glob Stud Law Rev.* 2010;9(4):721–742.
14. Hope T, Savulescu J, Hendrick J. An introduction to law. In: Hope T, Savulescu J, Hendrick J (eds.) *Medical Ethics and the Law: The Core Curriculum.* London: Churchill Livingston. 2003:39–49.
15. Minister of Health. *Patient's Charter.* Healthcare Standards Directorate. Malta: Ministry of Health, 2016.
16. Pantai Medical Centre Sdn Bhd. Orthopaedic Surgery Informed Consent: Document MRF. *0050-10-15.* 2015.

10 Future Considerations

Alaaeldin Azmi Ahmad

CONTENTS

INTRODUCTION

The coronavirus pandemic has heightened global attention to public health and highlighted the increasing linkages, through disease and/or health management, between different parts of the world. It has also brought into sharp focus the endemic health disparities at the institutional level between developing and advanced economies. Though early-onset scoliosis (EOS) is not an infectious disease and not prone to the same epidemiological considerations as the novel coronavirus, it is, nonetheless, a global health problem for which vast institutional disparities exist between different parts of the world (because complex surgical problems, such as EOS, require significant resources to manage effectively) and for which health institutions in advanced economies can collaborate with local institutions in countries with limited resources to aid in bridging this gap.

In fact, though the pandemic has highlighted weaknesses in the epidemiological foundations in advanced countries, in the global health approaches toward developing countries, there has historically been an almost singular focus on infectious diseases as well as problems such as malnutrition to the detriment of areas such as complex surgical intervention. Therefore, whereas great strides have been made in developing countries to reduce the extent of infectious diseases and malnutrition, among other preventable problems, there remains much to be wanted from global health initiatives that focus on surgical interventions. This is partly because of the complexity of surgeries such as EOS and partly to the myth that surgery in regions with limited resources cannot be cost effective and/or

that it only serves a small part of the total global burden of diseases [1].

The marginalisation of surgery in the global health approach to developing countries has slowly started to change over the past decade, due, in part, to improvements in the epidemiological status of these countries as well as the continuing rise of a globalised middle class in many of those regions. These developments reduce the incidence of infectious diseases, malnutrition, and child mortality and increases the need for surgery dealing with rising incidence of trauma and managing long-term debilitating congenital conditions, even if they are not life-threatening. Therefore, surgery is increasingly becoming a priority in the programmes run by global health organisations for decreasing the disparity of health services globally, and with recognition of spinal disorders as a cause of increasing burden of disability on people living in low- and middle-income countries [2].

EOS is a spine disorder that affects children 10 years of and younger that, if not treated early and appropriately, would cause severe morbidity in the long run, if not death, due to its effect on the cardiopulmonary system in these children.

The science of EOS management has evolved relatively late, primarily over the past two decades, along with improved understanding of the effect of a deformed spine on the pulmonary function and of long-term complications with surgical fusion techniques. Nonetheless, much of this progress has been limited to advanced countries, while countries with limited resources continue to face a severe shortage of EOS surgery services. What little progress has been made in these regions is the result of the exceptional work of a limited number of surgeons who were able to develop their own EOS management skills despite financial and institutional constraints, and who have worked hard to instill this service in their countries and to transfer their expertise through training to younger surgeons. However, this remains a limited mode of knowledge production and transfer.

We believe that there will be major change in the availability of this service during the next decade for several reasons:

- Increasing prioritisation of spine surgery in global surgery initiatives in poor countries, with rising adoption and support of global spine programmes by major orthopaedic societies.
- A greater role of artificial intelligence (AI) in the training programmes for spine surgeons; if utilised in global training programmes, this can allow local surgeons to improve their EOS management skills under appropriate monitoring by experts and without the financial burden of frequent travel.
- The success of a small number of local experts in establishing EOS services has also motivated young spine surgeons to become involved EOS practice and to use training by these experts to better manage these complicated cases within the context they are living in. More broadly, the dissemination of EOS management services, albeit limited, with successful results, has also encouraged health authorities in these countries to invest more resources to maintain this service.

Next, we discuss the role of health globalisation and training programme centres in low- and middle- income countries in improving EOS services in regions with limited resources.

CHANGE IN HEALTH GLOBALISATION POLICIES

There is now wide international acceptance of the role of surgery in the public health safety net and that surgery does not take away from other services but adds to them. It can improve general medical care, complements related healthcare facilities such as radiology, laboratory, pathology services, and improves the trust between health institutions and the community [3]. Furthermore, there has been a shift in understanding the aim of global surgery. In the past, the main aim was to provide service relief through short-term volunteer missions, but now there is increasing attention to the role of global surgery in improving the local quality of care for people in low- and middle-income countries [4]. Accordingly, global organisations' plans have changed from organising short-term missions and paying for expensive implants to focussing on the resources necessary to achieve an evidence-based spine care delivery system that is patient-centred and that considers the patient and community needs and priorities [5].

The shift in focus in global surgery organisations from purely volunteer-driven efforts to an educational experience can be tailored and adapted to meet the needs of local surgical trainees as well as providers in host institutions. Academic institutions in advanced countries can partner with institutions in resource-limited countries to facilitate bridging the gap in surgical workforce and to help with the training needs of these countries.

From an international health perspective, is imperative that all efforts abroad focus time and resources toward programmes with an emphasis on local education, empowerment, and sustainable initiatives. This includes invested interests in the education of local staff members and mentoring models both abroad and at home. Continued mentoring is essential to empower the healthcare team to independently manage these complicated spine patients. With an increased focus on international health within the medical community, follow-up and continuity is imperative to ensure we are honoring our oath to 'do no harm'.

Multiple reports suggest the cost-effectiveness of subspecialty surgery, including paediatric spine surgery [6, 7, 8], and we must recognise the successes of particular organisations and programmes as examples and standards of how such care can be offered capably, responsibly, and successfully, even in the most resource-constrained setting. For example, the Scoliosis Research Society (SRS) started a paediatric spine deformity programme in Ecuador that performed 28 spine deformity cases over 10 years, and with only two complications, pseudarthrosis and post-operative delayed paraplegia, both resolved after reoperations [9]. The programme was effective in achieving good SRS questionnaire (SRS-22r) scores and improving health-related quality of life (HRQoL). The central vision of the programme was to empower the Ecuadorian staff to develop a long-term, sustainable programme to meet the needs of Ecuadorian children with complex spinal deformity. Major persistent obstacles included securing a financial commitment from the hospital as well as the ability to mentor a surgeon to develop a self-sustaining programme. Specific orthopaedic mentorship efforts have included training and teaching sessions in Ecuador, observation and involvement in the operating room, and SRS- and industry-sponsored training in the United States. After years of mentorship, there are a few Ecuadorian surgeons who are now able to independently perform multilevel posterior spinal fusion and instrumentation (PSFI).

Despite the presence of successful trials for global organisations in implementing paediatric spine deformity surgery in some low- and middle-income countries, such as Ecuador with the SRS and Kolkata, India with Straight Spine, most programmes actually fail to achieve long-term stability and independence for a variety of reasons, including inappropriate or incomplete training. When local staff are given inappropriate or incomplete training, there can easily develop a feeling among the staff that they have been 'used and abused'. Furthermore, though subspecialty surgical care requires significant physical materials, there is often little thought about the long-term supply of these materials, leading to supply-chain problems later down the road. The disappointment sometimes goes the other way: in some cases, communities will accept outside input in areas with minimal need, with the hope that the providers will eventually bring something of more benefit to the community. This can lead to disappointment in the minds of the global providers and a feeling of being used for ulterior motives.

TRAINING PROGRAMMES

A decade ago, if a doctor in a limited-resource country wanted to acquire paediatric spine training, he or she would have to go to a centre, usually in a developed country, and stay for at least 1 year to get a fellowship as a spine surgeon or as a paediatric orthopaedic surgeon dealing mainly with the spine. The trained surgeon would then return to his or her country, trying to implement the skills he or she learned during the fellowship. Obviously, this is a time and financially consuming process, and it is not easy to overcome all the obstacles related to landing a position, travelling, and implementing the procedures learned back in the home country with minimal resources. Trainees from low- and middle-income countries also often face a highly regulated set of conditions when visiting high-income countries, which focus on patient safety and liability protection for the host institution. Consequently, the participation of visiting trainees from LMICs is usually limited to observation only, with few opportunities for practical experience [10]. All of these factors, combined with the limited pool of highly skilled surgical teaching staff in the home country that often necessitates external travel, have contributed to the truncation of training opportunities for young paediatric spine surgeons from countries with limited resources.

Today, one important evolving innovation that can help overcome some of these obstacles is internet-based electronic learning (e-learning), which is becoming an integral part of medical courses in many countries [11] and that can be used to impart training skills to doctors in limited-resource countries without the need for travel and in-person fellowships abroad. More generally, blended learning (BL), defined as a technology-aided teaching approach that integrates components of face-to-face and online learning [12], can stimulate international education collaboration and connect skilled spine surgeons who can jointly contribute to the efforts to address local shortages of high-level spine training capacity. Recent literature suggests that BL produces better outcomes to traditional teaching methods in clinical disciplines [13, 14] and achieves an improvement in theoretical knowledge combined with high acceptance [15]. In low- and middle-income countries, BL is facilitated through improving technical infrastructure (e.g. internet and videoconferencing facilities) and advancing staff professional development in BL.

A study done by Alpaslan Senkoylu et al. [16] discusses the applicability of BL in a paediatric spine deformity course programme in particular, with orthopaedic and neurosurgeons as the main participants. The course included 11 lectures within the online part and six case discussions in the face-to-face part. The quiz scores were improved significantly in contrast to traditional face-to-face learning only. Though further research is needed, this preliminary study suggests the likely efficiency of the BL format in spine deformity training for the orthopaedic and neurosurgeon specialist.

Artificial intelligence (AI) also includes the advantages of electronic simulation training. Complex spine surgeries, including EOS cases and severe deformed paediatric spine require a high level of proficient surgical skills for any surgeon dealing with these problems. Traditional methods of surgical training involve practise in the operating room by observation, assisting, and lastly doing the procedure with monitoring. This traditional pathway is competitive and not easy to access for the orthopaedic surgeon who did not acquire enough training in paediatric spine during his or her residency, compounding the previously mentioned difficulties about acquiring a fellowship and travelling for the local young doctor. By contrast, computer-based simulations in BL can overcome some of these problems, as they evolve as a teaching tool to improve the surgical skills related to highly technical procedures as a precursor to real operating room involvement. There is preliminary evidence that simulations are potentially even more effective than traditional methods. A study [17] comparing virtual simulation training (using immersive touch simulator) and traditional training (including verbal and visual cues to action) for novice doctors putting pedicle screws in lumbar spine through posterior approach shows the average number of errors per screw in the simulation group was 0.96 versus 2.08 in the nonsimulation group.

For spine surgeons in developing countries, virtual simulation enables the practitioner to train in a virtual workspace and to rehearse before surgery without the need to go through difficulties of travelling and of procuring hands-on experience in centres in developed countries. Virtual simulation training is also valuable in giving performance feedback to the trainer and trainee, as the trainee can repeat the procedure multiple times until he or she can master the technique, and the trainer can assess which methods work best for communicating the necessary knowledge.

AVAILABILITY OF HIGHLY EXPERIENCED SURGEONS IN LMICS

Two decades ago, there were very few experienced EOS surgeons in LMICs, with the bulk of surgeries offered through short-term missions spearheaded by global health organisations and experts. However, there is now a small but growing presence of a number of experts in EOS management based in LMICs who have been able to provide EOS services to the local population while innovating ways to work around the problem of limited resources.

One of the major innovations revolved around the problem of high implant and instrument expenses in a constrained financial context. This book recounts some of the experiences of these experts in developing surgical methods in accordance with the basic laws in EOS management that are safe, reliable, and maintain growth, while overcoming the burden of frequent surgeries with regular spinal implants that are more affordable than those traditionally used. As a result of these innovations, local industries and companies have been motivated to produce implants and instruments with vouchers compatible with the economy status in these areas.

Another venue of innovation is big data collection. Big data in surgery can be defined as the amalgamation and integration of various data sources along the patient pathway to produce a rich matched data set. Technological advances have led to the generation of large amounts of data, both in surgical research and practise that need to be analysed to maximise the patient healthcare. This is done with ease in developed countries with the availability of personal tracking systems, specialised analytical skills, and technological infrastructure. By contrast, collecting patient data in LMICs is hard because of limited institutional infrastructure. In this context, data is now increasingly gathered by local experts through the use of personally available technologies such as the smartphone, which contains applications used in clinical assessment and x-ray measurements for scoliosis [18].

The success of a small number of local experts in establishing EOS services has also motivated young spine surgeons to become involved in EOS practise and to use training by these experts to better manage these complicated cases within the context they are living in. More broadly, the dissemination of EOS management services, albeit limited, with successful results, has also encouraged health authorities in these countries to invest more resources to maintain this service [19]. In addition, it encourages global organisations to become involved in spine education and research programmes, in collaboration with said local experts, and to gradually replace the short-term mission services – which can be performed by the local expert instead – with long-term resource-rich training programmes. Last but not least, the proliferation of EOS services, through a combination of local and global work, raises awareness about this medical condition and about the importance of seeking surgical intervention for children early on [20]. Within the next 10 years we hope to have EOS services included in numerous centres dealing with paediatric orthopaedic and/or spine surgery, along with the necessary implants from the local companies and the dissemination of knowledge through training, fellowship programmes, and BL programmes to empower the local surgeon to manage EOS children with the resources he or she has.

CONCLUSION

We are now in the age of digital knowledge, and the means of electronic communication have become increasingly important after the coronavirus epidemic. This has led to increased interest from local and international institutions dealing with spine programmes in education and training through online activities (webinars, Zoom meetings, etc.) as well as the hands-on training with virtual and augmented reality techniques. There is also increased interest in dealing with the big data in LMICs, especially with the help of technologies such as smart phones that can, to some extent, overcome the resource limitations in these regions. As a result of the above, there is an unprecedented opportunity for surgeons in limited-resource settings to obtain training opportunities and exchange information with the most advanced global and regional centres. The potential of organising the big data through simple tools available within limited-resource regions will promote research with universal standards.

REFERENCES

1. Bae JY, Groen RS, Kushner AL. Surgery as a public health intervention: Common misconceptions versus the truth.
2. Murray CJ, Vos T, Lozano R, et al. Disability-adjusted life years (DALYs) for 291 diseases and injuries in 21 regions, 1990–2010: A systematic analysis for the Global Burden of Disease Study 2010. *The Lancet.* 2012;380(9859):2197–223.
3. DeVries CR, Price RR. *Global Surgery and Public Health: A New Paradigm.* Jones & Bartlett Publishers; 2012.
4. Murray CJ, Vos T, Lozano R, et al. Disability-adjusted life years (DALYs) for 291 diseases and injuries in 21 regions, 1990–2010: A systematic analysis for the Global Burden of Disease Study 2010. *The Lancet.* 2012;380(9859):2197–223.
5. Chou L, Ranger TA, Peiris W, et al. Patients' perceived needs of health care providers for low back pain management: A systematic scoping review. *The Spine Journal.* 2018;18(4):691–711.
6. Davis MC, Than KD, Garton HJ. Cost effectiveness of a short-term pediatric neurosurgical brigade to Guatemala. *World Neurosurgery.* 2014;82(6):974–9.
7. Chen AT, Pedtke A, Kobs JK, et al. Volunteer orthopedic surgical trips in Nicaragua: A cost-effectiveness evaluation. *World Journal of Surgery.* 2012;36(12):2802–8.
8. Gosselin RA, Gialamas G, Atkin DM. Comparing the cost-effectiveness of short orthopedic missions in elective and relief situations in developing countries. *World Journal of Surgery.* 2011;35(5):951–5.
9. Fletcher AN, Schwend RM, The Ecuador Pediatric Spine Deformity Surgery Program. An SRS-GOP site, 2008–2016. *Spine Deformity.* 2019;7(2):220–7.
10. Mshelbwala PM, Azzie GR, Nwomeh BC. Developing educational opportunities for trainees on both sides. *InAcademic Global Surgery.* 2016:117–25. Springer, Cham.
11. Shantikumar S. From lecture theatre to portable media: Students' perceptions of an enhanced podcast for revision. *Medical Teacher.* 2009;31(6):535–8.

12. Bonk CJ, Graham CR. *The Handbook of Blended Learning: Global Perspectives, Local Designs*. John Wiley & Sons; 2012.

13. Liu Q, Peng W, Zhang F, et al. The effectiveness of blended learning in health professions: Systematic review and meta-analysis. *Journal of Medical Internet Research*. 2016;18(1):e2.

14. Carbonaro M, King S, Taylor E, et al. Integration of e-learning technologies in an interprofessional health science course. *Medical Teacher*. 2008;30(1):25–33.

15. Back DA, Haberstroh N, Antolic A, et al. Blended learning approach improves teaching in a problem-based learning environment in orthopedics-a pilot study. *BMC Medical Education*. 2014;14(1):17.

16. Senkoylu A, Senkoylu B, Budakoglu I, et al. Blended learning is a feasible and effective tool for basic pediatric spinal deformity training. *Global Spine Journal*. 2020:2192568220916502.

17. Gasco J, Patel A, Juan O-B, et al. Virtual reality spine surgery simulation: An empirical study of its usefulness. *Neurological Research*. 2014;36(11):968–73.

18. Robertson GA, Wong SJ, Brady RR, et al. Smartphone apps for spinal surgery: Is technology good or evil? *European Spine Journal*. 2016;25(5):1355–62.

19. Meara JG, Leather AJ, Hagander L, et al. Global surgery 2030: Evidence and solutions for achieving health, welfare, and economic development. *Lancet*. 386(9993):569–624.

20. DeVries CR, Price RR. *Global Surgery and Public Health: A New Paradigm*. Jones & Bartlett Publishers; 2012.

Index

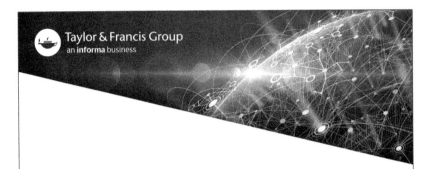